ROYAL VICTORIA HOSPITAL
WOMEN'S PAVILION LIBRARY

Pelvic Inflammatory Disease

We dedicate this book to our wives and families, for their continued love and support: Rhea Sweet, children Jennifer, Andrew, and Eric, and grandchildren Hanna, Emily, Benjamin, Paige, Samantha, Morgan, Dylan, Jordan, and Tanner; Ronit Wiesenfeld, and children Rachel, Maia, Jacob, and Shira.

Pelvic Inflammatory Disease

Edited by

Richard L. Sweet MD
Department of Obstetrics and Gynecology
University of California, Davis
UC Davis Medical Center
Sacramento, CA, USA

Harold C. Wiesenfeld MD, CM
Department of Obstetrics, Gynecology and
Reproductive Sciences
University of Pittsburgh School of Medicine
Magee-Womens Hospital
Pittsburgh, PA, USA

WOMEN'S PAVILION LIBRARY
ROYAL VICTORIA HOSPITAL
687 PINE AVENUE WEST
MONTREAL, CANADA
H3A 1A1

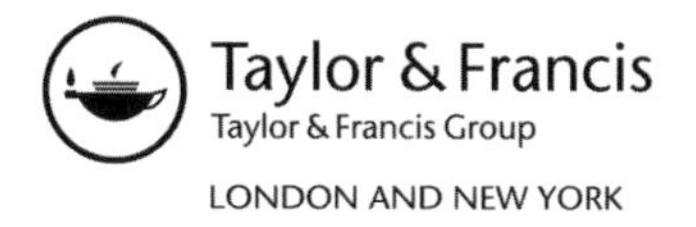

LONDON AND NEW YORK

© 2006 Taylor & Francis, an imprint of the Taylor & Francis Group
Taylor & Francis Group is the Academic Division of Informa plc

First published in the United Kingdom in 2006 by Taylor & Francis, an imprint of Informa plc, 2 Park Square, Milton Park, Abingdon, Oxon OX14 4RN

Tel.: +44 (0) 207 017 6000
Fax.: +44 (0) 207 017 6699
E-mail: info.medicine@tandf.co.uk
Website: http://www.tandf.co.uk/medicine

All rights reserved. No part of this publication may be reproduced, stored in a retrieval system, or transmitted, in any form or by any means, electronic, mechanical, photocopying, recording, or otherwise, without the prior permission of the publisher or in accordance with the provisions of the Copyright, Designs and Patents Act 1988 or under the terms of any licence permitting limited copying issued by the Copyright Licensing Agency, 90 Tottenham Court Road, London W1P 0LP.

Although every effort has been made to ensure that all owners of copyright material have been acknowledged in this publication, we would be glad to acknowledge in subsequent reprints or editions any omissions brought to our attention.

Although every effort has been made to ensure that drug doses and other information are presented accurately in this publication, the ultimate responsibility rests with the prescribing physician. Neither the publishers nor the authors can be held responsible for errors or for any consequences arising from the use of information contained herein. For detailed prescribing information or instructions on the use of any product or procedure discussed herein, please consult the prescribing information or instructional material issued by the manufacturer.

A CIP record for this book is available from the British Library.

Library of Congress Cataloging-in-Publication Data
Data available on application

ISBN 1-84214-289-5
ISBN 978-1-84214-289-9

Distributed in North and South America by

Taylor & Francis
2000 NW Corporate Blvd
Boca Raton, FL 33431, USA

Within Continental USA
Tel: 800 272 7737; Fax: 800 374 3401
Outside Continental USA
Tel: 561 994 0555; Fax: 561 361 6018
E-mail: orders@crcpress.com

Distributed in the rest of the world by
Thomson Publishing Services
Cheriton House
North Way
Andover, Hampshire SP10 5BE, UK
Tel.: +44 (0)1264 332424
E-mail: salesorder.tandf@thomsonpublishingservices.co.uk

Composition by Tek-Art, Croydon, Surrey

Printed and bound in the UK by CPI Bath

Contents

Contributors

Jennifer Botte MD
Department of Obstetrics and Gynecology,
Women & Infants Hospital,
Providence, RI, USA

Mitchell D. Creinin MD
Department of Obstetrics, Gynecology & Reproductive Sciences,
University of Pittsburgh School of Medicine,
Magee-Womens Hospital, Pittsburgh, PA, USA

Anne B. Lichtenwalner DVM PhD
Visiting Scholar, Department of Obstetrics & Gynecology,
University of Washington Medical Center,
Seattle, WA, USA

Dorothy L. Patton PhD
Department of Obstetrics and Gynecology,
University of Washington Medical Center,
Seattle, WA, USA

Jeffrey F. Peipert MD MPH
Department of Obstetrics and Gynecology,
Division of Research,
Women & Infants Hospital,
Providence, RI, USA

Matthew F. Reeves MD
Department of Obstetrics, Gynecology & Reproductive Sciences,
University of Pittsburgh School of Medicine,
Magee-Womens Hospital, Pittsburgh, PA, USA

David E. Soper MD
Department of Obstetrics and Gynecology,
Medical University of South Carolina,
Charleston, NC, USA

Richard L. Sweet MD
Department of Obstetrics and Gynecology,
University of California, Davis, UC Davis Medical Center,
Sacramento, CA, USA

Andrea Ries Thurman MD
Department of Obstetrics and Gynecology,
Medical University of South Carolina,
Charleston, NC, USA

Cheryl K. Walker MD
Department of Obstetrics and Gynecology
University of California, Davis, UC Davis Medical Center,
Sacremento, CA, USA

Harold C. Wiesenfeld MD CM
Department of Obstetrics, Gynecology & Reproductive Sciences,
University of Pittsburgh School of Medicine,
Magee-Womens Hospital,
Pittsburgh, PA, USA

Preface

Pelvic inflammatory disease (PID) remains one of the major health issues adversely affecting women worldwide. Not only are there substantial medical and economic costs attributable to acute illness, but long-term sequelae such as tubal factor infertility, ectopic pregnancy, and chronic pelvic pain also create an even greater public health burden and cost.

The impetus for writing this book was the desire to impart to health care providers the most up to date knowledge about PID, in the hope of ameliorating the suffering this disease causes women worldwide. To accomplish this, we have included chapters by leading researchers on the epidemiology and risk factors, microbiology, pathogenesis, pathologic findings and treatment of PID. In addition, the role of post-procedural upper genital tract infections and the diagnosis and management of tubo-ovarian abscess are considered.

Increasing importance has been attributed to subclinical PID, which is as common as clinically apparent infection. Moreover, just as clinically apparent disease, subclinical PID appears to adversely affect the future fertility of women. Because of the importance of recognizing this problem, up to date new information concerning subclinical PID is included.

Early diagnosis and treatment of acute PID have been shown to be important steps in decreasing the long term sequelae of PID. However, the optimum approach is primary prevention of acute PID and the sexually transmitted infections (STIs) which account for as much as two-thirds to three-quarters of PID. Thus, a chapter on prevention of PID and future horizons has been included.

It is the editors sincere hope that, by providing a comprehensive resource book on PID, we will empower clinicians with a knowledge base that will ameliorate the adverse impact of PID on the reproductive health of women.

Richard L. Sweet MD
Harold C. Wiesenfeld MD, CM

1. Epidemiology

Jennifer Botte and Jeffrey F. Peipert

INTRODUCTION

Pelvic inflammatory disease (PID) is an enormous problem in women's health, affecting millions of women worldwide. Each year in the United States alone, more than 1 million women develop acute pelvic inflammatory disease. The disease has both significant short-term and potentially devastating long-term complications. Women who develop PID are at risk for infertility, ectopic pregnancies, and chronic pelvic pain. More than 100 000 women become infertile each year and 150 women die as a consequence of PID.[1] In addition to these medical outcomes, PID creates an enormous financial burden on healthcare systems. Estimates of the cost of PID in the United States, including outpatient visits, hospital admissions, and surgical procedures done for sequelae of PID, reach as high as 4 billion dollars annually.[2] The lifetime cost of treatment for each person diagnosed with PID is estimated to be greater than \$3000.[3]

In order to accurately diagnose and treat this disease, clinicians must have a sound foundation of knowledge regarding the epidemiology of PID. In this chapter, we will review the incidence/prevalence of PID, and factors that are associated with an increased or decreased risk for developing PID.

DEFINITIONS

Epidemiology is the study of disease occurrence in populations. The epidemiology of pelvic inflammatory disease is complex and requires an understanding of individual and group transition dynamics.[4] In order to explain the transmission of sexually transmitted diseases (STDs), Anderson and May[5] proposed a simple formula as follows:

$$R_0 = \beta c D$$

where R_0 refers to the number of new infections that occur, on average, from an individual with an STD. R_0 must be greater than 1.0 for an infection to spread in a population. β is the probability of transmission from one individual to another, and reflects the concept that some infections are easier to transmit than others. Several biologic features are incorporated into probability of transmission, β: ID_{50} (the number of organisms that are required for infecting 50% of persons exposed), the site of transmission (e.g. anal vs vaginal intercourse), and immunity all play a role. In the above formula, c is the number of new sexual partners. The duration of infectiousness (D) is how long an individual remains infectious and is determined by the biologic nature of the infection and whether people receive treatment.

The greater the values for β (probability of transmission), c (number of new partners), and D (duration of infectiousness), the greater the value for R_0 and the greater the spread of the disease. Consider how this equation can be applied to pelvic inflammatory disease. Prevention and control efforts could focus on:

- decreasing β, by reducing high-risk sexual practices (e.g. unprotected intercourse)
- decreasing c, by limiting the number of partners among sexually active individuals
- decreasing D, by improving access to health care for infected individuals and their partners.

Screening programs also reduce the duration an individual is infectious through efficient detection when asymptomatic and treatment.

PELVIC INFLAMMATORY DISEASE: INCIDENCE AND TRENDS

Our knowledge regarding the epidemiology of PID is limited by several factors, the most important one being the absence of clear and unambiguous data regarding the incidence and prevalence of the disorder. The *incidence* of a disease is the number of new cases that occur during a specified period of time in a population at risk for developing the disease. *Prevalence* is the number of affected persons in a population at a specified time. Prevalence is usually expressed as a number divided by a specific number of persons in the population (e.g. 5 cases per 1000 persons). Incidence and prevalence of PID are difficult to ascertain; available figures are rough estimates at best. PID is a difficult diagnosis to make, with a relatively high frequency of both false-negative and false-positive diagnoses. In addition, while infections with *Neisseria gonorrhoeae* and *Chlamydia trachomatis* are reportable infections with highly sensitive and specific diagnostic tests, there is no reliable test for the diagnosis of PID. Many cases of PID are misdiagnosed as other disorders (false-negative diagnosis) and thus not captured. Many other cases are misdiagnosed as PID when the symptoms are actually due to endometriosis, gastrointestinal disorders, or other etiologies of acute pain (false positives).

There is sparse data regarding the global epidemiology of PID. However, we can extrapolate from other STDs. In 1995, the World Health Organization (WHO) estimated the number of four important curable STDs that occurred in the world: *Treponema pallidum* (12 million); *N. gonorrhoeae* (62 million); *C. trachomatis* (89 million); and *Trichomonas vaginalis* (170 million).[6] The total number (333 million) was a substantial increase compared with 298 million in 1990. The large majority of curable STDs occurred in the developing world: South and Southeast Asia (116 million, 49%); sub-Saharan Africa (50 million, 21%); Latin America (23 million, 10%). These estimates ignore population sizes. Startling discrepancies in incidence rates remain between the developing and industrialized world when population sizes are considered. The annual incidence of acquiring a curable STD in different populations is as follows: Western Europe (1–2%); North America (2–3%), Latin America (7–14%), South and Southeast Asia (9–17%), and sub-Saharan Africa (11–35%).[7] The actual incidence of PID in these geographic areas is not known, but may correlate with other curable STDs.

Reasons for this disparity between the developing and industrialized worlds can be found by examining the Anderson–May equation. General features that are more common in developing countries include poorer access to healthcare facilities, lack of availability to antimicrobials and preventive contraceptive practices (e.g. condoms), possibly increased numbers of sex partners, and poor socioeconomic status and nutrition that can affect immunologic status.

Compared with other industrialized countries, the United States has rates of STDs that are several-fold higher than other countries. In fact, the rates in some geographic areas exceed those in some developing countries.[8] There are several postulated reasons for the disparity between the United States and other industrialized countries. Many nations have made concerted efforts to lower their rates of STDs through intensive prevention and control programs. For example, in 1970 Sweden had a rate of gonorrhea of 481 per 100 000, compared with a rate of 297 per 100 000 in the United States. In 1995, the rate in Sweden dropped to 3 per 100 000, compared to 150 per 100 000 in the United States.[9] It is clear that intensive prevention and control programs can be successful.

Specific statistics addressing PID incidence in the United States are derived from hospital discharge surveys, outpatient surveys, and self-reporting. Many studies are based on diagnosis codes using the International Classification of Diseases (ICD-9). However, these diagnostic codes have not been carefully evaluated for validity. In addition, upper genital tract infections are often treated with ambulatory (outpatient) therapy. Thus, many cases go unreported. PID can be asymptomatic (silent PID) or very mildly symptomatic. As a result, many patients go undiagnosed. For these reasons, the current estimates may underestimate PID incidence and prevalence.

INCIDENCE ESTIMATES IN THE UNITED STATES, CANADA, AND SWEDEN

From 1979 to 1988, more than 270 000 women were hospitalized for PID annually. There were 1.2 million office visits for PID made during this same time period.[10] National Hospital discharge surveys from 2001 report only 28 000 women treated as inpatients for PID. Data from the National Center for Health Statistics and the National Survey of Family Growth reported a decline in rates of PID from 14% in 1982 to 8% in 1995.[11,12] Canada also saw a significant decline in hospitalizations for PID. Between 1984 and 1994, the rate of admission for PID declined from 386 per 100 000 women of reproductive age to 125.[13] US surveillance data for PID hospitalizations were recently published by the Centers for Disease Control and Prevention (CDC) (Figure 1.1). A steady decline in PID hospitalizations is noted between the early 1980s and mid-1990s, when the number of hospitalizations reached a plateau.

The apparent decrease in diagnosed cases of PID raises a number of questions. The trend may reflect the increasing tendency to treat patients with PID as outpatients, and thereby decrease the number of reported inpatient cases of PID. However, outpatient visits for PID have also declined. The CDC reports a significant decrease in initial doctor's office visits for PID over a 10-year period. In 1993, 407 000 visits were made by patients with this diagnosis, and in 2003, 123 000 visits were made (Figure 1.2).[1] The difference may be accounted for by changing trends in sexually transmitted infections. Swedish data reflect similar trends. In a 25-year study from Sweden, hospital admissions for PID decreased steadily from 1987 to 1994. Infections with *C. trachomatis* decreased from 28.4% in 1985 to 7.7% in 1994, whereas infections with *N. gonorrhoeae* also dramatically decreased during this period.[9,14]

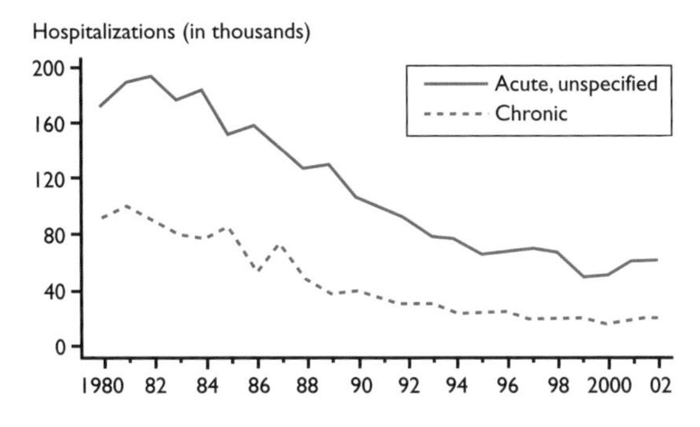

Figure 1.1 Pelvic inflammatory disease hospitalizations of women 15–44 years of age: United States, 1980–2002. Note: the relative standard error for the estimates of the overall total number of PID cases range from 6% to 18%. *Source*: Centers for Disease Control and Prevention. Sexually Transmitted Disease Surveillance, 2003. Atlanta, GA: US Department of Health and Human Services, September 2005. http://www.cec.gov/std/stats

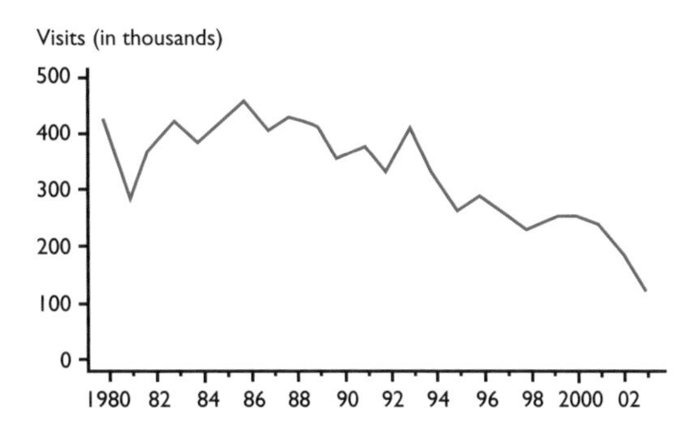

Figure 1.2 Initial visits to physician's offices for pelvic inflammatory disease by women 15–44 years of age: United States, 1980–2003. *Source*: Centers for Disease Control and Prevention. Sexually Transmitted Disease Surveillance, 2003. Atlanta, GA: US Department of Health and Human Services, September 2005. http://www.cec.gov/std/stats

INFECTIONS WITH *CHLAMYDIA TRACHOMATIS* AND *NEISSERIA GONORRHOEAE*

Infections with *N. gonorrhoeae* and *C. trachomatis* are clearly important predecessors of many cases of PID. One must understand the epidemiology of these two infections to have a complete picture of the epidemiology of PID.

CHLAMYDIA TRACHOMATIS

Chlamydial infection is a leading cause of pelvic inflammatory disease. It is estimated that every year, more than 3 million chlamydial infections occur in the United States. In 2002, there were over 800 000 reported cases.[1] A graph from the CDC's Chlamydia Surveillance Report 2003 depicts the rising incidence of genital chlamydial infections (Figure 1.3).[1] In 2003, the median state-specific chlamydia positivity

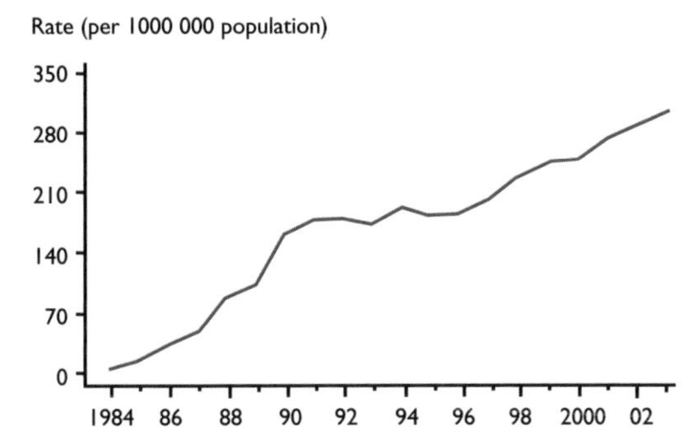

Figure 1.3 Rates of genital chlamydial infection in the United States, 1984–2003. *Source*: Centers for Disease Control and Prevention. Sexually Transmitted Disease Surveillance, 2003. Atlanta, GA: US Department of Health and Human Services, September 2005. http://www.cec.gov/std/stats

rate among 15- to 24-year-old women screened during family planning visits was 5.9% (range = 2.8–18.9%).[1] In nearly all states, chlamydia positivity was greater than the Healthy People 2010 goal of 3.0%.[15] This data may be an underestimate, however, because it reflects only those women seeking care. It is also likely to be affected by the sensitivity of different types of diagnostic tests used throughout the country (EIA, DNA probe assay, DNA amplification).[1] In addition, not all women seen in medical offices and clinics are screened for chlamydia. Given the tendency of chlamydial infections to be asymptomatic, selective screening policies result in under-diagnosis and under-reporting.

Chlamydia has been isolated as often as 20–40% of the time from the cervix or upper genital tract from women diagnosed with PID.[16] In a study of 537 women at risk for pelvic infection, Hillier and colleagues performed vaginal smears, cervical cultures and endometrial biopsies on all participants. Seventy-seven women had histologic endometritis. Of the women with endometritis, 21.5% tested positive for *C. trachomatis*, whereas 11.1% were positive for *N. gonorrhoeae*.[17] In a study of women with signs and symptoms of PID, those women testing positive for *C. trachomatis* or *N. gonorrhoeae* had an odds ratio (OR) of 4.3 of having histologically confirmed endometritis.[18]

Many women presenting with tubal factor infertility have antibodies to *C. trachomatis*. Only some of these seropositive women report a history of chlamydial infection, likely due to asymptomatic infection.[19] Chlamydia was first linked to tubal occlusion and thus to upper genital tract infection in 1979. Investigators showed that women with tubal occlusion had higher serum antibody titers for chlamydia than those with patent tubes. In a meta-analysis in 1997, this relationship persisted.[20]

NEISSERIA GONORRHOEAE

PID occurs in 10–20% of gonorrhea infections[21–23] and is the most common complication of such infections.[24] Infection with *N. gonorrhoeae* can result in overt PID or asymptomatic (subclinical) PID. In a 2002 cross-sectional study of women with lower genital tract infection who were asymptomatic, 26% of women diagnosed with gonorrhea had histologic evidence of endometritis.[25] In another study by Hillier and colleagues, a group of women who were clinically suspected of having PID underwent endometrial biopsies. Gonorrhea cultures were positive more often in women with a histologic diagnosis of endometritis than in those without (OR = 5.7; 95% confidence interval (CI) 1.8–17.5). Chlamydial infection was also more likely in this group (OR = 4.8).[26] In women enrolled in the PEACH study with suspected PID, testing positive for *N. gonorrhoeae* or *C. trachomatis* was associated with a 4.4-fold increased risk of histologic evidence of endometritis (95% CI 2.9–6.6).[27]

TRENDS IN INFECTIONS WITH *NEISSERIA GONORRHOEAE* AND *CHLAMYDIA TRACHOMATIS*

In the United States, the incidences of gonorrhea and chlamydial infections are probably more accurate than are those for PID, because providers often screen for these STDs and are required to report positive cases. Reported cases of gonorrhea and chlamydial infections are helpful in tracking PID, because they are so closely linked to the disease. One would then expect that the prevalence of PID would mimic that of these STDs.

Reported rates of gonorrhea in the United States declined from 1985 to 1996, at which time the incidence began to increase (Figure 1.4). A similar trend was seen in Finland between 1981 and 1990, during which time the rate of new infection decreased from

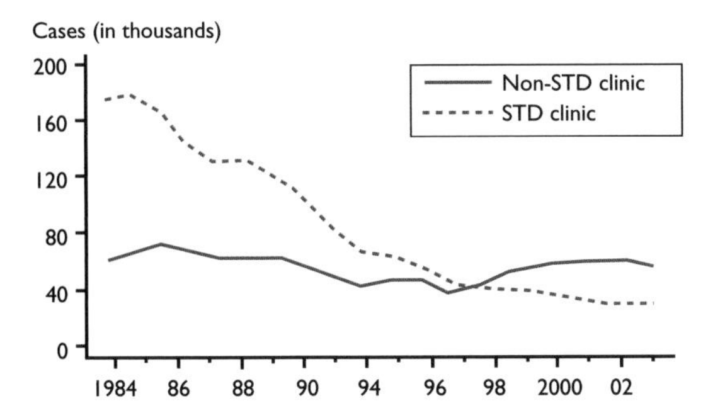

Figure 1.4 Reported cases of gonorrhea by reporting source: United States, 1984–2003. Note: prior to 1996, the sexually transmitted disease (STD) clinic source of report corresponded to public (clinic) source of report, and the non-STD clinic category corresponded to private source of report. After 1996, as states began reporting morbidity data electronically, the specific source of report (i.e. STD clinic) became available from an increasing number of states. *Source*: Centers for Disease Control and Prevention. Sexually Transmitted Disease Surveillance, 2003. Atlanta, GA: US Department of Health and Human Services, September 2005. http://www.cec.gov/std/stats

171/100 000 to 55/100 000. Other Nordic countries reported rates at least twice as high during that same time period.[28] In the United States, the incidence has increased by nearly 9% since 1996.[1]

The reported increase in chlamydial infections in the United States has been attributed to the expansion of chlamydial screening programs. According to the US Preventive Services Task Force, there is good evidence that screening women at risk for *C. trachomatis* infection can prevent adverse reproductive sequelae by reducing the rate of PID.[1] The strongest evidence to support screening in women is from a randomized trial of 2607 women at a health maintenance organization in Seattle.[29] This trial evaluated the effectiveness of screening and treating unmarried, asymptomatic women (aged 18–34 years old) at high risk for infection. Participants were considered high risk based on a scoring system that included young age (<25 years old), black race, nulligravidity, douching, and two or more partners in the past year. Participants were randomly assigned to one group that received screening and treatment (when indicated) for chlamydia or to a second group that received routine care (no routine chlamydial screening). By the end of the follow-up period, there were 9 verified cases of PID in the screened group (8 per 10 000 women-months of follow-up) and 33 cases in the usual care (not screened) group (18 per 10 000 women-months; relative risk 0.44, 95% CI 0.20–0.90). Thus, screening for *C. trachomatis* infection in sexually active young women (<25 years old) and other women at high risk is recommended and supported by level I evidence.[29]

TRENDS IN LONG-TERM SEQUELAE OF PELVIC INFLAMMATORY DISEASE

Although the decreasing rates of chlamydial infection account somewhat for the significantly smaller numbers of PID cases over time, they do not do so entirely. If the overall incidence of PID has decreased, one would expect to see significant decreases in the long-term sequelae of PID, such as infertility and ectopic pregnancy. A 1996 Swedish study showed a strong relationship between chlamydial infection and the sequelae of PID. The authors reviewed more than 100 000 chlamydia cultures obtained between 1985 and 1995, 5.4% of which were positive for chlamydia. They also looked at more than 50 000 pregnancies during that time period, 1.8% of which were ectopic. The rates of both chlamydial infection and ectopic pregnancies were shown to decrease during that decade, and the rates of PID were shown to correlate with that of chlamydial infection.[30] These data support the role of chlamydial screening in prevention of PID and its sequelae.

It is estimated that PID is the source of 50% of cases of infertility and 30% of ectopic pregnancies.[31] Both would be expected to decrease in light of the significantly fewer cases of PID. Unfortunately, this does not seem to be the case. The CDC reported a rise in ectopic pregnancies from 1970 through 1989; the rate increased from 4.5 to 16.0 ectopic pregnancies per 1000 reported pregnancies. Ectopics accounted for less than 2% of all pregnancies during this period of time, but complications of ectopic pregnancy comprised 13% of all pregnancy-related deaths. Deaths from ectopics have significantly decreased, accounting for only 3.5 deaths per 10 000 ectopics. This is a 10-fold decrease since 1970.[32] Rates of ectopic pregnancy peaked in 1989, and then began to

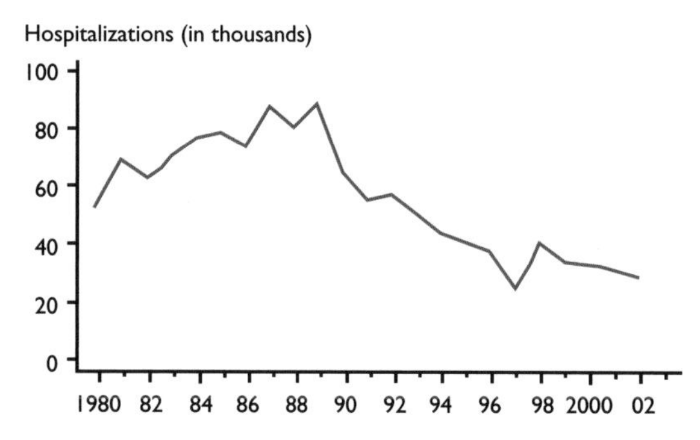

Figure 1.5 Hospitalizations for ectopic pregnancy in women 15–44 years of age: United States, 1980–2002. Note: some variations in 1981 and 1988 estimates may be due to changes in sampling procedures. The relative standard error for these estimates ranges from 8% to 12%. *Source*: Centers for Disease Control and Prevention. Sexually Transmitted Disease Surveillance, 2003. Atlanta, GA: US Department of Health and Human Services, September 2005. http://www.cec.gov/std/stats

decrease (Figure 1.5). The rates are lower, but the change is not as significant as the change in reported PID cases. At the same time, rates of infertility have remained essentially unchanged, with 2.1 million cases in 1995 compared with 2.4 million in 1982.[33] This further adds to the concern that PID remains under-diagnosed and untreated.

RISK FACTORS FOR PELVIC INFLAMMATORY DISEASE

The epidemiology of PID is unique. Unlike an infectious disease that is caused by one particular microbiologic agent, PID is a syndrome that can result from a number of different etiologic pathways.[34] The majority of cases of PID are the result of ascending spread of STD pathogens from the lower genital tract to the upper genital tract. However, PID can be the result of a mechanical insult (e.g. endometrial instrumentation) or a perturbation of normal vaginal flora and ascending spread into the endometrium and/or fallopian tubes.[25,35] Risk factors will vary depending on the

Table 1.1 Risk factors associated with STD acquisition, the development of PID, and the development of PID sequelae

Risk variable	Acquisition of STD	Development of PID	Development of PID sequelae
Demographic/social indicators			
Age	+	+	–
Socioeconomic status	+	+	•
Marital status	+	+	•
Residence, rural/urban	+	•	•
Individual behavior/practices			
Sexual behavior			
Number of partners	+	•	•
Age at first sexual intercourse	+	•	•
Frequency of sexual intercourse	+	•	•
Rate of acquiring new partners	+	•	•
Contraceptive practice			
Barrier	–	–	–
Pills	+	–	•
Intrauterine device	•	+	+
Healthcare behavior			
Evaluation of symptoms	+	+	+
Compliance with treatment instructions	+	+	+
Sex partner referral	+	+	+
Others			
Douching	•	+	•
Smoking	+	+	•
Substance abuse	+	•	•
Menstrual cycle	+	+	•

STD = sexually transmitted diseases; PID = pelvic inflammatory disease.
Variable may be associated with increased risk (+) or decreased risk (–), or no association reported (•).
Source: Padian NS, Washington AE. Risk factors for pelvic inflammatory disease and associated sequelae. In: Landers DV, Sweet RL, eds. Pelvic Inflammatory Disease. New York: Springer-Verlag, 1997: 21–9. (With kind permission of Springer Science and Business Media.)

etiologic pathway. Because the majority of PID is believed to be sexually transmitted, most of this chapter will focus on this etiologic pathway. Padian and Washington provided a delineation of risk factors associated with STD acquisition, the development of PID, and the development of PID sequelae (Table 1.1).[34] This delineation may be helpful as risk factors for PID are considered.

Many different factors may place a woman at increased (or decreased) risk of disease acquisition. Risk factors include characteristics that may not be alterable (e.g. age, race/ethnicity, etc.), biologic factors (e.g. vaginal ecosystem), a variety of behaviors (e.g. sexual history, sexual practices, contraception, seeking heath care, partner notification, drug abuse, etc.), and contextual factors (e.g. urban setting, social networks, etc.). Women with multiple sexual partners, or whose partners have had multiple sexual partners, are certainly at increased risk of acquiring STDs and developing PID. Use of contraceptives and type of contraceptive (e.g. barrier vs hormonal method) may affect the likelihood of development of PID, as could the existing vaginal microflora (e.g. lactobacilli-predominant vs anaerobic/bacterial vaginosis flora). We will review the existing evidence regarding each of these factors and the relationship to upper genital tract infection.

AGE

Young women are at higher risk for developing PID. The largest number of PID cases occurs in women between the ages of 15 and 25 years old. PID rates are low in patients over the age of 35 years old.[36–40] It is estimated that one in eight adolescent girls will develop PID.[41] In contrast to the 1:8 risk of acquiring PID in adolescents, the risk is 1:80 for women 24 years of age.[42] Incidences of both STDs and PID decrease significantly with increasing age beyond the age of 24 years old. Younger age, even among adolescents, is associated with an increased risk of PID. A case–control study of 123 sexually active adolescent girls evaluated risk factors for PID. Questionnaires were given to both adolescent girls with PID and those without, and it was noted that the group with PID had a greater difference in age between adolescents and their partners.[43] A retrospective study in Sydney concluded that women aged 15–19 years old were at higher risk than older women.[44]

Some investigators have suggested that age may be a risk marker for PID, rather than a risk factor.[31] Eschenbach noted that age was not associated with PID when gonorrhea and chlamydia were controlled for in the analysis.[45] It was suggested that young age is related to PID through increased rates of these two STDs.

Risk of STDs and PID in young women may be elevated due to a number of different factors: anatomic changes (cervical ectopy), sexual frequency and practices, and lack of barrier contraceptive use. Adolescent girls and young women tend to have increased cervical ectopy, with a greater amount of columnar epithelium exposed and therefore a larger surface area for infectious organisms to attach.

Age also affects risk for acquisition of sexually transmitted infections: not only are younger women more likely to acquire a sexually transmitted infection when exposed, due to biologic factors as previously discussed, but they are also more likely to be exposed. The exposure rates are higher in young women due to behavioral factors, including engaging in unprotected sex and having multiple sexual partners. Girls aged 15–19 years old have the highest rate of gonorrhea infection.[16] A study of female army recruits found that women under age 25 were more likely than older women to test positive for chlamydia (OR = 2.7).[46] A retrospective study in Washington State found young age to be the greatest predictor of initial and repeat chlamydial infections.[47] The US Preventive Services Task Force recommends screening for chlamydia in women under age 25 due to their increased risk of acquiring infection.[48] In a study evaluating criteria for screening women for chlamydia, age-based criteria worked best. Only 59–71% of women were screened to detect 84–92% of infections in the population. There is concern that young women with lower genital tract infection are more likely to develop PID than older women due to their longer time at risk and higher rate of repeat infections.[47]

A woman's age at the time of first sexual intercourse affects her risk of developing PID. In a case–control study of inner-city adolescents, Suss and colleagues reported that younger age at first intercourse was associated with acute PID. This study also noted that the age difference between the patient and her partner was also a significant risk factor for PID.[43] A study of Pakistani women further elucidated the role of age at first intercourse. They found an OR for developing PID of 2.3 for women married before age 21 compared with women married later.[49]

There also may be a hormonal explanation for the association of young age and risk of PID. Younger women, especially adolescents, often have anovulatory cycles with persistently elevated levels of estrogen. Well-estrogenized endocervical mucus facilitates the penetration of bacteria from the cervix to the uterus and fallopian tubes. This is in contrast to an ovulatory woman who is producing appropriate levels of both estrogen and progesterone. Progesterone thickens the cervical mucus, making it tenacious and highly impermeable to bacteria.[50]

RACE/ETHNICITY

There is strong evidence for an association between race/ethnicity and STDs/PID. African-American women are the highest-risk group.[1] The increased risk of PID is explained somewhat by differential rates of gonorrhea and chlamydial infection in different racial/ethnic groups. For example, rates of gonorrhea and syphilis are 30 times higher in African-Americans

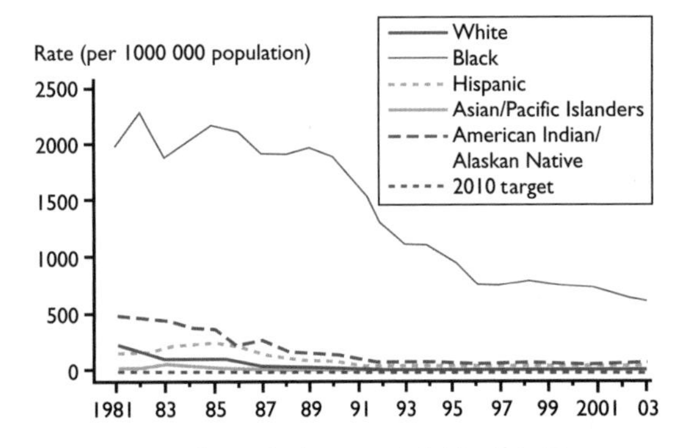

Figure 1.6 Rates of gonorrhea by race and ethnicity: United States, 1981–2003 and the Healthy People 2010 target. Note: the Healthy People 2010 target for gonorrhea is 19.0 cases per 100 000 population. *Source*: Centers for Disease Control and Prevention. Sexually Transmitted Disease Surveillance, 2003. Atlanta, GA: US Department of Health and Human Services, September 2005. http://www.cec.gov/std/stats

than in whites.[1] A graph from the gonorrhea rates by race and ethnicity depicts the discrepancy between rates of gonorrhea infections in blacks and other ethnicities (Figure 1.6).[1] In 2003, results of a study screening over 23 000 female army recruits were published. The prevalence of chlamydial infection was 9.5% overall, 16% in African-Americans and 5.4% in whites.[46] Approximately 8% of more than 60 000 women interviewed by the National Survey of Family Growth reported a previous diagnosis of PID, whereas 10.6% of surveyed African-American women reported this diagnosis.[33]

The changes in the rates of gonorrhea over time also differ by racial/ethnic groups. In African-Americans, the rates of gonorrhea decreased by 18.9% between 1999 and 2003 (808.4 to 655.8 cases per 100 000 population). However, gonorrhea among whites increased 22.5% (32.7 cases per 100 000 in 2003). Asian/Pacific Islanders increased 17.5% (22.8 per 100 000 in 2003), Hispanics increased 11.0% (71.1 per 100 000 in 2003), and American Indian/Alaska Natives increased 5.5% (103.5 per 100 000 in 2003). In 2003, the gonorrhea rate among African-Americans was 20 times greater than the rate for whites. This is down from 30 times greater in 1999.[1]

In the most recent CDC surveillance report, rates of chlamydial infection in the United States are also significantly increased among African-American females compared with whites. The rate of chlamydial infection in African-American women is 7 times higher than the rate in white women (1633.1 and 217.9 per 100 000 respectively). Chlamydial infection rates in African-American males were 11 times higher than among white males (584.2 and 52.9 per 100 000, respectively). These marked differences in STD rates in African-Americans can explain, in part, the higher rates of PID among black women.[1]

A number of other factors have been postulated as reasons for the African-American race as a risk factor for PID. Access to health care may affect the reported prevalence of infection. African-Americans are more likely to attend public health clinics, public hospitals, and emergency rooms to obtain treatment, and are therefore more likely to be tested and reported. Black women are also more likely to be exposed to infected black men than white women.[51]

SOCIOECONOMIC STATUS

Our understanding of the epidemiology of PID and STDs has evolved significantly over the past two decades. Increasing attention has focused on underlying socioeconomic and cultural determinants of STDs, and on dynamic patterns of spread of infection through sexual networks and through populations.[52] Lower socioeconomic status (SES) has often been cited as a risk factor for PID. In a case–control study of women admitted for PID, patients were more likely than controls to have fewer years of education, and were more likely to receive public assistance.[53]

The association between SES and PID is in part the result of differential rates of STDs in lower SES groups. Consider gonococcal incidence for example. Reports have demonstrated that census tracts representing the lowest SES quartile accounted for the majority of reported gonorrhea.[54] As gonorrhea and PID rates decline in some local areas, the morbidity becomes concentrated in low-SES core groups residing in low-SES areas.[55] In a study of gonorrhea morbidity in cities in the United States with greater than 200 000 population, six factors were accounted for 75% of the variation in morbidity: population density, percent households with female heads, city government general expenditures per capita, violent crime rate, percent of families below poverty level, and percent births to mothers younger than 20.[56]

GEOGRAPHY

A woman's geographic place of residence may also put her at risk for acquiring lower and therefore upper genital tract infection. In the Unites States, the CDC's Gonococcal Isolate Surveillance Project described a higher rate of gonoccocal infections among women in southeastern states.[57] Data from the CDC in 1999 also show a higher prevalence of chlamydia in southern and southeastern states. In fact, 7 of the 10 states with the highest rates of chlamydial infections were located in the south.[1] A study of 27 000 female army recruits found that women from southern states had a higher prevalence of chlamydial infection.[46]

The relationship between geography and risk for PID has been tied to rates of STDs. In 2003, the South had the highest rates of gonorrhea among the four regions in the country. However, rates of gonorrhea in the South have declined from 195.1 per 100 000 population in 1999 to 149.8 in 2003. In contrast, the rates of gonorrhea in the West have increased by 25% from 51.3 per 100 000 population to 64.0 in 2003. Rates in the Northeast (91.1 in 2003) and Midwest (136.3 in 2003) have shown minimal change since 1999.[1]

Urban populations also appear to be at higher risk compared with more rural populations. A population-based chlamydia registry in Washington State revealed that women living in rural areas were less likely than those in urban area to develop chlamydial infection.[47] It is not clear if geographic location and urban vs rural residence is associated with health care availability, sexual practices, or differences in health education.

PRIOR INFECTION

Women with a prior history of gonorrhea, chlamydial infection, or PID have an increased risk for a subsequent episode. Relative risks of PID in women with a previous infection with *N. gonorrhoeae* or *C. trachomatis* range from 1.7 to 2.5.[58,59] In the Women's Health Study, women with a history of gonorrhea had a two-fold increased risk of PID compared with women without a history of gonorrhea (OR = 1.8; 95% CI 1.4–2.3). Flesh and colleagues noted that a patient with PID was 2.3 times more likely than a patient without PID to have a prior episode of PID.[60] It is estimated that nearly 25% of women with acute PID will develop a second episode of PID due to reinfection or inadequate treatment. Repeat infections have important public health significance, as infertility rates increase dramatically with each episode of PID. Westrom reported that the rate of infertility due to tubal occlusion increased from 11% after one episode of PID to over 50% with three or more episodes of PID.[61]

BEHAVIORAL FACTORS

Unlike demographic factors, which are not easily changed, there are modifiable behavioral factors that are also related to a woman's risk of developing PID. Women with multiple sexual partners are at risk for acquiring STDs, and therefore at increased risk for the development of PID. There are other alterable behaviors that may affect the risk of acquiring upper genital tract disease. These factors include douching, sexual practices, and choice of contraception.

NUMBER OF SEXUAL PARTNERS

Women with multiple sexual partners are at increased risk for developing lower and upper genital tract infection.[58,62,63] Multiple sexual partners or partners with multiple partners increases a woman's at risk for acquiring STDs. The number of recent sexual partners has been associated with cervical *N. gonorrhoeae* and *C. trachomatis* infection.[64–66] A case–control study of women hospitalized for PID found that women with four or more recent sexual partners were three times as likely to develop PID as women with only one recent partner.[62] In the 1995 National Survey of Family Growth, women with 10 or more lifetime partners were twice as likely to report a history of PID as women with only 2 or 3 lifetime partners.[12] The rate of acquiring new partners is also associated with PID.[34] A new sexual partner within the prior month is also associated with PID acquisition.[67] A study of women with lower genital tract infection revealed that those women who were also diagnosed with endometritis reported a higher number of lifetime partners (9.2 vs 6.2).[68] Having multiple sexual partners is also linked with long-term sequelae of PID. A meta-analysis by Mol and colleagues found that women with a history of ectopic pregnancy were also more likely to have a history of more than one sexual partner.[69]

SEXUAL PRACTICES

The risk of acquiring PID has been related not only to the number of sexual partners but also to sexual practices. There is some evidence that women with one recent partner, but frequent sexual intercourse, have an increased risk of developing disease.[58,62,67,70] A case–control study[62] showed that women with one partner who had intercourse six or more times per week were 3.2 times more likely to develop PID than similar women with one partner who reported having intercourse less than once per week.

CONTRACEPTION

Contraceptive practices may be an alterable behavior that can decrease a woman's risk of pelvic inflammatory disease. It is difficult to separate the association of contraceptives and PID from behaviors and attitudes that may influence contraceptive choice. For example, women who use barrier contraceptives may be at higher (or lower) risk for STDs (e.g. greater number of sexual partners) than women who use hormonal methods. Women who use no contraceptive method tend to take greater risks and have poor healthcare utilization, which can then increase the rates of STDs and PID. Thus, it is important to critically evaluate the literature that demonstrates an association between contraception and STDs/PID. Investigators must control for other important confounding variables (e.g. age, sexual history, race/ethnicity, healthcare behaviors, etc.) Contraceptives also may alter the rate of STD acquisition, for example by increasing the surface area of cervical columnar cells (ectropion), or they may prevent ascent of organisms into the upper genital tract by altering the characteristics of cervical mucus.

BARRIER METHODS

Consistent use of barrier methods of contraception, including male condoms, the diaphragm, and the cervical cap, can prevent lower tract infection and the development of PID.[71,72] Male condoms, when used consistently and correctly, are very effective in preventing numerous STDs, including the human immunodeficiency virus (HIV).[73] In fact, when used consistently and correctly, the male (latex) condom is the most effective method for protecting against STDs and HIV.[73] A report of the effectiveness of condoms for prevention was released by the NIH in 2000. The report provided the following key findings:

- even 100% consistent use of condoms does not eliminate the risk of STDs

- gonorrhea and chlamydial transmission are reduced by approximately 50% with 100% condom use.[74]

Barrier methods of contraception were first shown in the literature to decrease the risk of PID in 1982. This retrospective study found that women who used barrier methods of contraception were 0.6 times as likely to be hospitalized for PID.[75] The mechanism for the prevention of PID with condom use is most likely through the prevention of STDs and lower genital tract infection. In addition, by eliminating or reducing the quantity of sperm, a potential vector for upper tract spread is reduced. In a more recent report of 684 sexually active women with suspected PID, Ness and colleagues noted that persistent use of condoms during the study reduced the risk of PID recurrence, chronic pelvic pain, and infertility.[76] Given the potential for condoms to reduce STDs and adverse sequelae associated with STDs, it is important to identify factors associated with consistent condom use (or lack thereof) and the risk of being exposed to an STD pathogen (i.e. number of unprotected coital acts).

In contrast, a study of women at risk for lower genital tract infection compared women with lower genital tract infection alone versus women with lower genital tract infection and endometritis. The group with endometritis were 4.7 times more likely to report using barrier methods of contraception (95% CI 1.5–14.9) than the group without endometritis.[68] In the PEACH study, the use of barrier methods was associated with histologic endometritis.[77] It is difficult to interpret these conflicting results. One possibility is that inconsistent barrier method use may be a risk marker of higher-risk sexual behaviors. Another possibility is that the control or reference groups in these studies (women with lower genital tract infection or women with signs and symptoms of PID, but no endometritis) are not ideal control groups to address the association of condoms and PID.

In summary, whereas some studies have found a reduction of bacterial STDs with the consistent use of male condoms, there is sparse longitudinal data demonstrating this reduction.[74] Thus, there is some controversy surrounding the use of condoms as primary prevention of STDs and PID. However, most experts would agree that the body of evidence supports a reduction of risk of STDs and PID with the consistent and correct use of male condoms.[72,78]

FEMALE-CONTROLLED BARRIER METHODS

There is limited evidence that female-controlled barrier methods, such as the contraceptive sponge or diaphragm, can help prevent STDs and possibly PID. Rosenberg and colleagues recently reported that women using the sponge or diaphragm had significantly lower rates of both gonorrhea and trichomoniasis than women using condoms. As compared with women using no contraceptive or those with tubal ligation, rates of these STDs were at least 65% lower.[79] An advantage of female-dependent methods is the avoidance of relying on the male partner for consistent condom use. It is possible that female-controlled barrier methods may prevent more STDs than condoms, because women may use them more consistently than men use condoms.[80]

Numerous research initiatives are currently under way to develop new barrier methods of prevention: both chemical and mechanical.[81] Microbicides are chemicals or compounds used to fight off potential pathogens and to prevent STD/HIV transmission. Many potential products are in various stages of development and are being tested at this time for safety, acceptability, and efficacy.[82] Preliminary studies have found that microbicides are acceptable to many women, and thus may play an important role in the prevention of STDs and HIV in the future.[83,84]

SPERMICIDES

Some studies have demonstrated a protective effect of a barrier method when used with a spermicidal agent that has antibacterial properties.[85–88] Roddy reported that nonoxynol-9, the most commonly used spermicide, did not protect women against acquisition of HIV, gonorrhea, or chlamydia.[89] In a Cochrane systematic review, Wilkinson and colleagues concluded that there is good evidence that nonoxynol-9 does not protect against STD acquisition, and there is some evidence that it may be harmful by increasing the rate of genital ulceration.[90]

HORMONAL CONTRACEPTION

Oral contraceptive pills (OCPs) have been postulated to decrease the risk of PID. Early reports revealed that use of OCPs reduced the risk of developing PID by 40–60%[67] when compared with women who did not use contraception. In women with chlamydial infection, the risk of PID was reduced by 70%; however, the risk of PID was not reduced in women with gonorrhea.[67] A case–control study of women hospitalized for PID revealed a 60–80% reduction in the risk of PID for women using OCPs for more than 1 year compared with women who did not use OCPs. However, there were few women in this study using current low-dose OCPs.[91] The protective effect of OCPs on chlamydial PID, but not gonococcal, Gram-negative, or anaerobic PID, suggests that OCPs may alter the immune response to chlamydia and reduce the inflammation in the fallopian tubes. This concept is consistent with the findings that OCP users have less severe damage to the fallopian tubes when PID is diagnosed laparoscopically, compared with women using an intrauterine device (IUD) or using no contraception.[92] It is important to remember that the hormonal formulation of the OCPs used in many early studies of PID contained higher doses of steroids than OCPs used today.

This protective role of hormonal contraceptives was not demonstrated in the PEACH study, where no relationship was found between women who developed upper genital tract infection and the use of OCPs.[77] Some authors have reported no effect of OCPs on PID development and have expressed concern that the medication masks symptoms.[93] Questions raised by conflicting results of retrospective trials are often best addressed by prospective studies. In 2001, a group of 948 HIV-1-negative female sex workers in Kenya were followed prospectively. Women were initially screened for HIV, gonorrhea, chlamydia, syphilis, trichomonas, bacterial vaginosis, and vaginal candidiasis. Over a follow-up period of more than 1 year, women were rescreened and asked about their sexual practices. Women using OCPs were found to be at increased risk for cervical chlamydial infections and decreased risk for bacterial vaginosis. Women using DMPA (depot medroxyprogesterone acetate) were at increased risk for cervical chlamydial infection, but at decreased risk for PID, bacterial vaginosis, and trichomonas infection.[94] The increased risk of chlamydial infection among OCP users has been reported in the past,[95,96] but the findings of the decreased risks associated with DMPA use are new to the literature.

Mechanisms have been proposed to account for the change in risk with hormonal contraception. OCP users often have an increased area of cervical ectopy, and thus an increased area for chlamydial infection. At the same time, progesterone results in thickening of the cervical mucus, limiting the ability of infectious organisms to infect the upper genital tract. Some authors have proposed that the decrease in menstrual blood flow decreases retrograde flow, making the tubes a less desirable place for organisms to infect. There is obviously a complex interaction among hormonal contraceptive use, age, sexual behavior, cervical ectopy, cervical infection with gonorrhea and chlamydia, and ascending infection.

INTRAUTERINE DEVICE

In the past, the IUD earned a reputation for increasing the risk of pelvic inflammatory disease. More recent randomized trial data[97,98] and reviews of the medical literature[99] have established that the risk of upper tract infection and infertility among IUD users is quite low. Early studies from the 1960s to 1980s reported a two- to four-fold increased risk of PID with IUD use compared with women using other contraceptive methods or no method. Results from the Women's Health Study revealed that Dalkon Shield IUD users were at excessive risk for PID.[100] Five years later, analysis of the data showed that women with one sexual partner, and therefore at low baseline risk for acquiring PID, were at no increased risk if they had an IUD in place.[101] A few years following this study, analysis of the WHO's IUD clinical trial data showed an increased risk of PID during the first 20 days following insertion. During the 8 years of follow-up, the risk was not significantly increased for women with IUDs compared with women without IUDs after this initial peri-insertional period.[97] The timing of infection has led to the hypothesis that the infection following insertion of IUDs is probably due to contamination of the endometrial cavity during the procedure.[97]

Some experts believe that the rate of PID in IUD users can be decreased by screening for *N. gonorrhoeae* and *C. trachomatis* prior to insertion, and by recognizing early signs of infection such as abnormal vaginal discharge, vaginal bleeding, and mild abdominal pain.[24] However, there are limited data to support this assertion. One trial that specifically evaluated the use of prophylaxis prior to IUD insertion found that the rate of PID in IUD users was far lower than expected and prophylaxis did not significantly reduce the risk of PID.[98] According to this trial and a meta-analysis, the routine use of antibiotic prophylaxis is unwarranted.[98,102] It is important to note that in many of these trials of antibiotic prophylaxis, patients were usually screened for cervical infection prior to IUD insertion. In a randomized trial in Kenya, with relatively high prevalences of gonorrhea and chlamydial infection and no prior screening, prophylaxis reduced the risk of both PID and unplanned IUD-related clinic visits by one-third, although the PID reduction was not statistically significant ($p = 0.17$).[103]

Most studies addressing the association of PID and IUD use have assessed the use of copper or inert IUDs. Limited data suggest that progesterone-containing IUDs may reduce the rate of PID compared with copper and non-medicated IUDs.[104]

TUBAL LIGATION

Although tubal sterilization does not protect against sexually transmitted diseases,[85,86] it has been shown to reduce the spread of organisms from the lower genital tract to the peritoneal cavity and thus protect against PID. This protection is incomplete, however, as suggested by rare case reports of PID and tubo-ovarian abscess in women who have undergone sterilization.[105,106]

DOUCHING

Women diagnosed with PID report frequent douching more commonly than controls, even after statistical adjustment for gonorrhea and chlamydial infections.[107] Ness and colleagues noted that frequent and recent douching was associated with histologic endometritis or upper genital tract infection with gonorrhea or chlamydia.[108] Other investigators have noted a link between douching and PID and a link between douching and ectopic pregnancy and/or infertility.[109,110] Thus, douching may modify the vaginal flora, which in some way may enhance ascending invasion of bacteria into the upper genital tract.

CIGARETTE SMOKING

Smoking has been implicated as a risk factor for infection with *N. gonorrhoeae* and *C. trachomatis*, and in some studies smoking has been associated with PID.[111,112] In the Women's Health Study, there was a two-fold increased risk of PID in current smokers and former smokers.[111] Women who smoke also appear to be at risk for PID-related complications such as infertility and ectopic pregnancy. After adjusting for gravidity, race, IUD use, and douching, Chow et al found a two-fold increased risk of ectopic pregnancy in women who smoked.[113] Phipps et al noted a 60% increased risk of tubal infertility in current smokers compared with non-smokers.[114] It is unclear whether cigarette smoking alters cervical mucus to facilitate ascending infection or if smoking is simply a risk marker for other high-risk behaviors.

BIOLOGICAL FACTORS: VAGINAL MICROFLORA

The alteration of vaginal flora seen in bacterial vaginosis (BV) has been implicated in an increased risk for PID. While the relationship between cervical infection with *N. gonorrhoeae* or *C. trachomatis* and PID is clearly documented, the evidence for BV as a risk factor for PID is somewhat controversial. The 100- to 1000-fold increase in bacterial numbers found in BV may allow a variety of bacteria to ascend into the upper genital tract with frequent sexual intercourse. In addition, the more alkaline vaginal pH found in BV may be more conducive to cervical and ascending infection.

Women with BV have a three-fold increased risk of post-abortal PID than women without BV. This increased rate was reduced in a randomized trial of therapy for BV.[115] In one study of 117 patients with histologically confirmed endometritis, the presence of anaerobic Gram-negative rods was associated with an OR of 2.6 compared with those without anaerobic Gram-negative rods.[26] Korn and colleagues performed an endometrial biopsy in a group of women who tested negative for gonorrhea and chlamydia and had no signs of PID. Those with BV at baseline were much more likely to have histologic evidence of endometritis than those with normal vaginal flora (OR = 15). More recently, a cross-sectional study of 556 high-risk women found subclinical PID on endometrial biopsy in 15% of women with BV (OR = 2.7). Those women testing positive for *N. gonorrhoeae* or *C. trachomatis* had higher rates of endometritis: 26% and 27%, respectively.[25] Given the association between BV and sexual activity, it is clear that sexual history is a confounding factor in the relationship between BV and PID. In a study of 116 patients with suspected upper genital tract infection, women with BV had an OR of 3.0 for having objective evidence of upper genital tract infection (histologic endometritis or laparoscopic salpingitis) even after controlling for sexual history and other confounding variables.[116]

In contrast to the findings above, in a recent observational cohort study of 1179 women, Ness and colleagues found no relationship between baseline BV and the development of PID.[76] However, in the group of patients at greatest risk (women with two or more sexual partners in the previous 2 months), there was an association found between BV and PID.[76] Additional research is clearly needed to sort out the relationship between BV, incidence of STDs, and ascending upper genital tract infection.

SURGICAL PROCEDURES

Surgical procedures are implicated in approximately 10–15% of cases of PID.[117] Example procedures include dilation and curettage, outpatient endometrial sampling, hysteroscopy, hysterosalpingogram, pregnancy termination, sonohysterogram, and IUD insertion. Any procedure that violates the protective cervical mucus barrier can result in upper tract infection. Among women undergoing therapeutic abortion, those with evidence of BV have been found to have a three-fold increased risk of post-abortal endometritis. A randomized trial found that preoperative treatment of BV reduced the risk of post-abortal infection.[115]

SUMMARY

Pelvic inflammatory disease continues to be a common and serious infectious disease in reproductive-age women. Recent data suggest that the incidence of PID may be on the decline in the United States and some other developed countries. However, rates of tubal factor infertility do not appear to be dramatically decreasing. This suggests that under-diagnosis and under-recognition may be commonplace. Important risk factors for PID include young age, African-American race, early age of intercourse, multiple sexual partners, previous episode or history of STD/PID, douching, and lack of barrier contraception. Efforts at prevention of PID include routine screening of young and high-risk women, rapid recognition and treatment of lower genital tract infection, and encouraging behavioral change to modify an individual's risk. Prevention trials will evaluate new female-controlled barrier methods and microbicides in an effort to prevent lower and upper genital tract infection.

REFERENCES

1. Centers for Disease Control and Prevention. Sexually Transmitted Disease Surveillance 2003. Last update: September 2004. Accessed: December 31, 2004. http:www.cdc.gov/std/stats
2. Van Voorhis WC, Barrett LK, Sweeney YT et al. Repeated *Chlamydia trachomatis* infection of *Macaca nemestrina* fallopian tubes produces a Th1-like cytokine response associated with fibrosis and scarring. Infect Immun 1997;65(6):2175–82.
3. Yeh JM, Hook EW 3rd, Goldie SJ. A refined estimate of the average lifetime cost of pelvic inflammatory disease. Sex Transm Dis 2003;30(5):369–78.
4. Schmid GP. Epidemiology of sexually transmitted infections. In: Faro S, Soper DE, eds. Infectious Diseases in Women. Philadelphia: WB Saunders, 2001:395–402.
5. Anderson RM, May RM. Epidemiological parameters of HIV transmission. Nature 1988;333(6173):514–19.
6. Gerbase AC, Rowley JT, Heymann DH, et al. Global prevalence and incidence estimates of selected curable STDs. Sex Transm Infect 1998;74(Suppl 1):S12–6.

7. Dallabetta GA, Laga M, Lamptey PR. Control of STDs. Arlington, VA: AIDSCAP/Family Health International.
8. Piot P, Islam MQ. Sexually transmitted diseases in the 1990s. Global epidemiology and challenges for control. Sex Transm Dis 1994;21(2 Suppl):S7–13.
9. The Institute of Medicine. The Hidden Epidemic: Confronting Sexually Transmitted Diseases. Washington, DC: National Academy Press, 1997.
10. Rolfs RT. Epidemiology of pelvic inflammatory disease: Trends in hospitalizations and office visits 1979–1988. In: Proceedings of the CDC and NIH Joint Meeting: Pelvic Inflammatory Disease: Prevention, Management, and Research in the 1990s. Bethesda, MD, September 4–5, 1990.
11. National Center for Health Statistics. Reproductive Health. Last update: June 22, 2004. Accessed: December 31, 2004. www.cdc.gov/nchs/fastats/reproduc.htm
12. National Center for Health Statistics. National Survey of Family Growth. Vital Health Statistics. Last update: June 22, 2004. Accessed: December 31, 2004. www.nichd.nih.gov/about/cpr/dbs/res national5.htm
13. Kurtz R, Doherty J. Hospitalizations for pelvic inflammatory disease in Canada, 1983/84–1993/94. Division of STD Prevention and Control, Bureau of HIV/AIDS and STD, LCDC, 1998.
14. Kamwendo F, Forslin L, Bodin L, Danielsson D. Decreasing incidences of gonorrhea- and chlamydia-associated acute pelvic inflammatory disease. A 25-year study from an urban area of central Sweden. Sex Transm Dis 1996;23(5):384–91.
15. Centers for Disease Control and Prevention. Healthy People 2010. Sexually Transmitted Diseases. Last update: September 2004. Accessed: December 31, 2004. http://www.healthypeople.gov/document/html/volume2/25stds.htm# Toc489706322
16. Center for Disease Control and Prevention. Tracking the Hidden Epidemics: Trends in STDs in the United States 2000. Last update: 2001. Accessed: December 31, 2004. http://www.cdc.gov/nchstp/dstd/Stats Trends/Trends2000.pdf
17. Yudin MH, Hillier SL, Wiesenfeld HC, et al. Vaginal polymorphonuclear leukocytes and bacterial vaginosis as markers for histologic endometritis among women without symptoms of pelvic inflammatory disease. Am J Obstet Gynecol 2003;188(2):318–23.
18. Peipert JF, Ness RB, Blume J, et al. Clinical predictors of endometritis in women with symptoms and signs of pelvic inflammatory disease. Am J Obstet Gynecol 2001;184(5):856–63; discussion 63–4.
19. Cates W Jr, Wasserheit JN. Genital chlamydial infections: epidemiology and reproductive sequelae. Am J Obstet Gynecol 1991;164(6 Pt 2):1771–81.
20. Mol BW, Lijmer J, Dijkman B, et al. The accuracy of serum chlamydial antibodies in the diagnosis of tubal pathology: a meta-analysis. Fertil Steril 1997;67(6):1031–6.
21. Emmert DH, Kirchner JT. Sexually transmitted diseases in women. Gonorrhea and syphilis. Postgrad Med 2000;107(2):181–4, 9–90, 93–7.
22. Eschenbach DA, Buchanan TM, Pollock HM. Polymicrobial etiology of acute pelvic inflammatory disease. N Engl J Med 1975;293:166–71.
23. Holmes KK, Eschenbach DA, Knapp JS. Salpingitis: overview of etiology and epidemiology. Am J Obstet Gynecol 1980;138:893–900.
24. Hook EW, Handsfield HH. Gonococcal infections in the adult. In: Holmes KK, Sparling PF, Mardh PA, et al, eds. Sexually Transmitted Diseases, 3rd edn. New York: McGraw-Hill, 1999:457.
25. Wiesenfeld HC, Hillier SL, Krohn MA, et al. Lower genital tract infection and endometritis: insight into subclinical pelvic inflammatory disease. Obstet Gynecol 2002;100(3):456–63.
26. Hillier SL, Kiviat NB, Hawes SE, et al. Role of bacterial vaginosis-associated microorganisms in endometritis. Am J Obstet Gynecol 1996;175(2):435–41.
27. Peipert J, Ness RB, Blume J. Clinical predictors of endometritis in women with symptoms and signs of pelvic inflammatory disease. Am J Obstet Gynecol 2001;184:856–64.
28. Hiltunen-Back E, Rostila T, Kautiainen H, et al. Rapid decrease of endemic gonorrhea in Finland. Sex Transm Dis 1998;25(4):181–6.
29. Scholes D, Stergachis A, Heidrich FE, et al. Prevention of pelvic inflammatory disease by screening for cervical chlamydial infection. N Engl J Med 1996;334(21):1362–6.
30. Egger M, Low N, Smith GD, et al. Screening for chlamydial infections and the risk of ectopic pregnancy in a county in Sweden: ecological analysis. BMJ 1998;316(7147):1776–80.
31. Westrom L, Eschenbach DA. Pelvic inflammatory disease. In: Holmes KK, Mardh PA, Sparling PF, Lemon SM, eds. Sexually Transmitted Diseases. New York: McGraw-Hill, 1999.
32. Goldner TE, Lawson HW, Xia Z, Atrash HK. Surveillance for ectopic pregnancy – United States, 1970–1989. MMWR CDC Surveill Summ 1993;42(6):73–85.
33. Abma J, Chandra A, Mosher W, et al. Fertility, family planning, and women's health: new data from the 1995 National Survey of Family Growth. National Center for Health Statistics. Vital Health Stat 1997:23(19):1–114.
34. Padian NS, Washington AE. Risk factors for pelvic inflammatory disease and associated sequelae. In: Landers DV, Sweet RL, eds. Pelvic inflammatory disease. New York: Springer-Verlag, 1997:21–9.
35. Korn AP, Bolan G, Padian N, et al. Plasma cell endometritis in women with symptomatic bacterial vaginosis. Obstet Gynecol 1995;85:387–90.
36. Forslin L, Falk V, Danielsson D. Changes in the incidence of acute gonococcal and nongonococcal salpingitis. Br J Vener Dis 1978;54:247–50.
37. Rees E, Annels EH. Gonococcal salpingitis. Br J Vener Dis 1969;45:205–15.
38. McCormack WM, Stumacher RJ, Johnson K. Clinical spectrum of gonococcal infection in women. Lancet 1977;i:1182–5.
39. Arya OP, Mallinson H, Goddard AD. Epidemiological and clinical correlates of chlamydial infection of the cervix. Br J Vener Dis 1981;57:118–24.
40. Hobson D, Karayiannis P, Byng RE. Quantitative aspects of chlamydial infection of the cervix. Br J Vener Dis 1980;56:156–62.
41. Shafer MA, Sweet RL. Pelvic inflammatory disease in adolescent females. Epidemiology, pathogenesis, diagnosis, treatment, and sequelae. Pediatr Clin North Am 1989;36(3):513–32.
42. World Health Organization. Pelvic inflammatory disease in non-gonococcal urethritis and other selected sexually transmitted diseases of public health importance. WHO Techn Rep Ser 1981;660:89.
43. Suss AL, Homel P, Hammerschlag M, et al. Risk factors for pelvic inflammatory disease in inner-city adolescents. Sex Transm Dis 2000;27(5):289–91.
44. Marks C, Tideman RL, Estcourt CS, et al. Assessment of risk for pelvic inflammatory disease in an urban sexual health population. Sex Transm Infect 2000;76(6):470–3.
45. Eschenbach DA. Epidemiology of acute pelvic inflammatory disease. Banff; Canada: International Society for STD Research, 1991.
46. Gaydos CA, Howell MR, Quinn TC, et al. Sustained high prevalence of Chlamydia trachomatis infections in female army recruits. Sex Transm Dis 2003;30(7):539–44.
47. Xu F, Schillinger JA, Markowitz LE, et al. Repeat *Chlamydia trachomatis* infection in women: analysis through a surveillance case registry in Washington State. Am J Epidemiol 2000;152:1164–70.

48. US Preventive Services Task Force. Screening for chlamydial infection: recommendations and rationale. Am J Prev Med 2001;20((3S)):90–4.
49. Sajan F, Fikree FF. Does early age at marriage influence gynaecological morbidities among Pakistani women? J Biosoc Sci 2002;34(3):407–17.
50. Enhorning G, Huldt L, Melen B. Ability of cervical mucus to act as a barrier against bacteria. Am J Obstet Gynecol 1970;108:532–7.
51. Quinn RW, O'Reilly KR, Khaw M. Gonococcal infection in women attending the venereal disease clinic in Nashville Davidson County Metropolitan Health Department 1984. South Med J 1988;81:851.
52. Aral SO, Holmes KK. Social and behavioral determinants of the epidemiology of STDs: industrialized and developing countries. In: Holmes KK, Sparling PF, Mardh PA, Lemon SM, eds. Sexually Transmitted Diseases. New York: McGraw-Hill, 1999:39–76.
53. Jossens MO, Eskenazi B, Schachter J, Sweet RL. Risk factors for pelvic inflammatory disease. A case control study. Sex Transm Dis 1996;23(3):239–47.
54. Rice RJ, Roberts PL, Handsfield HH, Holmes KK. Sociodemographic distribution of gonorrhea incidence: implications for prevention and behavioral research. Am J Public Health 1991;81(10):1252–8.
55. Aral SO, Wasserheit JN. Social and behavioral correlates of pelvic inflammatory disease. Sex Transm Dis 1998;25(7):378–85.
56. Zaidi AA. Socio-demographic factors associated with gonorrhea rates in the United States: an ecologic analysis. Seville, Spain: International Society for STDs Research, 1997.
57. Centers for Disease Control. Gonococcal Isolate Surveillance Project Annual Report, 2002.
58. Eschenbach DA, Harnish JP, Holmes KK. Pathogenesis of acute pelvic inflammatory disease: role of contraception and other risk factors. Am J Obstet Gynecol 1977;128:838–50.
59. Lee NC, Rubin GL, Grimes DA. Measures of sexual behavior and the risk of pelvic inflammatory disease. Obstet Gynecol 1991;77(3):425–30.
60. Flesh G, Weiner JM, Corlett RC Jr, et al. The intrauterine contraceptive device and acute salpingitis: a multifactor analysis. Am J Obstet Gynecol 1979;135(3):402–8.
61. Westrom L. Incidence, prevalence, and trends of acute pelvic inflammatory disease and its consequences in industrialized countries. Am J Obstet Gynecol 1980;138(7 Pt 2):880–92.
62. Lee NC, Rubin GL, Grimes DA. Measures of sexual behavior and the risk of pelvic inflammatory disease. Obstet Gynecol 1991;77:425–30.
63. Flesh G, Weiner JM, Corlett RC. The intrauterine device and acute salpingitis: a multifactor analysis. Am J Obstet Gynecol 1979;135:402–8.
64. D'Costa LJ. Prostitutes are a major reservoir of sexually transmitted disease in Nairobi, Kenya. Sex Transm Dis 1985;12:64–9.
65. Handsfield HH. Criteria for selective screening for *Chlamydia trachomatis* infection in women attending family planning clinics. JAMA 1986;255:1730–5.
66. Schachter J, Stoner E, Moncada J. Screening for chlamydial infections in women attending family planning clinics. West J Med 1983;138:375–9.
67. Wolner-Hanssen P, Eschenbach DA, Paavonen J. Decreased risk of symptomatic chlamydial pelvic inflammatory disease associated with oral contraceptive use. JAMA 1990;263:54–9.
68. Nelson DB, Ness RB, Peipert JF, et al. Factors predicting upper genital tract inflammation among women with lower genital tract infection. J Womens Health 1998;7:1033–40.
69. Ankum WM, Mol BWJ, van der Veen F, Bossuyt PMM. Risk factors for ectopic pregnancy: a meta-analysis. Fertil Steril 1996;65(6):1093–9.
70. Lidegaard O, Helm P. Pelvic inflammatory disease: the influence of contraceptive, sexual, and social life events. Contraception 1990;41:475–83.
71. Kelaghan J, Rubin GL, Ory HW, Layde PM. Barrier-method contraceptives and pelvic inflammatory disease. JAMA 1982;248(2):184–7.
72. Stone KM, Timyan J, Thomas EL. Barrier methods for the prevention of sexually transmitted diseases. In: Holmes KK, Sparling PF, Mardh PA, et al, eds. Sexually Transmitted Diseases, 3rd edn. New York: McGraw-Hill, 1999:1307–21.
73. Stone KM, Timyan J, Thomas E. Barrier methods for the prevention of sexually transmitted diseases. In: Holmes KK, Sparling PF, Mardh PA, et al, eds. Sexually Transmitted Diseases, 3rd edn. New York: McGraw-Hill, 1999.
74. National Institute of Allergy and Infectious Diseases. Scientific evidence on condom effectiveness for sexually transmitted disease (STD) prevention. US Department of Health and Human Services; 2001.
75. Kelaghan J, Rubin GL, Ory HW, Layde PM. Barrier-method contraceptives and pelvic inflammatory disease. JAMA 1982;248:184–7.
76. Ness RB, Hillier SL, Kip KE, et al. Bacterial vaginosis and risk of pelvic inflammatory disease. Obstet Gynecol 2004;104(4):761–9.
77. Ness RB, Soper DE, Holley RL, et al. Hormonal and barrier contraception and risk of upper genital tract disease in the PID Evaluation and Clinical Health (PEACH) study. Am J Obstet Gynecol 2001;185(1):121–7.
78. Sexually transmitted diseases treatment guidelines 2002. Centers for Disease Control and Prevention. MMWR Recomm Rep 2002;51(RR-6):1–78.
79. Joint Programme on HIV/AIDS. Epidemic Update 2002;23.
80. Faundes A, Elias C, Coggins C. Spermicides and barrier contraception. Curr Opin Obstet Gynecol 1994;6(6):552–8.
81. Schwartz JL, Gabelnick HL. Current contraceptive research. Perspect Sex Reprod Health 2002;34:310–16.
82. Van Damme L, Jespers V, Van Dyck E, Chapman A. Penile application of dextrin sulphate gel (Emmelle). Contraception 2002;66(2):133–6.
83. Coetzee N, Blanchard K, Ellertson C, et al. Acceptability and feasibility of Micralax applicators and of methyl cellulose gel placebo for large-scale clinical trials of vaginal microbicides. Aids 2001;15(14):1837–42.
84. Darroch JE, Frost JJ. Women's interest in vaginal microbicides. Fam Plann Perspect 1999;31(1):16–23.
85. Austin H, Louv WC, Alexander WJ. A case–control study of spermicides and gonorrhea. JAMA 1984;251(21):2822–4.
86. Quinn RW, O'Reilly KR. Contraceptive practices of women attending the Sexually Transmitted Disease Clinic in Nashville, Tennessee. Sex Transm Dis 1985;12(3):99–102.
87. Louv WC, Austin H, Alexander WJ, et al. A clinical trial of nonoxynol-9 for preventing gonococcal and chlamydial infections. J Infect Dis 1988;158(3):518–23.
88. Cook RL, Rosenberg MJ. Do spermicides containing nonoxynol-9 prevent sexually transmitted infections? A meta-analysis. Sex Transm Dis 1998;25(3):144–50.
89. Roddy RE, Zekeng L, Ryan KA, et al. A controlled trial of nonoxynol 9 film to reduce male-to-female transmission of sexually transmitted diseases. N Engl J Med 1998;339(8):504–10.
90. Wilkinson D, Ramjee G, Tholandi M, Rutherford G. Nonoxynol-9 for preventing vaginal acquisition of sexually transmitted infections by women from men (Review). The Cochrane Collaboration 2002(1):1–15.
91. Panser LA, Phipps WR. Type of oral contraceptive in relation to acute, initial episodes of pelvic inflammatory disease. Contraception 1991;43(1):91–9.

92. Wolner-Hanssen P, Svensson L, Mardh PA, Westrom L. Laparoscopic findings and contraceptive use in women with signs and symptoms suggestive of acute salpingitis. Obstet Gynecol 1985;66(2):233–8.
93. Ness RB, Keder LM, Soper DE. Oral contraceptives and the recognition of endometritis. Am J Obstet Gynecol 1997;176:580.
94. Baeten JM, Nyange PM, Richardson BA, et al. Hormonal contraception and risk of sexually transmitted disease acquisition: results from a prospective study. Am J Obstet Gynecol 2001;185(2):380–5.
95. Washington AE, Aral SO, Wolner-Hanssen P, et al. Assessing risk for pelvic inflammatory disease and its sequelae. JAMA 1991;266(18):2581–6.
96. Cottingham J, Hunter D. *Chlamydia trachomatis* and oral contraceptive use: a quantitative review. Genitourin Med 1992;68(4):209–16.
97. Farley TMM. Intrauterine devices and pelvic inflammatory disease: an international perspective. Lancet 1992;339:785.
98. Walsh T, Grimes D, Frezieres R, et al. Randomized controlled trial of prophylactic antibiotics before insertion of intrauterine devices. IUD Study Group. Lancet 1998;351:1005–8.
99. Grimes DA. Intrauterine device and upper-genital-tract infection. Lancet 2000;356:1013–19.
100. Lee NC, Rubin GL, Ory HW, Burkman RT. Type of intrauterine device and the risk of pelvic inflammatory disease. Obstet Gynecol 1983;62:1–6.
101. Lee NC, Rubin GL, Borucki R. The intrauterine devices and pelvic inflammatory disease revisited: new results from the Women's Health Study. Obstet Gynecol 1988;77:1–6.
102. Grimes DA, Schulz KF. Prophylactic antibiotics for intrauterine device insertion: a meta-analysis of the randomized controlled trials. Contraception 1999;60:57–63.
103. Sinei SK, Schulz KF, Lamptey PR, et al. Preventing IUCD-related pelvic infection: the efficacy of prophylactic doxycycline at insertion. Br J Obstet Gynaecol 1990;97(5):412–19.
104. Toivonen J, Luukkainen T, Allonen H. Protective effect of intrauterine release of levonorgestrel on pelvic infection: three years' comparative experience of levonorgestrel- and copper-releasing intrauterine devices. Obstet Gynecol 1991;77(2):261–4.
105. Levgur M, Duvivier R. Pelvic inflammatory disease after tubal sterilization: a review. Obstet Gynecol Surv 2000;55(1):41–50.
106. Green MM, Vicario SJ, Sanfilippo JS, Lochhead SA. Acute pelvic inflammatory disease after surgical sterilization. Ann Emerg Med 1991;20(4):344–7.
107. Scholes D, Daling JR, Stergachis A, et al. Vaginal douching as a risk factor for acute pelvic inflammatory disease. Obstet Gynecol 1993;81(4):601–6.
108. Ness RB, Soper DE, Holley RL, et al. Douching and endometritis: results from the PID Evaluation and Clinical Health (PEACH) study. Sex Transm Dis 2001;28(4):240–5.
109. Daling JR, Weiss NS, Schwartz SM, et al. Vaginal douching and the risk of tubal pregnancy. Epidemiology 1991;2(1):40–8.
110. Zhang J, Thomas AG, Leybovich E. Vaginal douching and adverse health effects: a meta-analysis. Am J Public Health 1997;87(7):1207–11.
111. Marchbanks PA, Lee NC, Peterson HB. Cigarette smoking as a risk factor for pelvic inflammatory disease. Am J Obstet Gynecol 1990;162(3):639–44.
112. Buchan H, Villard-Mackintosh L, Vessey M, et al. Epidemiology of pelvic inflammatory disease in parous women with special reference to intrauterine device use. Br J Obstet Gynaecol 1990;97(9):780–8.
113. Chow WH, Daling JR, Weiss NS, Voigt LF. Maternal cigarette smoking and tubal pregnancy. Obstet Gynecol 1988;71(2):167–70.
114. Phipps WR, Cramer DW, Schiff I, et al. The association between smoking and female infertility as influenced by cause of the infertility. Fertil Steril 1987;48(3):377–82.
115. Larsson PG, Platz-Christensen JJ, Thejls H, et al. Incidence of pelvic inflammatory disease after first-trimester legal abortion in women with bacterial vaginosis after treatment with metronidazole: a double-blind, randomized study. Am J Obstet Gynecol 1992;166(1 Pt 1):100–3.
116. Peipert J, Montagno A, Cooper A. Bacterial vaginosis as a risk factor for upper genital tract infection. Am J Obstet Gynecol 1997;177(5):1184–7.
117. Jacobson L, Westrom L. Objectivized diagnosis of acute pelvic inflammatory disease. Diagnostic and prognostic value of routine laparoscopy. Am J Obstet Gynecol 1969;105(7):1088–98.

2. Microbiology

Richard L. Sweet

BACKGROUND

Pelvic inflammatory disease (PID) is one of the most common and important complications of sexually transmitted infections among non-pregnant reproductive-age women.[1] According to the Centers for Disease Control and Prevention (CDC), PID is a spectrum of upper genital tract infections that includes any combination of endometritis, salpingitis, pyosalpinx, tubo-ovarian abscess, and pelvic peritonitis.[2] Salpingitis is the most important component of the PID spectrum due to its association with long-term sequelae.[3] Acute PID and acute salpingitis are often used interchangeably. In this chapter, the term PID will be used.

For many locales, PID is not a reportable disease and precise figures on the incidence and prevalence of acute PID in the United States and most other nations of the world are not available. Thus, multiple indirect sources have been utilized to estimate these figures, including hospital discharge data, emergency room visits, patient surveys, physician office visits, and extrapolations from gonorrhea and chlamydia incidence figures. Further complicating the situation is the recent recognition that up to two-thirds of the cases of PID go unrecognized.[1,3] In the 1970s and 1980s, approximately 1 million cases of acute PID were diagnosed annually in the United States,[4,5] with an estimated yearly cost of $5.5 billion.[6] Thirty percent of diagnosed cases of acute PID were hospitalized in that era.[7] Since the peak in the 1980s, both the estimated cases of acute PID and hospitalization rates for acute PID have declined.[1,8] By the year 2000, approximately 780 000 cases of clinical acute PID were being diagnosed annually and the number of hospitalized cases had fallen from 289 086 in 1981 to 113 903 in 1996, a 57% decline.[8] As noted above, these figures do not take into account "unrecognized" or "subclinical" PID, which is probably as common if not even more common than clinically diagnosed acute PID.[1,3,9,10]

PID is a major public health concern, primarily due to its associated long-term consequences and the resultant adverse effect on the reproductive health of women.[1,11] One-fourth of women with at least one episode of acute PID go on to develop long-term sequelae.[12,13] These include tubal factor infertility, ectopic pregnancy, and chronic pelvic pain.[11,13–18] More recently, similar sequelae have been ascribed to "unrecognized" or "subclinical" PID.[9,19] Eschenbach has estimated that PID causes 30% of infertility, 50% of ectopic pregnancies, and numerous cases of chronic pelvic pain.[20] The latter often leads to surgical intervention, including total hysterectomy and bilateral salpingo-oophorectomy.

In order to prevent the significant medical and economic consequences associated with acute PID, prevention and treatment plans must be developed that are based upon an understanding of the microbiologic etiology and pathogenesis of acute PID. However, several factors have confounded our ability to determine the microbial etiology of acute PID.

First, most studies assessing the etiology of acute PID have relied on specimens obtained from the lower genital tract (predominantly cervical) rather than the upper genital tract (endometrial cavity and fallopian tubes), which is the actual site of infection.[1] Secondly, the majority of studies have focused on the sexually transmitted pathogens, *Neisseria gonorrhoeae* and *Chlamydia trachomatis* and failed to use techniques appropriate for determining the presence of additional potential pathogens such as anaerobic and facultative bacteria or genital mycoplasmas. Thirdly, only rare attempts have been undertaken to determine whether viral agents, such as cytomegalovirus or herpes simplex virus, are present in women with acute PID. Lastly, the lack of validated and standardized criteria for the diagnosis of acute clinical PID and "subclinical" PID has further compromised our ability to ascertain the microbial etiology of acute PID.

Whether the recently described entity of "subclinical" or "unrecognized" PID is associated with similar putative microorganisms as acute clinically apparent PID remains to be fully elucidated. Initial retrospective studies, suggesting that subclinical PID is an important cause of tubal factor infertility, demonstrated serologic evidence of prior chlamydial or gonococcal infection in 23–91% and in over 60%, respectively, despite an absence of a prior known history of acute PID in nearly two-thirds of these women.[21–25] More recent studies have demonstrated an association between subclinical PID and chlamydial and gonococcal cervicitis and bacterial vaginosis (BV).[10,26,27]

ETIOLOGY AND PATHOGENESIS: GENERAL CONCEPTS

Until the late 1970s, acute PID was believed to be a monoetiologic infection with *N. gonorrhoeae* as the primary etiologic agent.[1] However, subsequent studies established that the etiology of acute PID was polymicrobic in nature,[28–35] with a wide variety of microorganisms recovered from the upper genital tract of women with acute PID. Among these microorganisms are *N. gonorrhoeae, C. trachomatis*, genital mycoplasmas (*Mycoplasma hominis* and *Ureaplasma urealyticum*), anaerobic and aerobic/facultative bacteria from the endogenous flora of the vagina and cervix such as *Prevotella* species (*P. bivia*), black-pigmented Gram-negative anaerobic rods, *Peptostreptococcus* species, *Gardnerella vaginalis, Escherichia coli, Haemophilus influenzae*, and aerobic streptococci.[1]

Of particular importance are those studies that assessed the recovery of microorganisms from the upper genital tract of women with acute PID (Table 2.1). In general, *C. trachomatis* and/or *N. gonorrhoeae* were recovered from approximately one-third to one-half of PID cases, whereas non-gonococcal non-chlamydial microorganisms account for up to two-thirds of PID. These findings are consistent with those reported by our group in a large series (n = 589) of hospitalized acute PID cases where *N. gonorrhoeae* and/or *C. trachomatis* were recovered from 65% of cases whereas in 30% only anaerobic and/or facultative bacteria were present.[41] In addition, anaerobic and/or facultative

Table 2.1 Recovery of microorganisms from the upper genital tract of patients with acute PID

Study	No. of patients	*Chlamydia trachomatis*	*Neisseria gonorrhoeae*	Anaerobic and facultative bacteria
Sweet[34,36,37,a]	380	68 (18%)	172 (45%)	267 (70%)
Wasserheit[35]	23	11 (44%)	8 (35%)	11 (44%)
Heinonen[31]	25	10 (40%)	4 (16%)	17 (68%)
Paavonen[30]	35	12 (34%)	4 (11%)	24 (69%)
Brunham[32]	50	21 (42%)	8 (16%)	10 (20%)
Soper[33]	84[b]	1 (1.2%)	32 (38%)	12 (13%)
	51[c]	6 (7.4%)	49 (98%)	16 (32%)
Hillier[39]	85[b]	3 (4%)	16 (19%)	43 (50%)
	178[c]	23 (13%)	44 (25%)	168 (94%)
	278[d]	27 (9.9%)	37 (13.4%)	170 (61%)
Haggerty[40]	45[c,e]	12 (26.5%)	15 (33.3%)	NA[f]

[a]Includes patients in Landers et al.[38]
[b]Fallopian tube/cul-de-sac.
[c]Endometrial cavity.
[d]Women with clinically diagnosed acute PID.
[e]Women with histologic acute endometritis.
[f]NA = not available as total (anaerobic Gram-negative rods 31.7%, anaerobic Gram-positive cocci 22%, *Gardnerella vaginalis* 30.5%).

bacteria were recovered from the upper genital tract in nearly 50% of patients with *C. trachomatis* and/or *N. gonorrhoeae*. Thus, non-gonococcal non-chlamydial bacteria were present in nearly two-thirds of acute PID cases.[41]

The overwhelming majority of PID cases occur as the result of intracanalicular spread of microorganisms that ascend from the vagina and/or endocervix to reach the endometrial cavity and fallopian tubes.[1,40,42] Approximately 10–20% of women with untreated gonococcal or chlamydial cervicitis develop acute PID.[1,3,43,44] However, a few studies have noted higher rates, with up to 40% of women not treated for *N. gonorrhoeae* or *C. trachomatis* or who have been exposed to men with gonococcal or chlamydial urethritis developing clinical symptoms of PID.[45,46] Utilization of endometrial biopsy to detect histologic acute endometritis has demonstrated substantial percentages of subclinical ascending infection of the upper genital tract in women with gonococcal and/or chlamydia cervicitis and BV.[10,26,39,40,42,47,48]

For acute PID to develop, microorganisms from the lower genital tract must ascend through the internal cervical os into the endometrial cavity, through the uterotubal junction and into the fallopian tubes.[3,49,50] This intracanalicular spread of microorganisms is associated with a continuum of infection both microbiologically and histologically that includes the cervix, endometrium, and fallopian tubes.[3,51] The endocervical canal and cervical mucus plug are the major barriers protecting the upper genital tract from microorganisms present in the vagina and cervix.[49,52] Infection of the cervix with *C. trachomatis, N. gonorrhoeae*, and/or other microorganisms could result in damage to the endocervical canal or breakdown of the cervical mucus plug, leading to ascending infection.[49] In addition, damage to the normal clearance mechanisms for microorganisms associated with ciliated epithelial cells in the endometrium and fallopian tube might facilitate ascendance of microorganisms.[49] Conversely, Soper et al proposed that bacterial vaginosis may facilitate ascent of sexually transmitted disease (STD) organisms and aerobic bacteria through enzymatic degradation of cervical mucus by proteolytic enzymes associated with the BV-associated bacteria.[33] This complex interaction of STD organisms and the endogenous flora of the vagina and cervix is portrayed in Figure 2.1.

The unique anatomy and physiology of women may also facilitate ascending infection with *N. gonorrhoeae, C. trachomatis*, and/or endogenous bacteria from the vagina.[49,50] Young age is a major risk factor for PID. Cervical ectopy occurs more commonly in adolescents and results in a larger target area for attachment of *C. trachomatis*.[53,54] Other specific age-related changes in cervical mucus or endocervical defense mechanisms could also play a role in facilitating ascending infection.[49] Hormonal fluctuations associated with the menstrual cycle determine the potential for ascending infection via their effect on cervical mucus. At midcycle, when estrogen levels are high and progesterone low, cervical mucus may facilitate ascendance of infection, whereas after ovulation high progesterone levels make the mucus thick and less penetrable to bacteria.[49,50] In addition, at the time of menses, the cervical mucus plug is lost and microorganisms from the vagina and cervix can more easily ascend

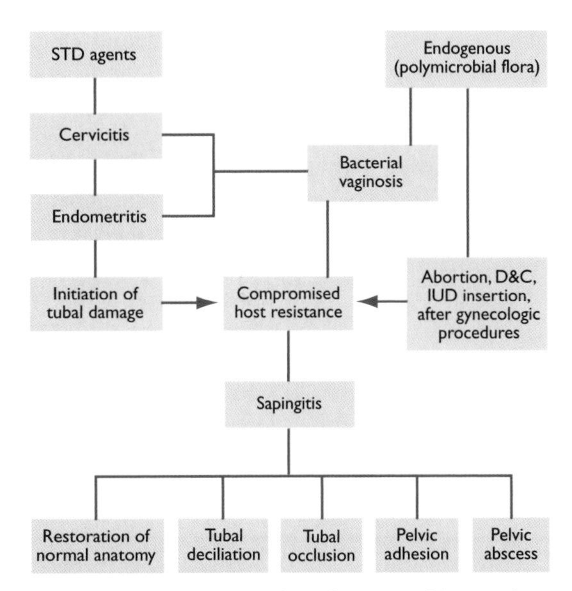

Figure 2.1 Possible interrelation of sexually transmitted disease and endogenous organisms in the pathogenesis of pelvic inflammatory disease. (Reprinted with permission from Sweet RL, Gibbs RS. Infectious Diseases of the Female Genital Tract, 4th edn. Philadelphia: Lippincott, Williams and Wilkins, 2002.)

into the uterine cavity. As a consequence, the majority of symptomatic chlamydial and gonococcal PID cases have their onset during or just after the menses.[55–57] Lastly, retrograde menstruation has been proposed as a mechanism by which microorganisms from the endometrial cavity may be propelled into the fallopian tubes.[49]

Whether combination oral contraceptives decrease or increase the risk for PID is controversial.[49,58] Women who use oral contraceptives may be at increased risk for cervical chlamydial infection.[53,54,58] However, most studies demonstrate that both the incidence of PID as well as the clinical and laparoscopic severity of PID are reduced in patients using oral contraceptives.[49,59–63] In-vitro studies have demonstrated that progesterone inhibits the growth of *N. gonorrhoeae*.[64–67] However, animal models have shown that estrogen and progesterone appear to facilitate the growth of *C. trachomatis* and ascension of *C. trachomatis* into the upper genital tract.[49] As a result of these studies, Rice and Schachter voiced concern that oral contraceptives may mask the signs and symptoms of ascending infection, leading to an increase of subclinical cases that are also associated with long-term sequelae.[49] More recently, Ness and colleagues, using histologic endometritis as a surrogate for PID, confirmed that such may be the case.[68]

The host immune system protects against infection through rapid and efficient clearance of microorganisms. However, the resultant inflammatory response, paradoxically, may lead to tissue damage or persistent infection.[49] For example, secretory immunoglobulin A (IgA) antigonococcal antibody inhibits attachment of *N. gonorrhoeae* to epithelial cells but interferes with phagocytosis of bacteria by polymorphonucleocytes (PMNs). Similarly, oxygen metabolites such as hypochlorite, superoxide anion, and hydrogen peroxide, which are produced when PMNs phagocytose bacteria, may cause tissue damage to the mucosal surface of the genital tract.[69] In addition, the cell-mediated immune response to *C. trachomatis* may also result in a pathogenic mechanism, leading to tissue damage.[49]

Recent attention has focused on genetic factors that control our response to microbial pathogens and influence our susceptibility to infectious diseases.[70–72] Initial attention has addressed genetic variations that control and regulate the immune responses to infectious agents. These immunogenetic polymorphisms protect subgroups of individuals from specific infectious agents.[70] Moreover, they determine whether the host mounts an effective immune response to pathogens, under-responds, leading to overt infection, or over-responds, initiating immune cascades that may result in more severe infections.[70] Of particular interest are the polymorphisms that occur in the genes encoding cytokines and chemokines, their receptors, or their inhibitors. These variations in genes determines whether the host initiates a proinflammatory (Th1) or anti-inflammatory (Th2) cytokine response.[70–72] In addition, the major histocompatibility complex (MHC; HLA system), consisting of the three major classes of HLA (Class I, Class II, and Class III), plays a significant role in developing and regulating the immune response to pathogenic microorganisms.[70]

NEISSERIA GONORRHOEAE

Gonorrhea, with over 350 000 cases reported in 2002, is the second most commonly reported communicable disease in the United States. Assuming a 50% under-reporting, an estimated 700 000 cases of gonorrhea occur annually in the United States.[73] The causative agent for gonorrhea is the Gram-negative diplococcus *N. gonorrhoeae*. Man is the only known natural host for *N. gonorrhoeae*. The organism has a predilection for infecting columnar or pseudostratified epithelium and thus the mucosal surfaces of the urogenital tract are the most common sites for gonococcal infection.[74]

Traditionally, non-tuberculous acute PID was divided into gonococcal and non-gonococcal disease. The separation was based solely on the recovery of *N. gonorrhoeae* from the endocervix of patients with acute PID. Studies utilizing endocervical cultures implicated the gonococcus as the causative agent in 33–81% of the cases of acute PID.[28,45,75–84] More recent studies with specimens also obtained from the abdominal cavity (culdocentesis) and/or fallopian tubes (laparoscopy) demonstrated similar recovery rates for *N. gonorrhoeae* from the endocervix (39%) but lower rates from the abdominal cavity/fallopian tubes (18% of total patients), with only 43% of patients with *N. gonorrhoeae* isolated from the cervix having the gonococcus in the abdominal cavity/fallopian tubes (Table 2.2). Generally, in populations with high endemic rates of gonorrhea, a high proportion of acute PID is associated with *N. gonorrhoeae*.[4] Thus, in many areas of the United States, *N. gonorrhoeae* has been recovered in 40–50% of acute PID cases.[4] As demonstrated by Westrom, in areas where the incidence of gonorrhea decreased, the proportion of PID cases associated with *N. gonorrhoeae* has also decreased.[85] Thus, in Sweden, without endemic gonorrhea, *N. gonorrhoeae* is recovered in less than 5% of acute PID cases.[85]

Recently, the PEACH study (the largest prospective cohort of acute PID in the United States) reported that among 831 women with clinical signs and symptoms of mild-to-moderate acute PID, *N. gonorrhoeae* was isolated in 170 (21.2%).[86] However, among a subgroup (n = 274) with acute PID confirmed by histologic endometritis, *N. gonorrhoeae* was isolated in only 11 (4%).[87]

Other recent, but smaller, studies have attempted to define the microbiology of acute PID utilizing a combination of cervical and endometrial cultures. Bukusi et al recovered *N. gonorrhoeae* from 44 (27%) of 162 women in Nairobi, Kenya with suspected acute PID.[88] Histologic endometritis confirmed the clinical diagnosis of PID in 63 (39%), with *N. gonorrhoeae* present in 25 of the patients (40%).[88] Eckert et al recovered *N. gonorrhoeae* from 67 (33%) of 106 women with acute PID confirmed by histologic endometritis and/or laparoscopic documentation of acute salpingitis.[89] *N. gonorrhoeae* was recovered from 56 (69%) of 81 cases of acute salpingitis and from 11 (44%) of histologic endometritis cases.[89] Haggerty and

Table 2.2 Isolation of *Neisseria gonorrhoeae* and *Chlamydia trachomatis* from the endocervix and abdominal cavity/fallopian tubes in women with acute pelvic inflammatory disease

Study	Number of patients	Cervical infection		Abdominal/tubal Infection	
		N. gonorrhoeae	*C. trachomatis.*	*N.gonorrhoeae*	*C. trachomatis*
Eschenbach et al,[28] 1975	204	90 (44%)	20/100 (20%)	7/54 (13%)	1/54 (2%)
				7/21 (33%)[a]	
Monif et al,[147] 1976	17	16 (94%)	ND	10 (62%)	ND
Eilard et al,[132] 1976	22	7 (32%)	6 (27%)	1/7	1/6
Mardh et al,[133] 1977	53	11 (17%)	19 (36%)	1/14 (7%)	6/20 (30%)
				1/2 (50%)[a]	6/7 (86%)[a]
Cunningham et al,[76,148] 1978	104	56 (54%)	ND	30 (29%)	ND
				30/56 (54%)[a]	
Thompson et al,[83] 1980	30	24 (80%)	3 (10%)	10 (33%)	3 (10%)[a]
				10/24 (42%)[a]	
Henry-Suchet et al,[149] 1980	39	18 (46%)	2 (5%)	1/4 (25%)	4 (24%)
				0/4	4/6 (67%)
Sweet et al,[29] 1980	39	19 (49%)	2 (5%)	8/35 (23%)	0/35
				8/19 (42%)[a]	0/2[a]
Gjonnaess et al,[134]1982	65	5 (8%)	26/56 (46%)	0/65	5/31 (16%)
				0/5[a]	4/5 (80%)[a]
Livengood et al,[145] 1992	23	9 (39%)	6 (26%)	6 (26%)	1 (4%)
				6/9 (67%)[a]	1/6 (17%)[a]
Soper et al,[150] 1992	36	25 (69%)	6 (17%)	12 (37%)	0
				12/25 (48%)[a]	0/6
Bevan et al,[146] 1995	104	14 (13%)	37 (36%)	3 (3%)	13 (13%)
				3/14 (21)[a]	13/37 (35)[a]
Totals	714	275 (39%)	131/479 (27%)	89/493 (18%)	40/363 (11%)
				77/178 (43%)[a]	28/69 (41%)[a]

[a]Isolation (%) *of C. trachomatis* or *N. gonorrhoeae* from abdomen of those with *C. trachomatis* or *N. gonorrhoeae* from the endocervix.

colleagues reported on 278 women from the PEACH study who had complete endometrial histologic and culture data at entry.[40] They noted that *N. gonorrhoeae* was present in 34 (12.2%) of all subjects. However, among the 45 women with histologic acute endometritis, *N. gonorrhoeae* was recovered from 15 (33.3%). In a study comparing patients with acute and subclinical PID, Wiesenfeld and coworkers isolated *N. gonorrhoeae* from the cervix in 80 (49%) of 168 women with acute PID and 15 (21%) of 75 women with subclinical PID and from the endometrium in 5 (9%) and 2 (3%) of acute PID and subclinical PID, respectively.[90]

As noted above, the usual route of infection for *N. gonorrhoeae* is direct intracanalicular ascending spread from the endocervix along the endometrial surface, through the uterotubal junction to the fallopian tube mucosal surface with resultant endosalpingitis. Thus gonococcal PID appears to be a continuum from cervicitis to endometritis to salpingitis.[51,89] Interestingly, the majority of women with gonococcal cervicitis do not develop acute subclinical PID.[3,10,45,46] The mechanisms by which *N. gonorrhoeae* causes acute PID probably include both human host and gonococcal factors.[49]

The environment of the lower genital tract is influenced by the menstrual cycle, which may play a significant role in the breakdown of local host mechanisms that normally prevent the ascent of microorganisms from the endocervix. It was found that 66–77% of the patients with gonococcal salpingitis present at the end of, or just after, the menstrual period.[46,56,57] In a laparoscopy study of acute PID, Sweet et al demonstrated an even more dramatic relationship between the menses and gonococcal salpingitis.[82] Although the recovery of *N. gonorrhoeae* from the cervix was most frequent within the first 7 days of the menstrual cycle, it was recovered from the cervix throughout the menstrual cycle. On the other hand, *N. gonorrhoeae* was isolated from the fallopian tubes only within the first 7 days after the onset of menses. During the menstrual period, the loss of the cervical mucus plug allows microorganisms from the endocervix and vagina to gain access to the endometrial cavity. The bacteriostatic effect of cervical mucus is lowest at the onset of menses. Additionally, the endometrium, which may offer local protection against bacterial invasion, has been sloughed. Moreover, menstrual blood from the endometrial cavity is an excellent culture medium. It had been postulated that the gonococci either migrate into the fallopian tubes or are carried there with refluxed menstrual blood. An alternative mechanism, suggested by Toth et al, may be the transport of *N. gonorrhoeae* via attachment to sperm;[91] however, no in-vivo studies have demonstrated that such a mechanism exists or that sperm can actually bring bacteria into the upper genital tract.

Nowicki et al hypothesized that contact of gonococci with menstrual blood containing serum rich in human compliment C1q may be a mechanism that increases the virulence of *N. gonorrhoeae* and contributes to the onset of PID.[92–94] These authors suggested that C1q-mediated resistance to complement killing of *N. gonorrhoeae* represents a mechanism of gonococcal virulence.[94]

Isolation rates of *N. gonorrhoeae* from the fallopian tubes in patients with laparoscopically confirmed acute salpingitis are inversely related to the duration of symptoms.[36,95,96] Whether this observation is due to an inability of *N. gonorrhoeae* to survive in the upper genital tract in the face of endogenous bacteria ascending into the upper genital tract or that gonococcal infection produces rapid onset of severe symptoms leading quickly to patients seeking health care is unclear.[36]

Soper et al reported that while laparoscopy-confirmed PID patients ≤ 7 days from onset of menses were just as likely as patients with an interval of >7 days to have positive cultures for *N. gonorrhoeae* from the endocervix, the mean number of days from the first day of the last menstrual period was significantly shorter in patients with gonococcal salpingitis (12.1 ± 6.7 days) than in those with non-gonococcal salpingitis (30.0 ± 25.7).[97] In a subsequent study, Soper and coworkers did not confirm these findings, as there was no statistically significant difference noted between duration intervals.[33] However, in this study, the duration intervals were <24 hours, 24–48 hours, and >48 hours. Moreover, there was a trend favoring recovery of *N. gonorrhoeae* from tube/cul-de-sac isolates at the shorter intervals.

Studies utilizing human fallopian tube organ cultures have shown that as gonococci reach the endosalpinx, they become attached to mucosal epithelial cells, penetrate the epithelial cells, and cause cell destruction.[98–100] Within 2–7 days, ciliary motility is lost in fallopian tube organ cultures inoculated with *N. gonorrhoeae*. Gonococci selectively attach to and invade the nonciliated mucus-secreting cells of the fallopian tube epithelium.[99,100] Gregg et al have reported on the production by the gonococcus of an endotoxin (lipopolysaccharide) that damages ciliated cells in human fallopian tube organ culture systems.[101] Peptidoglycan, a second structural component of the surface of *N. gonorrhoeae*, has also been shown to damage the fallopian tube mucosa.[102]

Additional pathogenic mechanisms have been described for *N. gonorrhoeae*. Gonococci produce IgA proteases that break down secretory IgA, which binds to microorganisms and prevents their adherence to mucosal surfaces.[103] Consequently, adherence of gonococci to mucosal cells is facilitated. *N. gonorrhoeae* also produces extracellular products such as phospholipase and peptidase, which can lead to cellular damage.[49] Production of interferon-gamma (IFN-γ) is induced by *N. gonorrhoeae*. In turn, IFN-γ induces expression of MHC Class II IA antigens on epithelial cells, which leads to activation of both the humoral and cell-mediated immune response directed against these epithelial cells.[49] This immune response may be another mechanism by which *N. gonorrhoeae* destroys fallopian tube epithelial cells infected with the organism.[49,104] Grifo et al demonstrated that IFN-γ was present in the serum in 65% of women with acute PID compared with none of healthy female controls.[104]

Inherent properties of *N. gonorrhoeae* also determine its ability to produce acute PID. It has been postulated that different strains of gonococci exist and that a particular strain or strains may be associated with development of acute PID. This concept holds for disseminated gonorrhea, in which the strain producing disseminated disease varies by microbiologic susceptibility patterns and auxotypes (nutritional requirements) from the gonococci causing asymptomatic lower genital tract disease. Sweet and coworkers studied several potential virulence factors in paired fallopian tube/peritoneal cavity and endocervical isolates of *N. gonorrhoeae* obtained from patients with acute PID undergoing laparoscopy. Specifically, auxotypes, antimicrobial susceptibility, serum bactericidal activity, and colony phenotype were studied.[105,106] *N. gonorrhoeae* recovered from women with PID had significantly different auxotypes and antimicrobial susceptibility patterns compared with those from uncomplicated anogenital infection. *N. gonorrhoeae* causing acute PID were relatively more resistant to multiple antimicrobial agents, and the auxotype pattern most associated with acute PID was the prototrophic pattern (i.e. no extra amino acids required for growth), whereas the arginine, hypoxanthine, and uracil auxotype pattern was associated with uncomplicated lower genital tract gonorrhea. However, there was no difference among paired peritoneal cavity/cervical isolates of *N. gonorrhoeae* recovered from salpingitis patients relative to auxotypes and antimicrobial susceptibility patterns. The potential virulence factor that was significantly different in the paired fallopian tube/endocervical gonorrhea specimens was colony phenotype.[105] The organisms in the fallopian tubes of women with acute salpingitis tended to be the transparent colony phenotype, whereas those present in the cervix of the same women tended to be opaque. In previous studies, women cultured during the menstrual cycle, except during the time of the menses, had a preponderance of opaque organisms isolated, with a peak at the time of ovulation. The organisms usually recovered from the male urethra are heavily opaque, and the organisms recovered from women on oral contraceptives are opaque (women on oral contraceptives appear to be protected against the development of upper genital tract disease if they acquire gonorrhea).

Thus, epidemiologically and clinically, it appears that the transparent colony phenotypes may well be the virulent form of the gonococcus in the pathogenesis of acute salpingitis. In order to test this hypothesis, human fallopian tube and cervical organ culture explant systems were used to evaluate endocervical and fallopian tube attachment. At both the endocervix and fallopian tubes, the transparent colony phenotype of *N. gonorrhoeae* attaches more avidly to human fallopian tube tissue than their opaque colony phenotype counterparts.[107] It appears that something in the cervical milieu (hormones, pH, or an unidentified factor) may either select out the transparent colony phenotype or selectively drive the gonococci from opaque to transparent forms. The basic difference between the opaque and transparent colony phenotypes are proteins present in the outer cell membrane of the organism.

Over the past 30 years, our understanding of the pathogenic mechanisms of the gonococcus has been expanded.[108,109] Initially, Kellogg et al[110] demonstrated that there are differences in the virulence of *N. gonorrhoeae* associated with specific colony types. Kellogg colony types 1 and 2 (now called P+ colonies), which contain pili, are capable of producing infection, whereas types 3 and 4 (now called P– colonies), which do not contain pili, fail to cause infection.[110] The pili appear to facilitate attachment of gonococci to epithelial surfaces.[111,112] Also, other gonococcal surface structures in addition to pili are associated with pathogenesis.

Pathogenic neisseriae possess an extraordinary capability to vary their surface structures. Not only does this property protect the organism from the host immune response but also such variation affects the function of factors that interact with host cells. As a result, the gonococcus can interact with epithelial cells or phagocytic cells, adhere to cells, invade cells, or remain protected from serum factors inside a capsule of sialated lipopolysaccharide.[109] These surface structures and functions are determined by proteins present in the outer membrane of the gonococcus. The most prominent protein in the outer membrane is the porins protein (Por), previously designated protein I, which is an important cofactor in gonococcal invasion of epithelial mucosa cells.[109] It is also involved in the events leading to endocytosis of the gonococcus by mucosal cells.[111] The opacity-associated proteins designated Opa (formerly protein II) are a family of proteins that promote cell adhesion, thus setting the stage for cell invasion.[108,109,112] The Opa proteins are the determinant of colony phenotype, a characteristic first noted by James and Swanson[113] to be important in the pathogenesis of gonococcal infection. They demonstrated that transparent colonies (now known to be Opa-negative) are more associated with cultures from the endocervix than from the male urethra, particularly at the time of menses.[113] Draper et al[105] reported that transparent (Opa-negative) colonies were the virulent form recovered from the fallopian tubes of patients with laparoscopically confirmed PID. Colonies of *N. gonorrhoeae* containing Opa proteins (Opa-positive) appear opaque. One Opa protein (Opa_{50}) interacts with epithelial cell lines and promotes invasion, whereas the 10 remaining Opa proteins (Opa_{52}) mediate binding to phagocytic cells.[114] All pathogenic neisseriae contain a reduction modifiable protein (RMP) (formerly designated protein III).[108] Many blocking antibodies that prevent bacterial activity are directed against this antigen.[108] Thus, anti-RMP antibodies block access of other antibodies, including bactericidal immunoglobulin M (IgM), to their targets on the gonococcal surface. Rice et al[115] demonstrated that RMP is important for successful transmission of *N. gonorrhoeae* to sexual partners. This is the result of the presence of anti-RMP antibodies in genital secretions blocking the protective antibodies usually present in genital secretions.[108]

Additional gonococcal virulence factors include:

- lipopolysaccharides, which possess endotoxin activity, causing cytotoxic effects on the epithelium of the fallopian tube and the systemic findings of fever and toxicity[99]
- IgA protease, which is present in all gonococci and destroys the secretory IgA[108]
- iron-repressible proteins, which are involved in uptake of iron, an essential requirement for growth of gonococci.[108]

As noted by Westrom and Eschenbach, immunologic defense mechanisms induced by *N. gonorrhoeae* may provide some protection against recurrent gonococcal PID.[3] Buchanan and associates, utilizing principal outer membrane proteins to serotype the gonococcus, demonstrated the presence of nine serotypes of gonococci.[116] They noted that three of the serotypes (1, 2, and 8) were responsible for nearly 75% of gonococcal salpingitis. In addition, these investigators reported that reinfection with a similar serotype of gonococci results in cervical infection but not in fallopian tube infection, whereas reinfection with gonococci of a different serotype results in both cervical and fallopian tube infection. This finding suggests the presence of immunity of the fallopian tube site among previously infected women.

CHLAMYDIAL PELVIC INFLAMMATORY DISEASE

Chlamydial infection is the most commonly reported communicable disease in the United States, with over 834 000 cases of genital chlamydial infection reported to the CDC in 2002.[73] The causative agent, *C. trachomatis*, is the most common bacterial sexually transmitted organism in the United States, with an estimated 4 million new cases occurring annually.[117,118]

C. trachomatis is one of the four recognized species of *Chlamydia*. There are 15 serotypes of *C. trachomatis*, which are responsible for three major groups of infections. Serotypes L_1, L_2, and L_3 are the causative agents of lymphogranuloma inguinale. Serotypes A, B, Ba, and C are the putative agents for endemic blinding trachoma. The remaining serotypes (D, E, F, G, H, I, J, and K) are the oculogenital and sexually transmitted strains that cause acute PID. In addition, these strains cause inclusion conjunctivitis of the newborn, pneumonia of the newborn, urethritis, cervicitis, epididymitis, and Reiter's syndrome.[119]

C. trachomatis is an obligate intracellular bacterium.[120] Similar to *N. gonorrhoeae*, it has a predilection for columnar and pseudostratified epithelium of the urogenital tract. *C. trachomatis* has a unique and long growth cycle of 48–72 hours. Schachter[121] has divided the life cycle of chlamydiae into several steps:

1. initial attachment of the elementary body (infectious particle) to a host cell
2. entry into the host cell
3. morphologic change into the reticulate body (metabolical active form), with subsequent intracellular growth and replication
4. transformation of the reticulate bodies into the elementary bodies
5. release of the infectious elementary bodies.

Initiation of infection is dependent upon an initial step involving attachment of the metabolically inactive but infectious elementary body to a susceptible host cell. This probably involves a specific receptor–ligand interaction.[121] The host cells are generally nonciliated colummnar or cuboidal epithelia, such as those found in the conjunctiva, urethra, endocervix, and mucosa of the endometrium and fallopian tubes. Following attachment to the host cell, the elementary body is rapidly ingested by a phagocytic process similar to ordinary bacterial phagocytosis.[122] This process is an enhanced phagocytosis that is induced by the elementary body, which then is selectively taken up by the susceptible host cell. Chlamydia entry appears to occur via a mechanism similar to receptor-mediated endocytosis.[123] Intracellularly, the elementary bodies exit within a cytoplasmic vacuole in the phagosome, where they remain throughout their entire growth cycle. In this state, chlamydiae may be protected from host defense mechanisms, such as cellular lysosomes. Schachter[121] proposed that these two characteristics – induced phagocytosis and prevention of phagolysosomal fusion – are major virulence factors of chlamydia. In the next step of the growth cycle, the elementary body, approximately 8 hours after entry, undergoes reorganization into what is called a reticulate or initial body, which represents the metabolically active and dividing form of the organism. They divide for approximately 8–24 hours and then condense and reorganize to form new elementary bodies. Recognition of those characteristic cytoplasmic inclusions was the classic method for detection of chlamydiae. As the number of elementary bodies increases, infectivity increases. By 48–72 hours, the host cell bursts and liberates these infectious particles. The cycle then starts anew. The complete infectious cycle takes approximately 48–72 hours.

As an obligate intracellular bacterium, *C. trachomatis* is an extremely well-adapted human parasite that depends on the host cell for nutrients and energy.[120,121] Chlamydiae do not stain with the Gram stain, and in many respects resemble free-living Gram-netagive bacteria. They contain DNA and RNA, are susceptible to certain antibiotics, have a rigid cell wall, are similar in structure and content to Gram-negative bacteria, and multiply by binary fission. They differ from most bacteria but are similar to viruses in that they are obligate intracellular parasites. They may be regarded as bacteria that have adapted to an intracellular environment; thus, they need viable cells for their multiplication and survival.

Chlamydiae differ from free-living Gram-negative bacteria in lacking the peptidoglycan layer that resides between the outer and inner membranes of the cell wall and provides shape and rigidity to these bacteria.[124] However, elementary bodies are rigid as the result of covalent disulfide linkages among outer membrane proteins.[125] The outer membrane proteins involved in the disulfide linkage are the major outer membrane protein (MOMP), with a molecular weight of 60 kDa, and a 12 kDa cysteine-rich protein.[126] In addition to its role in maintaining the structural integrity of *C. trachomatis*, the MOMP is a transmembrane protein that functions as a poron, allowing ingress and egress of low-molecular-weight substances such as sugars and some antibiotics.[127] Chlamydiae also contain a lipopolysaccharide (LPS) similar to that present in the outer membrane of Gram-negative bacteria.[128]

It is generally held that chlamydial salpingitis – similar to the situation in gonococcal salpingitis – results from the intracanalicular spread of *C. trachomatis* from the endocervix to the endometrium and thence to the fallopian tube.[78,129,130] It is estimated that 10% of *C. trachomatis* cervical infections ascend to cause PID.[4] Ripa et al have shown that *C. trachomatis* in a grivet monkey model gains access to the fallopian tube mucosa as an ascending intracanalicular infection from the endocervix.[131] Toth et al have reported that *C. trachomatis* attaches to sperm and have suggested that sperm may well be the vector that facilitates spread of microorganisms, including chlamydia, into the upper genital tract.[91] However, actual attachment of *C. trachomatis* was not proven. Moreover, no study has demonstrated that sperm can carry *C. trachomatis* into the upper genital tract in vivo. Recently, an association between chlamydial salpingitis and menstruation, similar to that for *N. gonorrhoeae*, has been noted.[56] In this study, among the women who developed acute PID, 50% of chlamydial infection occurred within 7 days of the onset of menses. Thus, it appears that the pathogenesis of chlamydial salpingitis parallels that seen in gonococcal disease. No specific virulence factors that facilitate the development of acute PID have been identified for *C. trachomatis*.

C. trachomatis has been the focus of many investigations and is now firmly established as a major etiologic agent for acute PID. Recent studies have also suggested that *C. trachomatis* plays an important role in the etiology of subclinical PID.[1,3,10]

Scandinavian investigators were the first to demonstrate the important role of *C. trachomatis* in the etiology of acute PID[132–141] (Table 2.3). These studies reported the recovery of *C. trachomatis* from the cervix in 22–47% of women with acute PID. Of more significance, *C. trachomatis* was recovered from the fallopian tube(s) in 9–30% of women with visually confirmed acute PID.[132–134] Based on serologic assessment, Scandinavian studies demonstrated that *C. trachomatis* was associated with 23–62% of acute PID cases.[132–141]

Initial investigations in the United States failed to confirm a significant role for chlamydia in the etiology of acute PID. Eschenbach and coworkers isolated *C. trachomatis* from the peritoneal cavity in only one of 54 cases of acute PID, despite a 20% isolation rate of this organism from the cervix.[28] In the first laparoscopy study performed in the United States, Sweet and coworkers did not recover *C. trachomatis* from the fallopian tube exudate in 37 patients with laparoscopy-confirmed salpingitis.[34,82] Thompson et al isolated *C. trachomatis* from the culdocentesis aspirates in only 10% of women with acute PID.[83] In contradistinction, serologic data obtained from studies in the United States demonstrated a four-fold rise in chlamydial antibodies in approximately 20% of acute PID cases.[28,82] Thus, at that time, the evidence supporting chlamydia as a major etiologic factor for acute PID in the United States was indirect, based on endocervical isolation and serologic studies. Several

Table 2.3 *Chlamydia trachomatis* in acute pelvic inflammatory disease

Study	No. of patients	Isolation rate of *C. trachomatis*		
		Endocervix	Upper genital and peritoneal cavity	Four-fold rise in serum antibodies
Eilard et al[132]	22	6 (27%)	2 (9%)[a]	5 (23%)
Mardh et al[133]	53	19 (37%)	6/20 (30%)[a]	
Treharne et al[135]	143			88 (62%)
Paavonen et al[136]	106	27/26		19/72 (26%)
Paavonen[137]	228	68 (30%)		32/167 (19%)
Mardh et al[138]	60	23 (38%)		24/60 (40%)
Ripa et al[139]	206	52/156 (33%)		118 (57%)
Gjonnaess et al[134]	56	26 (46%)	5/42 (12%)[a]	26/52 (46%)
Moller et al[140]	166	37 (22%)		34 (21%)
Osser and Persson[141]	111	52 (47%)		37/72 (51%)
Eschenbach et al[28]	100	20 (20%)	1/54 (2%)[c]	15/74 (20%)
Sweet et al[82]	37	2 (5%)	0[a]	5/22 (23%)
Thompson et al[83]	30	3 (10%)	3 (10%)[a]	
Sweet et al[34]	71	10 (14%)	17 (24%)[d]	
Wasserheit et al[35]	22	10 (45%)	8 (36%)[d]	
Kiviat et al[143]	55	12 (22%)	12 (22%)[d]	
Brunham et al[32]	50	7 (14%)	4 (8%)[a]	20 (40%)
Landers et al[38]	148	41 (28%)	32 (22%)[d]	
Soper et al[33]	84[a]	13 (15%)	1 (1%)	
	51[b]		6 (51%) (12%)	
Kiviat et al[144]	69		16 (23%)	
Jossens et al[41]	580	129 (22%)	129 (22%)	
Hillier et al[39]	85[a]		3 (4%)	
	178[b]		23 (13%)	
Bevan et al[146]	104[j]	37 (35.5%)	10 (9.6%)[b]	27/72
			13 (12.5%)[a]	(37.5%)
Ness et al[86]	851		176 (22%)[e]	
Bukusi et al[88]	162		32 (20%)[e]	
	63[i]		18 (29%)[e]	
Eckert et al[89]	26[i]		6 (23%)[e]	
	83[j]		36 (43%)[e]	
Wiesenfeld et al[90]	168[g]	58 (36%)	32 (20%)	
	75[h]	25 (36%)	7 (10%)	

[a] Fallopian tube.
[b] Endometrial cavity.
[c] Culdocentesis.
[d] Fallopian tube and/or endometrial cavity.
[e] Endocervix and endometrial cavity.
[f] Study performed in Nairobi, Kenya.
[g] Acute PID.
[h] Subclinical PID.
[i] Histologic endometritis.
[j] Laparoscopy-confirmed salpingitis.

factors were proposed to explain the conflicting findings from Scandinavia and the United States. In Sweden, specimens for chlamydial cultures were obtained via biopsy or needle aspiration of the fallopian tube; in the United States, cultures were obtained from periotoneal fluid and/or tubal exudate. *C. trachomatis* is an intracellular organism, and thus fresh infected cells, such as obtained via biopsy, may be necessary to optimize recovery of the organism. In addition, the patient population studied were different: the Swedish investigators studied women with a milder disease than was usually hospitalized and enrolled in studies in the United States. In fact, it has been suggested by

Svensson and colleagues that patients with milder pelvic inflammatory disease are more likely to have *C. trachomatis* as the etiologic agent.[142] These investigators noted that the women with *C. trachomatis* as the causative agent were more likely to be afebrile and have longer-standing disease of milder type than women with gonococcal or nongonococcal, nonchlamydial disease. Paradoxically, at laparoscopy, those women with *C. trachomatis* infection based on serologic data had the most severe fallopian tube involvement and the highest estimated erythrocyte sedimentation rates (ESRs).[142] The Lund group of investigators also noted that acute PID patients with anaerobes recovered were more likely to be febrile, appeared to have more severe clinical symptoms and signs, and were prone to have associated inflammatory adnexal masses (L. Westrom, pers comm 1982).

More recent studies have suggested a definite role for *C. trachomatis* as an etiologic agent for acute PID in the United States (see Table 2.3). Sweet and coworkers in a study where specimens were obtained from the upper genital tract (endometrial cavity and/or fallopian tubes) provided direct evidence for the etiologic role of *C. trachomatis* in hospitalized women with acute PID.[34] They recovered *C. trachomatis* from 17 (24%) of 71 of these patients. Confirmation of a major role for *C. trachomatis* in the etiology of acute PID in the United States was provided by Wasserheit and colleagues, who demonstrated that 14 (61%) of 23 women with salpingitis and/or plasma cell endometritis had *C. trachomatis* identified in the upper genital tract.[35] Similarly, Kiviat et al[143] and Landers et al[38] both recovered *C. trachomatis* from the upper genital tract in 22% of PID patients. Jossens and coworkers, in a large study that included 580 hospitalized patients with acute PID, identified *C. trachomatis* in the upper genital tract in 129 (22%) patients.[41] Hillier et al recovered *C. trachomatis* from the endometrium in 23 (13%) of 178 patients with histologic endometritis and clinical acute PID.[39]

Bevan and coworkers noted that *C. trachomatis* was present in the genital tract in 40 (38.5%) of 104 women in the United Kingdom with acute salpingitis confirmed at laparoscopy.[146] In 13 (12.5%) laparoscopy-confirmed cases, *C. trachomatis* was recovered from swabs introduced into the fallopian tubes; among the 40 patients with chlamydia present in the cervix, it was present in the fallopian tube in nearly one-third of cases.[146] In the very large PEACH study, Ness et al reported isolation of *C. trachomatis* from the genital tract (endocervix or endometrial cavity) in 176 (22%) of 851 clinically diagnosed cases of acute PID.[86] In a more recent analysis of patients from the PEACH study, Haggerty and coworkers demonstrated that *C. trachomatis* was present in one-fourth of cases with histologic acute endometritis.[40] Bukusi et al, in a study from Nairobi, Kenya, recovered *C. trachomatis* from the genital tract (endocervix and endometrial cavity) in 32 (20%) of 162 women with clinically suspected acute PID.[88] Among patients with "confirmed" PID (e.g. histologic evidence of endometritis), *C. trachomatis* was present in 18 (29%) of 63 patients.[88] Eckert et al reported the isolation of *C. trachomatis* from the genital tract (endocervix or endometrial cavity) in 6 (23%) of 26 and 36 (43%) of 83 women with histologic endometritis and laparoscopy-confirmed acute salpingitis, respectively.[89] Most recently, Wiesenfeld et al noted that *C. trachomatis* was recovered from the endocervix in 58 (36%) and the endometrial cavity of 32 (20%) of 168 patients with clinically suspected acute PID.[90] Among women with subclinical PID (confirmed histologic acute endometritis), *C. trachomatis* was present in the endocervix of 25 (36%) and in the endometrial cavity of 7 (10%) of 75 cases, respectively.[90]

Results from laparoscopy studies (summarized in Tables 2.1–2.3) demonstrate recovery of *C. trachomatis* from the fallopian tubes/abdominal cavity in 76 (14%) of 544 patients with confirmed acute PID. Among patients with chlamydial cervical infection in these studies, *C. trachomatis* was isolated from the fallopian tubes/abdominal cavity in 41%. Generally, European studies from the 1970s and 1980s report isolation rates of *C. trachomatis* ranging from 25% to 50% in acute PID, whereas those from the United States showed lower rates of chlamydia.[3] Thus, current evidence strongly supports an important putative role for *C. trachomatis* in acute PID. This has major implications for clinical management, as is discussed in Chapter 9.

Epidemiologic studies have suggested that chlamydia plays a substantial role in infertility due to tubal obstruction and salpingitis.[129,149,151–159] These studies performed in a wide variety of populations and geographic areas have documented that women with tubal factor infertility are significantly more likely to have had previous systemic chlamydial infection as documented serologically than pregnant controls or nontubal factor infertility patients (Figure 2.2). A similar association with previous chlamydial infection and ectopic pregnancy has recently been demonstrated[154,160–163] (Figure 2.3). Thus, the two major sequelae of acute PID, namely tubal infertility and ectopic pregnancy, have been associated with prior chlamydial infection. Subsequently, these epidemiologic studies resulted in the concept of unrecognized (subclinical) PID, because about 50% of women with tubal factor infertility and serologic evidence of previous chlamydial infection had no history of being diagnosed or treated for acute PID.[129,149,151–159] While suggestive of a direct etiologic role in tubal infertility for *C. trachomatis*, such seroepidemiologic studies do not prove causation.

Subsequent investigations have provided a model for the pathogenesis of chlamydial salpingitis (including subclinical) and its sequelae.[164–170] Briefly, it is hypothesized that chlamydial PID is an immune-mediated disease resulting from immune responses to a chlamydial heat shock protein (Hsp): Hsp 60.[164–170] Thus, *C. trachomatis* elicits an inflammatory response similar to a delayed hypersensitivity reaction, with resultant damage to the fallopian tube. This hypersensitivity response is similar to the pathogenic mechanism by which *C. trachomatis* produces scarring and blindness in ocular trachoma.[171]

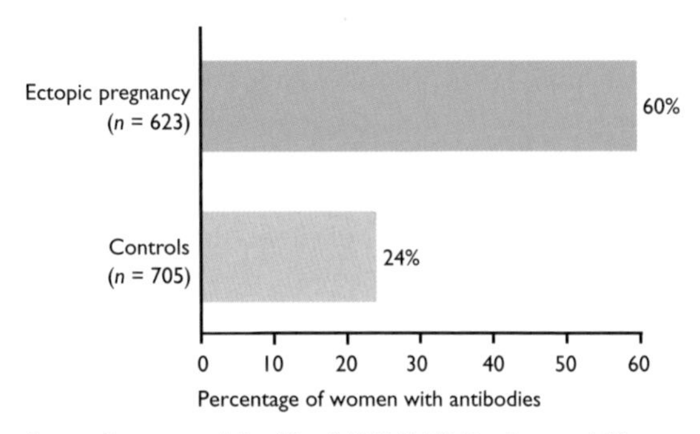

Sources: Svenson, et al. Fertil Steril 1985;44:313. Brunham, et al. Obstet Gynecol 1986;67:722. Hartford, et al. Fertil Steril 1987;47:118. Robertson, et al. Br J Obstet Gynaecol 1988;95:711. Walters, et al. Am J Obstet Gynecol 1988;159:942. Chaim, et al. Contraception 1989;40:59. Chow, et al. JAMA 1990;263:3164

Figure 2.3 Serologic studies demonstrating an association of previous infection with *Chlamydia trachomatis*, as determined by antichlamydial immunoglobulin G antibody and ruptured ectopic pregnancy. (Reprinted with permission from Sweet RL, Gibbs RS. Infectious Diseases of the Female Genital Tract, 4th edn. Philadelphia: Lippincott, Williams and Wilkins, 2002.)

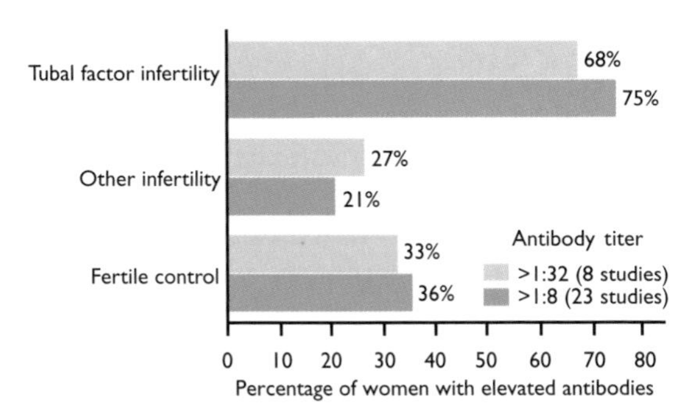

Figure 2.2 Serologic studies demonstrating an association of previous infection with *Chlamydia trachomatis* as determined by antichlamydial immunoglobulin G antibody and tubal factor infertility. (Reprinted with permission from Sweet RL, Gibbs RS. Infectious Diseases of the Female Genital Tract, 4th edn. Philadelphia: Lippincott, Williams and Wilkins, 2002.)

Further evidence supporting a role for *C. trachomatis* in the etiology of acute PID comes from animal model work, which has demonstrated the ability of chlamydia to produce acute salpingitis.[131,172–178] These have included use of several chlamydial strains: guinea pig inclusion conjunctivitis (GPIC) agent, the mouse pneumonia biovar of *C. trachomatis*, and human *C. trachomatis* in the guinea pig, mouse, and grivet monkey, respectively.[131,172–178]

As described above, chlamydial salpingitis results from the intracanalicular spread of *C. trachomatis* from the endocervix to the endometrium and thence to the fallopian tube.[78,129,130] Scanning and transmission electron microscopy has demonstrated that *C. trachomatis*, following ascent to the fallopian tube, attaches to the tubal epithelium and is engulfed via the process of endocytosis in a membrane-lined vacuole.[179] *C. trachomatis* replicates within the cell, where it is protected from recognition by the host immune system.[3] Ultimately, the elementary bodies, the infectious form of *C. trachomatis*, are released into the tubal lumen, where additional mucosal cells can be subsequently infected.[179] *C. trachomatis* replicates in both the ciliated and nonciliated mucosal cells in human fallopian/tube organ culture,[180] the oviducts of mice infected with mouse *C. trachomatis*,[181] and in a non-human primate model.[182]

In contradistinction to most bacterial infections, where tissue damage results from the direct effect of bacterial replication and inflammation, the damage and scarring associated with *C. trachomatis* appears to be the result of the host immune response to the infection.[164–171,176–178,183] Patton et al, in a monkey model, demonstrated that primary chlamydial infection is associated with mild-to-moderate inflammation with an influx of PMNs.[177] They further noted that this was a self-limited infection that peaks by 2 weeks and resolves within 5 weeks.[177] However, repeated inoculations with *C. trachomatis* resulted in an infection and inflammation characterized by the presence of mononuclear cells and formation of lymphoid follicles.[177] Unlike a self-limited infection with complete resolution, repeated infection in this monkey model produced extensive tubal scarring, distal tubal obstruction, and peritubal adhesions.[178] Such scarring of the fallopian tube subsequently leads to tubal infertility and/or ectopic pregnancy.[49]

Several interesting pieces of evidence support a role for the host immune system via the cell-mediated immune mechanism in the development of long-term sequelae secondary to chlamydial infection. Many investigations have provided data suggesting that chlamydial PID is a cell-mediated immune disease probably resulting from immune responses to chlamydial Hsp 60.[164–171,183] It has been hypothesized that this inflammatory immune response is similar to a delayed hypersensitivity reaction that results in damage to the fallopian tube. As noted by Moller et al, the histopathology of the inflammatory response in human fallopian tube tissue to the Hsp 60 protein is similar to that seen in blinding trachoma and genital tract models of infertility.[184] Wagar et al demonstrated that women with PID or ectopic pregnancy have antibodies against this protein.[185] Similarly, Brunham and coworkers noted that patients with tubal factor infertility had antibodies directed at the Hsp 60 antigen[186] and Witkin et al reported that induction of a cell-mediated immune response to the chlamydial Hsp 60 protein is a common feature of upper genital tract infection.[165] In addition, Patton et al demonstrated that *C. trachomatis* infection in monkeys induced delayed hypersensitivity, which is mediated by *C. trachomatis* Hsp 60.[167]

Ward noted that persistent and repeated chlamydial infections are particularly associated with pathologic disease.[187] IFN-γ plays a major role in the immune response to chlamydia and its subsequent inflammatory process.[187] It is responsible for induction of delayed chlamydial development and, as a result, restriction of chlamydial infection. However, delayed development leads to persistent expression of chlamydial Hsps, which share antigens not only with other bacterial Hsps but also with human Hsps.[187] According to Ward, the damage and scarring associated with chlamydial infection are dependent on four mechanisms of chlamydial disease:

- persistent chlamydial infection
- role of cytokines in chlamydial infection
- role of chlamydial Hsps in the pathogenesis of disease
- host genotype.

Whereas the normal chlamydial development cycle is a productive cycle of infection with release of infectious elementary bodies, persistent chlamydial infection is associated with incomplete chlamydial development and intermittent release of elementary bodies.[187] This incomplete growth cycle can be induced by either inappropriate antibiotic treatment (e.g. penicillin) or the cell-mediated immune response (e.g. IFN-γ, as discussed above). Such persistent ("latent") infection can subsequently revert back to infection and disease.[187]

Chlamydial infection induces production of a variety of cytokines, which lead to inflammation and scar formation.[188–190] The cytokines involved include tumor necrosis factor (TNF), interferon (IFN), and interleukins (ILs). As previously noted, the hallmark of chlamydial infection is an inflammatory process that is exacerbated by reinfection and subsequently results in tissue damage and scarring. Interaction of *C. trachomatis* with the cytokine network is a key element of this disease process. Chlamydial infection produces a cytokine response by direct infection of epithelial cells[191] and by interaction with cells of the immune system.[192] Rasmussen et al demonstrated that infection of cervical epithelial cells with *C. trachomatis* induced production of the proinflammatory cytokines IL-8, GRD-γ, granulocyte–macrophage colony-stimulating factor (GM-CSF), and IL-6.[191] Unlike the rapid and transient cytokine response induced by other invasive bacterial pathogens, chlamydia induces an epithelial cytokine response that is delayed until 20–24 hours after infection, persists throughout the chlamydial growth cycle, and requires bacterial protein synthesis. Rasmussen et al[191] proposed that the acute host response to chlamydia at the mucosal surface might be primarily initiated and sustained by epithelial cells, the target for chlamydial infection. Response to chlamydial infection by the cells of the immune system is a Th1-like response, with production of IL-2 and IFN-γ.[187] Although this Th1 response is crucial to resolving established chlamydial infection, as discussed earlier, it can also lead to persistent chlamydial infection and its associated adverse complications.

Hsps are a family of closely related proteins that are widely distributed in virtually all organisms and expressed when organisms are exposed to stress.[187,193,194] The major chlamydial Hsps (12, 60, and 75 kDa) are partially (40–50%) homologous with the human mitochondrial proteins Hsp 10, Hsp 60, and Hsp 70.[187] It has been postulated that the immune response to chlamydial Hsps, particularly Hsp 60, initiates (by antigenic mimicry) an autoimmune response against related human Hsps.[187] IFN-γ is central to this mechanism of pathogenesis.[193,194] Beatty and coworkers[195] reported that although treatment of chlamydial-infected cells with IFN-γ inhibited chlamydial development, it permitted expression of Hsp 60. Further, it appears that continued chlamydial Hsp 60 expression (secondary to the action of IFN-γ) initiates the chronic inflammatory responses associated with fibrosis and scarring characteristic of the sequelae of chlamydial infection (e.g. blinding trachoma, PID, infertility, and ectopic pregnancy).[187]

Witkin and coworkers demonstrated that peripheral blood monocytes from patients with acute PID produced increased levels of IL-1 and IL-6, cytokines capable of producing scarring and tissue damage.[196] Additional evidence for the role played by the cytokine response to chlamydial infection is provided by studies demonstrating the presence of IFN-γ in cervical secretions of women with chlamydial cervicitis[197] and in the sera of women with acute PID.[102] In addition to increases in cytokine production, the presence of IFN-γ induces expression of MHC Class II on epithelial cells.[3] Expression of MHC-II-bound antigens on epithelial cells of the fallopian tube, in turn, probably initiates a cell-mediated immune response directed against the epithelial cells infected with *C. trachomatis*, leading to destruction of the fallopian tube mucosal cells.[198]

In humans, several studies have demonstrated an association between antibody to chlamydial Hsps and the chronic sequelae of chlamydial infection, such as PID, infertility, ectopic pregnancy, and perihepatitis.[185,186,199–205] Wagar et al[185] and Brunham et al[186] reported that *C. trachomatis*-seropositive women with ectopic pregnancy had antibodies to a 57 kDa protein antigen of *C. trachomatis*. Wagar et al[185] documented that this protein antigen was a *C. trachomatis* Hsp 60 homologue. Witkin et al,[206] Peeling et al,[199] Eckert et al,[200] and Domeika et al[205] noted a significant association between the presence of antibodies to chlamydial Hsp 60 and PID. Similarly, Toye et al,[202] Arno et al,[203] and Witkin et al[207] demonstrated an association of antibodies to chlamydial Hsp 60 and tubal factor infertility. Money and coworkers[204] reported that antibodies to chlamydial Hsp 60 were associated with laparoscopically verified perihepataitis. Thus, it appears that the cell-mediated immune response to this antigen plays an important pathogenic role in *C. trachomatis*-associated sequelae to acute PID.

Host genotype appears to play an important role in determining the severity of human disease following chlamydial infection.[187] Kimani et al[208] studied 306 female sex workers in Nairobi, Kenya, 44 of whom developed chlamydial or combined chlamydial and gonococcal PID. These investigators reported that the MHC Class I HLA-A31 was independently associated as a risk factor for PID, with odds ratio (OR) = 5.6; 95% confidence interval (CI) 1.1–29.4. Recently, Cohen and coworkers[209] demonstrated an association of specific HLA Class II alleles with *C. trachomatis* microimmunofluorescence seropositivity among women with tubal infertility. They noted that among infertile women, DQA*0101 and DQB*0501 alleles were positively associated with *C. trachomatis* tubal infertility (OR = 4.9; 95% CI 1.3–18.6 and OR = 6.8; 95% CI 1.6–29.2, respectively).[209] These authors postulated that the DQ locus might modify susceptibility to, and pathogenicity of, *C. trachomatis* infection.

ANAEROBIC AND FACULTATIVE BACTERIA

The monoetiologic, sexually transmitted organism paradigm for the etiology of acute PID dramatically changed in the 1970s as it became apparent that the presence of pathogenic microorganisms in the endocervix was not absolute proof that such microorganisms were causally associated with upper genital tract infections such as acute PID. Investigations, that initially utilized transvaginal culdocentesis and subsequently laparoscopy to obtain cultures directly from the peritoneal fluid or fallopian tube exudate demonstrated a poor correlation between the cervical and intra-abdominal cultures. Despite isolation of *N. gonorrhoeae* from the endocervix of patients with acute PID, the gonococcus was recovered from only 6–70% of the peritoneal and/or tubal cultures.[28,29,74,79–81,94,138,139,210] Investigations in the late 1970s utilizing culdocentesis and appropriate anaerobic culture techniques resulted in the isolation of a variety of aerobic and anaerobic bacteria from the peritoneal fluid of patients with acute PID.[28,29,74,79–81,138,139,210] The organisms recovered most frequently in these studies were *N. gonorrhoeae* and anaerobic bacteria, including *Peptostreptococcus*, and *Bacteroides* and *Prevotella* species. A characteristic pattern evolved from these culdocentesis studies (Table 2.4). Although there was a high prevalence of *N. gonorrhoeae* (57%) in the cervix of these patients, less than one-fourth of the cases had *N. gonorrhoeae* as the only organism recovered from an intra-abdominal site. An additional one-fourth of the patients had a mixture of *N. gonorrhoeae* plus mixed anaerobic and aerobic bacteria (predominantly anaerobes). The other 50% of the patients did not have *N. gonorrhoeae*, but only a mixture of anaerobic and aerobic bacteria recovered from the abdominal cavity. Thus, the culdocentesis studies demonstrated that the etiology of acute PID was polymicrobic in nature and brought into question the exact role of *N. gonorrhoeae* in the pathogenesis of acute pelvic inflammatory disease. Several investigators[147,148,210] postulated that *N. gonorrhoeae*

Table 2.4 Isolation of *N. gonorrhoeae*, anaerobes, and aerobes from culdocentesis aspirates in acute pelvic inflammatory disease

Study	Number of patients	Culdocentesis		
		Endocervical *N. gonorrhoeae*	*N. gonorrhoeae* only	*N. gonorrhoeae* plus anaerobes and aerobes
Cunningham et al[76]	104	56 (54%)	12 (22%)	18 (32%)
Thompson et al[83]	30	24 (80%)	5 (21%)	5 (21%)
Eschenbach et al[28]	54	21 (39%)	6 (28%)	1 (5%)
Monif et al[147]	17	16 (94%)	5 (31%)	5 (31%)
Sweet et al[29]	26	13 (50%)	4 (31%)	4 (31%)
Chow et al[210]	20	13 (65%)		1 (5%)
Total	251	143 (57%)	32 (23%)	34 (24%)

initiates the process of acute PID, producing tissue damage and changes in the local environment, which in turn facilitates access to the upper genital tract for anaerobic and aerobic organisms from the normal flora of the cervix. On the other hand, other investigators[29,75,211] have suggested that not all PID is initiated with gonococcal infection and that, in fact, acute PID commences as an infection of polymicrobial etiology. At the other extreme, Soper et al have suggested that BV, an overgrowth of anaerobic and aerobic flora of the vagina, adversely affects the cervical mucus barrier and facilitates the ascent of *N. gonorrhoeae* into the upper genital tract.[33]

However, concern was expressed that microorganisms obtained from cul-de-sac fluid using an aspirated transvaginal approach did not accurately represent the microorganisms present in the fallopian tube. Sweet et al demonstrated a discrepancy between culdocentesis- and laparoscopy-procured fallopian tube isolates from females with acute PID.[82] Culdocentesis specimens yielded greater numbers of bacteria common to the vaginal flora than did the fallopian tube isolates. A subsequent investigation of 10 patients utilized cultures from the fallopian tube and the cul-de-sac obtained via laparoscopy and from the cul-de-sac obtained via transvaginal culdocentesis.[29] Close agreement between fallopian tube exudate and the cul-de-sac aspirate via laparoscopy was found, but there was a poor concordance with the culdocentesis results, suggesting that contamination occurs during transvaginal culdocentesis. Soper et al subsequently confirmed the finding that use of culdocentesis to obtain a microbiologic specimen from the peritoneal cavity is confounded by the problem of contamination with the vaginal flora.[212]

The optimum microbiologic sources for elucidating the etiology of acute PID are specimens obtained directly from the site of infection – the fallopian tubes and/or endometrial cavity. In 1980, Sweet and coworkers reported their results with cultures obtained directly from the fallopian tube in the first laparoscopy study of PID performed in the United States.[29,82] Although nearly 50% of the patients had *N. gonorrhoeae* recovered from the endocervix, the gonococcus was isolated from the fallopian tube in only 8 of 35 patients (23%). Among the acute PID patients with endocervical *N. gonorrhoeae*, only 24% had the gonococcus recovered from the fallopian tube. Anaerobic bacteria were the most frequent group of microorganisms recovered from the fallopian tube in these women with acute PID. In this initial work, *Ureaplasma urealyticum* was rarely recovered from the fallopian tube, whereas no isolates of *Mycoplasma hominis* or *C. trachomatis* were obtained. In Figure 2.4, the microbiologic results are summarized for cultures obtained from the upper genital tract (endometrial aspirates and/or fallopian tube specimens) of an additional 380 hospitalized women with acute PID.[34,36–38] *N. gonorrhoeae* and *C. trachomatis* were recovered from 45 and 18% of patients, respectively. However, nongonococcal, nonchlamydial bacteria (anaerobes and aerobes) were the most commonly isolated microorganisms, and were present in 70% of cases. Again, anaerobic bacteria were the predominant isolates. The nongonococcal,

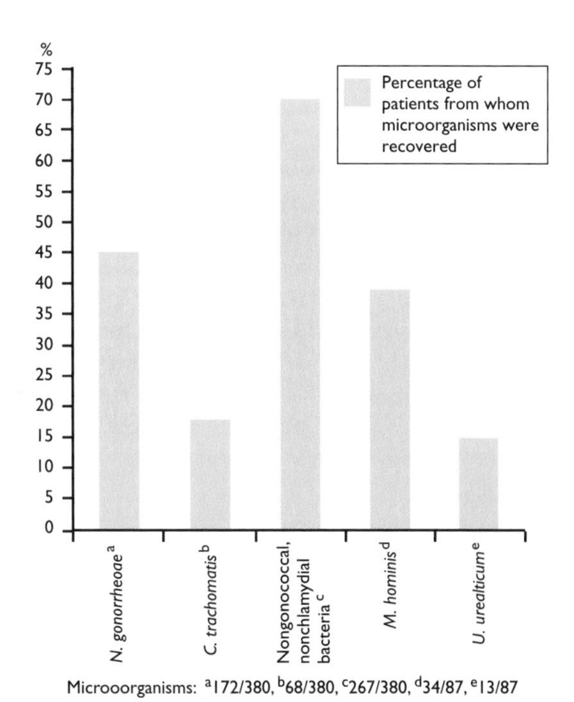

Figure 2.4 Summary of microbiologic results from hospitalized patients with acute PID.

nonchlamydial organisms identified are noted in Table 2.5. The most common included *Prevotella* (formerly *Bacteroides*) species, *Prevotella bivia*, *Prevotella disiens*, *Peptostreptococcus* species, *Gardnerella vaginalis*, group B streptococcus, and *Escherichia coli*. In a subsequent study we, demonstrated that in nearly one-third of hospitalized cases of acute PID, anaerobic and aerobic bacteria were the only microorganisms recovered from the upper genital tract and that among the two-thirds of patients with *N. gonorrhoeae* and/or *C. trachomatis* isolated, 50% also had anaerobic and aerobes recovered.[41] Thus, anaerobes and aerobes were associated with two-thirds of cases of acute PID.[41]

Frequent recovery of anaerobic and facultative (aerobic) bacteria from the upper genital tract of women with laparoscopy-confirmed acute PID has been confirmed by additional investigators in Scandinavia and the United States (see Table 2.1). Heinonen et al[31] reported that while *C. trachomatis* was the most common individual organism recovered from the fallopian tubes and endometrial cavity of patients with acute PID, nongonococcal nonchlamydial bacteria were the most commonly recovered group of microorganisms. In Finland, similar findings were reported by Paavonen and coworkers.[30] In Seattle, Wasserheit and colleagues demonstrated that anerobic and/or aerobic bacteria were recovered from the upper genital tract in 44% of patients with acute PID.[35] Brunham et al,[32] in a Canadian study, and Soper et al,[33] in a United States study, reported a lower recover of mixed anaerobic and facultative bacteria from the fallopian tubes with rates of 20% and 13%, respectively. However, Soper et al reported isolation of anaerobic and facultative organisms from the endometrial cavity in 31.4% of their laparoscopy-confirmed cases of PID.[33]

Hillier et al[39] investigated the microbiology in 178 women with clinically suspected acute PID; of these, all 178 had endometrial specimens obtained for microbiologic and histologic assessment and 85 cases were confirmed with laparoscopy. Whereas the endometrium yielded *N. gonorrhoeae* in 25% and *C. trachomatis* in 13% of patients, anaerobic and facultative bacteria were recovered from the endometrium in 94% of patients with a clinical diagnosis of PID. These organisms included *G. vaginalis*, *P. bivia*, black-pigmented anaerobic Gram-negative rods, *Fusobacterium* species, *Peptostreptococcus* species, and viridans streptococci. Among the nongonococcal, nonchlamydial bacteria, the most common were anaerobic Gram-negative rods (40%), especially *P. bivia* (28%) and black-pigmented rods (21%), *Peptostreptococcus* species (45%), and *G. vaginalis* (60%). Among the laparoscopy-confirmed cases of acute PID, anaerobic and facultative microorganisms were recovered from the fallopian tube or peritoneal fluid in 55% of patients. Although microorganisms were recovered less frequently from the fallopian tubes or peritoneal fluid, the microorganisms and their relative prevalences were similar in both sites. Similarly, in the patients (n = 117) with histologic endometritis, anaerobic Gram-negative rods (50%), *Peptostreptococcus* species (50%) and *G. vaginalis* (64%) were the most commonly recovered nongonococcal, nonchlamydial bacteria.

Recently, Haggerty et al[40] investigated the association between BV-associated microorganisms and histologic endometritis in a subgroup of 278 patients with complete endometrial histologic and culture data from the PEACH study. These investigators noted that in the majority (61%) of the women with clinically diagnosed PID, facultative or

Table 2.5 Nongonococcal nonchlamydial bacteria recovered from the upper genital tract of patients with acute salpingitis at San Francisco General Hospital (n = 188)

Prevotella (*Bacteroides*) species	88	*Gardnerella vaginalis*	121
Prevotella bivia	72	*Escheridia colischerichia*	25
Prevotella disiens	25	Nonhemolytic streptococci	49
Other *Prevotella* (*Bacteroides*)	99	Group B streptococci	29
Peptostreptococcus asaccharolyticus	93	Alpha-hemolytic streptococci	45
Peptostreptococcus anaerobius	71	Coagulase-negative staphylococci	72

anaerobic bacteria were recovered. Multiple microorganisms were the rule, with >1 microorganisms identified in the endometrium in 56% of cases. Anaerobic Gram-negative rods (e.g. *P. bivia*, *P. disiens*, and black-pigmented anaerobic Gram-negative rods) were present in 22% of women and anaerobic Gram-positive cocci (i.e. *Peptostreptococcus anaerobius* and *Peptostreptococcus asacharolyticus*) were present in 16%. In the subgroup with histologic acute endometritis, this finding was significantly associated with anaerobic Gram-negative rods (OR = 2.0; 95% CI 1.1–3.8), black-pigmented Gram-negative rods (OR = 3.1; 95% CI 1.4–7.0), and any anaerobic Gram-positive cocci (OR = 2.1, 95% CI 1.0–4.3). Even after excluding cases with endometrial *C. trachomatis* and/or *N. gonorrhoeae* infection, acute endometritis continued to be significantly associated with black-pigmented Gram-negative rods and anaerobic Gram-positive cocci. In summary, these authors of the largest study of PID undertaken in the United States demonstrated that the majority of PID cases have a nongonococcal, nonchlamydial etiology and that the BV-associated microorganisms were significantly associated with endometritis.[40] As a consequence of their findings, Haggerty et al recommended that all women with PID be treated with regimens that include metronidazole.[40] Eckert et al, in a proof-of-concept study of the antimicrobial treatment of subacute endometritis, noted a reduction of endometrial isolates from 28% to 11% with use of metronidazole in combination with treatment covering *C. trachomatis* and *N. gonorrhoeae*.[213]

Serologic data has also suggested that aerobic and anaerobic microorganisms are involved in the etiology of PID. Paavonen et al reported that significant enterobacterial common antigen and *Bacteroides fragilis* antibody titers were present in one-third of patients with PID.[214]

It is apparent that many of these nongonococcal, nonchlamydial microorganisms isolated from the upper genital tract of patients with acute PID have been implicated in BV, a complex synergistic alteration in the vaginal flora associated with *G. vaginalis*, members of the *Prevotella* (*Bacteroides*) species (especially *P. bivia*, *P. disiens*, and *P. capillosus*), *Peptostreptococcus* species, the mobile curved anaerobic rod *Mobiluncus* species, alpha-hemolytic streptococci, and *M. hominis*.[215–219]

BV is an imbalance in the microflora of the vagina in which the hydrogen peroxide-producing lactobacilli decrease in concentration while the anaerobic and facultative bacteria increase substantially.[220–224] During the past two decades, multiple investigators have demonstrated an association between BV and histologic endometritis and/or acute PID.[30,33,39,40,225–227] In addition, several have suggested that BV is an antecedent precursor for the development of nongonococcal, nonchlamydial PID.[33,225,227] Paavonen and coworkers noted that among 9 (29%) of 31 women with laparoscopy-confirmed acute PID, BV was present, compared with 0 of 14 controls.[30] In all 9 of these women, histologic endometritis was present on endometrial biopsy. Eschenbach initially proposed that BV might be an antecedent precursor in the lower genital tract for the development of nongonococcal, nonchlamydial PID.[75] Subsequently, Eschenbach et al demonstrated that women with BV were significantly more likely to have adnexal tenderness (4% vs 0.3%), uterine tenderness (4% vs 1%), cervical motion tenderness (3% vs 0.6%), and a diagnosis of PID (3% vs 0%) than control women without BV.[225] Hillier and colleagues reported that the BV-associated microorganisms (*Prevotella*, *Peptostreptococcus* species and *M. hominis*) were associated with histologic endometritis in confirmed cases of PID.[39] Even after controlling for the presence of chlamydial and gonococcal infection, recovery of BV-associated bacteria from the endometrial cavity was independently associated with histologic endometritis.[39] Soper et al demonstrated, in women with laparoscopy-confirmed PID, that BV was present in 61.8%.[33] Interestingly, all of the anaerobes recovered from the upper genital tract in their study were the BV-associated microorganisms.[33] Korn et al reported the presence of plasma cell endometritis in 22 women with BV compared with 1 (5%) of 19 controls.[226] Peipert and coworkers noted that objective evidence (histologic, microbiologic, or laparoscopic) of upper genital tract infection was present in 14 (56%) of 25 women with a clinical diagnosis of BV compared with 27 (30%) of 91 women without BV ($p = 0.015$).[47] Using logistic regression, the presence of BV was associated with a three-fold increased risk of upper genital tract infection (OR = 3.0; 95% CI 1.2–7.6). In a follow-up study, Korn et al demonstrated that plasma cell endometritis was present in 42% of women with BV vs 13% of controls (OR 6.5; 95% CI 1.7–3.5).[48]

In a thorough microbiologic evaluation of specimens obtained via endometrial biopsy and laparoscopy in patients with suspected acute PID, Hillier and colleagues[39] reported that the most frequently recovered microorganisms from the endometrium and the peritoneal fluid/fallopian tube were those associated with BV, including *G. vaginalis*, anaerobic Gram-negative rods, *Peptostreptococcus* species, *M. hominis*, and viridans streptococcus. These authors studied the relationship between BV-associated microorganisms (anaerobic Gram-negative rods, *M. hominis*, *Peptostreptococcus* species, *G. vaginalis*, and *Mobiluncus* species) and histologic endometritis after controlling for the presence of *N. gonorrhoeae* and *C. trachomatis*. Anaerobic Gram-negative rods, including *P. bivia*, black-pigmented species, and *M. hominis*, were more frequently recovered from the endometrial cavity of women with histologic endometritis than those without, among women with and without *N. gonorrhoeae* and *C. trachomatis*.[39] This association between BV-associated microorganisms and endometritis (independent of *N. gonorrhoeae* and *C. trachomatis*) was postulated as suggesting that BV-associated microorganisms in the endometrium increase the risk of endometritis among women with and without sexually transmitted disease pathogens.[39]

Bukusi et al demonstrated that among women with histologic endometritis, those with HIV-1 infection, especially those with significant immunosuppression, were more likely to have BV and less likely to have gonococcal or chlamydial infection.[88] These authors suggested that there was an increased risk of nongonococcal, nonchlamydial PID among HIV-infected immunosuppressed women and an increased role of BV-associated microorganisms in the pathogenesis of acute PID in HIV-infected women.[88] Among patients enrolled in the large PEACH study, Ness et al reported that BV was present in 59% of the women with clinically suspected acute PID.[86] Eckert et al, in a cross-sectional study, noted that 35 (37%) of 94 women with suspected clinical PID had BV. However, the prevalence of BV was 36%, 35%, and 39% for cases with neither endometritis or salpingitis, endometritis only, or salpingitis only, respectively.[89] Recently, Ness and colleagues from the PEACH study noted that bacterial vaginosis BV commonly is found in women with PID.[228] However, they found no overall increased risk of developing incident PID among women with BV after adjustment for confounding factors. Interestingly, dense growth of pigmented anaerobic Gram-negative rods in the 6 months before diagnosis did significantly increase a woman's risk of PID ($p = 0.04$).[228] Moreover, in the subgroup of women with ≥2 recent sexual partners, a significant association was demonstrated among BV, *G. vaginalis*, anaerobic Gram-negative rods, and PID.[228] Most recently, Haggerty and colleagues from the PEACH study reported that BV and anaerobic bacteria are associated with endometritis.[40] Among 278 cases of clinically suspected PID with complete endometrial histologic and microbiologic evaluation, BV was present in more than 50% overall and in 67% of those women with histologic acute endometritis. In addition, acute endometritis was significantly associated with bacterial vaginosis, endometrial dipthoroids, black-pigmented Gram-negative anaerobic rods, and anerobic Gram-positive cocci with ORs of 2.0–5.0.[40]

Interestingly, a higher incidence of BV has been noted in women wearing IUDs than among non-contraceptors or women using other contraceptive methods.[229,230] Such an association may play a role in the pathogenesis of nongonococcal, nonchlamydial PID. Several recent studies have confirmed this relationship among IUD use, endometritis, and BV.[39,89] Hillier et al noted a three-fold increase in endometritis compared with non-endometritis confirmed cases among women with clinically suspected PID.[39] Eckert et al reported that women with endometritis only 7 times more often had a current IUD (15% vs 2%; $p = 0.04$) than suspected clinical PID cases without either endometritis or salpingitis.[89] The association of current IUD use with endometritis held even after stratification for the presence or absence of current cervical infection with *N. gonorrhoeae* and/or *C. trachomatis* or BV.

The pathogenesis of nongonococcal, nonchlamydial PID has not been well studied or elucidated.[1] As noted previously, PID is a polymicrobial infection, with aerobic and anaerobic organisms inplicated.[2,3,36,231,232] As described above, a broad spectrum of facultative and anaerobic bacteria have been recovered alone or in combination with *N. gonorrhoeae* and/or *C. trachomatis* from the upper genital tract of women with acute PID.[3,28,29,36,39,148,227,231] Most commonly, these bacteria are components of the endogenous vaginal microflora. However, respiratory pathogens such as *Haemophilus influenzae*, *Streptococcus pneumoniae*, and group A beta-hemolytic streptococcus have been identified in the fallopian tubes of women with acute PID.[28,29,33,95] Typically, multiple bacteria are recovered from patients with acute PID. This finding formed the basis for the concept of "polymicrobial" etiology of PID initially coined by Eschenbach et al.[28]

The cervix and vagina of healthy women contain a multitude of aerobic and anaerobic bacteria.[233] How these organisms gain access to the upper genital tract to produce PID has not been clearly defined. As postulated for *N. gonorrhoeae*, they may reach the fallopian tube in menstrual blood reflux or attach to sperm and are then carried to the fallopian tubes. Eschenbach and Holmes have suggested that there may be a critical number of organisms needed to overwhelm local host defense mechanisms in the cervix, thereby allowing an infection to ascend to the upper genital tract.[44]

It seems that a continuum from the entity of BV, which is associated with significantly increased and very high colony counts of anaerobic bacteria and *G. vaginalis*, and nongonococcal, nonchlamydial acute PID exists. As described previously, many of the nongonococcal, nonchlamydial microorganisms recovered from the upper genital tract of women with acute PID are the same as the microorganisms associated with BV.[3,30,33,34,36,39,227,234] In addition to the microbiologic studies linking acute PID and BV, Eschenbach et al demonstrated that young women with BV were significantly more likely to have symptoms and signs associated with acute PID as well as to be diagnosed with acute PID than matched controls without BV.[225] As noted above, several investigations have confirmed an association between BV and histologic endometritis in women with clinical signs and symptoms of acute PID.[40,47,48,226,228] The hypothesis that the synergistic infection with anaerobes and *G. vaginalis* may be a third (in addition to *N. gonorrhoeae* and *C. trachomatis*) instance in which a lower genital tract infection ascends into the upper genital tract and produces acute PID needs to be confirmed. Even if such a hypothesis is not confirmed, it is apparent that nongonococcal, nonchlamydial bacteria are involved in the etiology and pathogenesis of acute salpingitis.[3,36,231,235] Westrom and Eschenbach noted our current inadequate state of knowledge as to how or in what circumstances endogenous vaginal bacteria produce infection in a healthy fallopian tube or if facultative and anaerobic bacteria can only infect fallopian tubes that have been "primed or compromised" by an earlier process.[3] Thus, whether the pathogenesis of nongonococcal, nonchlamydial acute PID involves an ongoing dynamic process initiated by ascending infection with *N. gonorrhoeae* and/or *C. trachomatis* followed by a superimposed polymicrobial stage or whether endogenous vaginal microorganisms ascend primarily into the upper genital tract to produce infection without preexisting cervical or upper genital tract infection with *N. gonorrhoeae* and/or *C. trachomatis* is debated. That aerobic/anaerobic bacteria arising from the endogenous vaginal flora can be primary pathogens was demonstrated by the laparoscopy study of Sweet and coworkers[96] where nongonococcal, nonchlamydial organisms caused acute salpingitis without antecedent infection with *N. gonorrhoeae* and/or *C. trachomatis*. Other investigations have also demonstrated the presence of facultative and anaerobic bacteria in the endometrium of patients with PID but without evidence of *N. gonorrhoeae* or *C. trachomatis*.[39,41] Clearly, some alteration to the normal cervical defense mechanism must occur to allow microorganisms from the cervix and vagina to gain access to the upper genital tract. Perhaps cervical infection with *N. gonorrhoeae* and/or *C. trachomatis* produces such a change. Soper et al suggested that BV might facilitate ascent of chlamydia and gonorrhea.[33] On the other hand, the metabolic byproducts and enzymes produced by vaginal bacteria could alter the cervical mucus and facilitate ascending infection.

GENITAL TRACT MYCOPLASMAS

The genital tract mycoplasmas *M. hominis*, *U. urealyticum*, and *M. genitalium* have been proposed as potential pathogens in the etiology of acute PID.[236–239] However, their role remains controversial. While *M. hominis* and *U. urealyticum* have been frequently recovered from the lower genital tract of women with PID, no difference exists between the prevalence of these mycoplasmas in the cervices of these patients and in sexually active control patients.[28,236] Most significantly, the genital tract mycoplasmas have been recovered infrequently (2–20%) from the peritoneal cavity and/or fallopian tubes of patients with salpingitis (Table 2.6).[28,82,237] *M. hominis* has been the primary focus of speculation as to a role of genital mycoplasmas in the etiology of PID. For *M. hominis*, Mardh and Westrom[237] reported a cervical isolation rate of 52%; Eschenbach et al[28] recovered *M. hominis* from lower genital tracts of 145 (72%) of 204 women with acute PID and Møller[238] recovered it from 91 (55%) of 166 PID cases. Serologic studies have also suggested a role for *M. hominis* in the etiology of acute PID.[28,236–239] These studies demonstrated that antibodies to *M. hominis* were present in one-fourth to one-half of women with acute PID. However, *M. hominis* is infrequently recovered from the fallopian tubes of women with acute PID (see Table 2.6). In addition to the low recovery rate from the fallopian tube, in-vitro studies with fallopian tube explant systems have failed to confirm that mycoplasmas may be pathogens in acute PID. Taylor-Robinson and Carney reported that despite proliferation of *M. hominis*, there was no apparent tubal damage produced.[240] This is in contradistinction to the circumstance with *N. gonorrhoeae* or *B. fragilis*, which when placed in a similar system produce extensive epithelial damages in which the tubal epithelium is completely destroyed.[98,242] However, it is important to recognize that the in-vitro fallopian tube explant system precludes the immune response and host defense mechanisms which may be important in the pathogenesis of acute salpingi-

Table 2.6 Evidence of genital mycoplasma infection among women with acute pelvic inflammatory disease

Study	Cervical isolation (%)	Tubal isolation (%)	Antibody titer change (%)
Mycoplasma hominis			
Sweet et al,[82] 1979	73	4	
Eschenbach et al,[28] 1975	72	4	20
Mardh and Westrom,[237] 1970	62	8	
Thompson et al,[83] 1980	60	17	
Møller et al,[238] 1983	55		30
Mardh et al,[239] 1981			40
Bevan,[146] 1995	38	0	
Ureaplasma urealyticum			
Eschenbach et al,[28] 1975	81	2	18
Mardh and Westrom,[237] 1970	56	4	
Sweet et al,[82] 1979	54	15	
Thompson et al,[83] 1980	33	20	
Henry-Suchet et al,[241] 1980	24	17	
Sweet et al,[96] 1981		9	

Reproduced with permission from Westrom L, Eschenbach D. Pelvic inflammatory disease. In: Holmes KK, Sparling PF, Mardh P-A, eds. Sexually Transmitted Diseases, 3rd edn. New York: McGraw-Hill, 1999:783–809.

tis. Møller and coworkers in the grivet monkey model demonstrated that *M. hominis* produces a parametritis rather than an acute salpingitis, and this could possibly explain the failure to recover mycoplasmas except in a few cases from the fallopian tubes.[243] Mardh et al in a study using scanning electron microscopy showed that *M. hominis* induced pathologic swelling in fallopian tube cilia in organ culture systems.[244] Although results obtained with serologic studies and cervical isolation approaches are suggestive, the role of *M. hominis* in the etiology of acute PID remains unclear. Most probably, *M. hominis* participates in acute PID as the result of its association with BV, rather than as a primary pathogen.

U. urealyticum has also been frequently recovered from the cervix of women with acute salpingitis (range 24–81%). However, the isolation rates of *U. urealyticum* from the fallopian tube were much less frequent (see Table 2.6). Eschenbach et al also demonstrated a significant increase of antibody to *U. urealyticum* in 20% of women with acute PID.[28] However, Møller et al were unsuccessful in their attempt to produce salpingitis in a monkey model with *U. urealyticum*[245] In general, the consensus opinion is that if there is any role in the etiology of acute PID for *U. urealyticum* it is minimal.[3,36]

More recently, attention has focused on a third genital tract mycoplasma, *M. genitalium*. This microorganism has been demonstrated in the cervix using polymerase chain reaction (PCR) amplification technology[246] and has induced acute salpingitis in animal models, including non-human primates.[247,248] However, no studies have been reported which demonstrate the presence of *M. genitalium* in tubal specimens from women with acute PID. Thus, its role in acute PID remains undetermined.[3]

OTHER MICROORGANISMS

There have been limited studies assessing the etiologic role of viruses in acute PID. A potential role has been suggested for the sexually transmitted disease viral agents – herpes simplex virus (HSV) II and cytomegalovirus (CMV). Laparoscopy studies in the United States by Sweet et al[82] and Wasserheit et al[35] failed to demonstrate the presence of HSV in the cervices or fallopian tubes of patients with acute PID. Investigators in Finland reported the recovery of HSV from the cervix and/or the upper genital tract of a few women with laparoscopy-confirmed acute PID.[249,250] Wasserheit et al noted that CMV was recovered from the cervices in 6 (28%) of 22 women with acute PID.[35] Moreover, they reported that CMV was associated with chlamydia cervicitis and postulated that chlamydial infection might reactivate latent CMV.

More recently, Clarke and coworkers reported that CMV was isolated from the cervix or endometrium of 30 (20.4%) of 147 women with PID and from the fallopian tubes or ovaries of 5 (22.7%) of 22 women with PID.[251] These authors demonstrated isolation of HSV from the cervix in 5 (3.4%) of 147 women with PID, but not from any endometrial or surgical specimens.[251] Based on their data, Clarke et al suggested that CMV, but not HSV, may contribute to the pathogenesis of PID in some patients.[251] A previous study by Clarke et al[252] demonstrated increased transmission or reactivation of CMV in association with concurrent infection by *N. gonorrhoeae* and/or *C. trachomatis*; they noted the rate of CMV cervical shedding was 14.3% among women with concurrent *C. trachomatis* or *N. gonorrhoeae* compared with only 4% among women without such infections.

Trichomonas vaginalis has been rarely recovered from the pelvis in women with acute PID.[3] Moodley et al assessed the association between the causative agents of vaginal discharge and PID among women attending an STD clinic in South Africa.[253] Among 119 women with clinical PID, patients with trichomoniasis had a significantly higher risk of PID than did women without *T. vaginalis* infection ($p = 0.03$).[253] When stratified by presence of HIV infection, the increased risk of PID with *T. vaginalis* was limited to the HIV-infected women.[253] Although interesting, these findings require confirmation, and the role of viral agents and protozoa in acute PID awaits further investigation.

REFERENCES

1. Sweet RL, Gibbs RS. Pelvic inflammatory disease. In: Infectious Diseases of the Female Genital Tract, 4th edn. Philadelphia: Lippincott, Williams and Wilkins, 2002: 368–412.
2. Centers for Disease Control. Pelvic inflammatory disease, 1993 Sexually Transmitted Diseases Treatment Guidelines. MMWR 1993;42:75.
3. Westrom L, Eschenbach DA. Pelvic inflammatory disease. In Holmes KK, Sparling PF, Mardh P-A, eds. Sexually Transmitted Diseases, 3rd edn. New York: McGraw-Hill, 1999: 783–809.
4. Washington AE, Cates W, Zadi AA. Hospitalizations for pelvic inflammatory disease. Epidemiology and trends in the United States, 1975 to 1981. JAMA 1984;251:2529–33.
5. Rolfs RT, Galaid E, Zaidi AA. Epidemiology of pelvic inflammatory disease: trends in hospitalizations and office visits, 1979–1988. In: Joint Meeting of the Centers for Disease Control and National Institutes of Health about Pelvic Inflammatory Disease Prevention, Management and Research in the 1990s. Bethesda, Maryland, September 4–5, 1990.
6. Washington AE, Katz P. Cost of and payment source for pelvic inflammatory disease: Trends and Projections, 1983 through 2000. JAMA 1991;266:2565–9.
7. Division of STD/HIV Prevention Annual Report 1989. Atlanta, GA: Centers for Disease Control, 1989.
8. Rein DB, Kassler WJ, Irwin KL, et al. Direct medical cost of pelvic inflammatory disease and its sequelae: decreasing but still substantial. Obstet Gynecol 2000;95:397–402.
9. Wolner-Hanssen, P, Kiviat NB, Holmes KK. Atypical pelvic inflammatory disease: subacute, chronic or subclinical upper genital tract infection in women. In: Holmes KK, Mardh P-A, Sparling PF, et al, eds. Sexually Transmitted Diseases. New York, McGraw-Hill, 1990: 615–20.
10. Weisenfeld HC, Hillier SL, Krohn MA, et al. Lower genital tract infection and endometritis: insight into subclinical pelvic inflammatory disease. Obstet Gynecol 2002;100:456–63.
11. Westrom L, Joesoef R, Reynolds G, et al. Pelvic inflammatory disease and fertility. A cohort study of 1844 women with laparoscopically verified disease and 657 control women with normal laparoscopic results. Sex Transm Dis 1992;19:185–92.
12. Westrom L. Incidence, prevalence, and trends of acute pelvic inflammatory disease and its consequences in industrialized countries. Am J Obstet Gynecol 1980;138:880.
13. Westrom L. Effect of acute pelvic inflammatory disease on fertility. Am J Obstet Gynecol 1975;122:876.
14. Brunham RC, Binns B, Guijon F, et al. Etiology and outcome of acute pelvic inflammatory disease. J Infect Dis 1988;158:510–17.
15. Safrin S, Schachter J, Dahrouge D, Sweet RL. Long-term sequelae of acute pelvic inflammatory disease. A retrospective cohort study. Am J Obstet Gynecol 1992; 166:1300–5.
16. Stacey CM, Munday PE, Taylor-Robinson D, et al. A longitudinal study of pelvic inflammatory disease. Br J Obstet Gynecol 1992;99:994–9.
17. Buchan H, Vessy M, Goldcard M, Fairweather J. Morbidity following pelvic inflammatory disease. Br J Obstet Gynecol 1993;100:558–62.
18. Chow JM, Yonekura ML, Richwald GA, et al. The association between *Chlamydia trachomatis* and ectopic pregnancy. A matched-pair, case-control study. JAMA 1990;263:3164–7.
19. Wiesenfeld HC, Krohn MA, Hillier SL, et al. Impaired fertility in women with subclinical PID. Abstract presented at Annual Meeting Infectious Diseases Society for Obstetrics and Gynecology. Hyannis, Massachusetts, August 7–9, 2003.
20. Eschenbach DA. Epidemiology of pelvic inflammatory disease. In: Landers DV, Sweet RL, eds. Pelvic Inflammatory Disease. New York: Springer-Verlag, 1997: 1–20.
21. Punnonen R, Terho P, Nikkanen V, Meurman O. Chlamydial serology in infertile women by immunofluorescence. Fertil Steril 1979;31:656–9.
22. Jones RB, Ardery BR, Hui SL, Cleary RE. Correlation between serum antichlamydial antibodies and tubal factor as a cause of infertility. Fertil Steril 1982;38:553–8.
23. Tjiam KH, Zeilmaker GH, Alberda AT, et al. Prevalence of antibodies to *Chlamydia trachomatis*, *Neisseria gonorrhoeae*, and *Mycoplasma hominis* in infertile women. Genitourin Med 1985;61:175–8.
24. Sellors JW, Mahony JB, Chernesky MA, Rath DJ. Tubal factor infertility: an association with prior chlamydial and asymptomatic salpingitis. Fertil Steril 1988;49:451–7.
25. World Health Organization Task Force on the Prevention and Management of Infertility. Tubal infertility: serologic relationship to post chlamydial and gonococcal infection. Sex Transm Dis 1995;22:71–7.
26. Korn AP, Bolan G, Padian N, et al. Plasma cell endometritis in women with symptomatic bacterial vaginosis. Obstet Gynecol 1995;85:387–90.
27. Paavonen J, Kiviat N, Brunham RC, et al. Prevalence and manifestations of endometritis among women with cervicitis. Am J Obstet Gynecol 1985;152:280–6.
28. Eschenbach DA, Buchanan T, Pollock HM, et al. Polymicrobial etiology of acute pelvic inflammatory disease. N Engl J Med 1975;293:166.
29. Sweet RL, Draper DL, Schachter J, et al. Microbiology and pathogenesis of acute salpingitis as determined by laparoscopy: what is the appropriate site to sample? Am J Obstet Gynecol 1980;138:985.
30. Paavonen J, Teisala K, Heinonen PK, et al. Microbiological and histopathological findings in acute pelvic inflammatory disease. Br J Obstet Gynecol 1987;94:454–60.
31. Heinonen PK, Teisala K, Punnonen R, et al. Anatomic sites of upper genital tract infection. Obstet Gynecol 1985;66:384–90.
32. Brunham RC, Binns B, Guijon F, et al. Etiology and outcome of acute pelvic inflammatory disease. J Infect Dis 1988;158:510–17.
33. Soper DE, Brockwell NJ, Dalton HP, Johnson D. Observations concerning the microbial etiology of acute salpingitis. Am J Obstet Gynecol 1994;170:1008–17.
34. Sweet RL, Schachter J, Robbie MO. Failure of beta-lactam antibiotics to eradicate *Chlamydia trachomatis* in the endometrium despite apparent clinical cure of acute salpingitis. JAMA 1983;250:2641–45.
35. Wasserheit JN, Bell TA, Kiviat NB, et al. Microbial causes of proven pelvic inflammatory disease and efficacy of clindamycin and tobramycin. Ann Int Med 1986;104:187–93.
36. Sweet RL. Pelvic inflammatory disease and infertility in women. Infect Dis Clin North Am 1987;1:199–215.
37. Sweet RL, Schachter J, Landers DV, et al. Treatment of hospitalized patients with acute pelvic inflammatory disease: comparison of cefotetan plus doxycycline and cefoxitin plus doxycycline. Am J Obstet Gynecol 1988;158:736–43.
38. Landers DV, Wolner-Hanssen P, Paavonen J, et al. Combination antimicrobial therapy in the treatment of acute pelvic inflammatory disease. Am J Obstet Gynecol 1991;164:849–58.
39. Hillier SL, Kiviat NB, Hawes SE, et al. Role of bacterial vaginosis-associated microorganisms in endometritis. Am J Obstet Gynecol 1996;175:435–41.
40. Haggerty CL, Hillier SL, Bass DC, Ness RB for the PID Evaluation and Clinical Health (PEACH) Study Investigators. Bacterial vagi-

nosis and anaerobic bacteria are associated with endometritis. Clin Infect Dis 2004;39:990–5.

41. Jossens MOR, Schachter J, Sweet RL. Risk factors associated with pelvic inflammatory disease of differing microbial etiologies. Obstet Gynecol 1994;83:989–97.
42. Centers for Disease Control. Pelvic inflammatory disease: guidelines for prevention and management. MMWR 1991;40:1–25.
43. Sweet RL. Diagnosis and treatment of acute salpingitis. J Reprod Med 1977;19:21.
44. Eschenbach DA, Holmes KK. Acute pelvic inflammatory disease: current concepts of pathogenesis, etiology, and management. Clin Obstet Gynecol 1975;18:35.
45. Platt R, Rich PA, McCormack WM. Risk of acquiring gonorrhea and prevalence of abnormal adnexal findings among women recently exposed to gonorrhea. JAMA 1983;250:3205–9.
46. Stamm WE, Guinan ME, Johnson C, et al. Effect of treatment regimens for Neisseria gonorrhoeae on simultaneous infection with *Chlamydia trachomatis*. N Engl J Med 1984;310:545–9.
47. Peipert JF, Montagno AB, Cooper AS, Sung CJ. Bacterial vaginosis as a risk factor for upper genital tract infection. Am J Obstet Gynecol 1997;177:1184–7.
48. Korn AP, Hessol NA, Padian NS, et al. Risk factors for plasma cell endometritis among women with cervical *Neisseria gonorrhoeae*, cervical *Chlamydia trachomatis*, or bacterial vaginosis. Am J Obstet Gynecol 1998;178:987–90.
49. Rice PA, Schachter J. Pathogenesis of pelvic inflammatory disease. JAMA 1991;266:2587–93.
50. Rice PA, Westrom LV. Pathogenesis and inflammatory response in pelvic inflammatory disease. In: Berger GS, Westrom LV, eds: Pelvic Inflammatory Disease. New York: Raven Press; 1992, 35–47.
51. Monif GRG. Gonococcal endometritis-salpingitis-peritonitis. Am J Obstet Gynecol 1977;129:711–14.
52. Odeblad E. The functional structure of human cervical mucus. Acta Obstet Gynecol Scand 1968;47(Suppl 1):57–9.
53. Svensson L, Westrom L, Mardh P-A. *Chlamydia trachomatis* in women attending a gynecological outpatient clinic with lower genital tract infection. Br J Vener Dis 1981;57:259–62.
54. Washington AE, Guve S, Schachter J, et al. Oral contraceptives, *Chlamydia trachomatis* infection, and pelvic inflammatory disease. JAMA 1985;253:2246.
55. Fullilove RE, Fullilove MT, Bower BP, Gross SA. Risk of sexually transmitted diseases among black adolescent crack users in Oakland and San Francisco, CA. JAMA 1990;263:851–5.
56. Sweet RL, Blankfort-Doyle M, Robbie MO, Schachter J. The occurrence of chlamydial and gonococcal salpingitis during the menstrual cycle. JAMA 1986;255:2062–4.
57. Nolan GJ, Osborne N. Gonococcal infection in the female. Obstet Gynecol 1973;42:156.
58. Washington AE, Goves S, Schachter J, Sweet RL. Oral contraceptives, *Chlamydia trachomatis* infection and pelvic inflammatory disease. JAMA 1985;124:2246–50.
59. Washington AE, Aral SO, Wolner-Hanssen P, et al. Assessing risk for pelvic inflammatory disease and its sequelae. JAMA 1991;266:2581–6.
60. Wolner-Hanssen P, Eschenbach DA, Paavonen J, et al. Decreased risk of symptomatic chlamydial pelvic inflammatory disease associated with oral contraceptive use. JAMA 1990;263:54–9.
61. Svensson L, Westrom L, Mardh P-A. Contraceptives and acute salpingitis. JAMA 1987;251:2553–5.
62. Wolner-Hansen P, Svensson L, Mardh P-A, et al. Laparoscopic findings and contraceptive use in women with signs and symptoms suggestive of acute salpingitis. Obstet Gynecol 1985;66:233–9.
63. Rubin GL, Ory HW, Layde PM. Oral contraceptives and pelvic inflammatory disease. Am J Obstet Gynecol 1982;140:630–5.
64. Koch ML. The bactericidal action of beta progesterone. Am J Obstet Gynecol 1950;59:168–71.
65. Morse SA, Fitzgerald TJ. Effect of progesterone on *Neisseria gonorrhoeae*. Infect Immun 1974;10:1370–7.
66. Salit IE. The differential susceptibility of gonococcal opacity variants to sex hormones. Can J Microbiol 1982;28:301–6.
67. Fitzgerald TJ, Morse SA. Alterations of growth, infectivity, and viability of *Neisseria gonorrhoeae* by gonadal steroids. Can J Microbiol 1976;22;286–94.
68. Ness RB, Keder LM, Soper DE, et al. Oral contraception and the recognition of endometritis. Am J Obstet Gynecol 1997;176:580–5.
69. Cross CE, Halliwell B, Borish ET, et al. Oxygen radicals and human disease. Ann Intern Med 1987;107:526–45.
70. Kotb M. Genetics of susceptibility to infectious diseases. Am Soc Microbiol News 2004;70:457–63.
71. Cook GS, Hill AV. Genetics of susceptibility to human infectious diseases. Nat Rev Genet 2001;2:967–77.
72. Holmes CL, Russell JA, Walley KR. Genetic polymorphisms in sepsis and septic shock: role in prognosis and potential for therapy. Chest 2003;124:1103–15.
73. Centers for Disease Control and Prevention. Summary of Notifiable Diseases, United States 2002. MMWR 2004;51:1–84.
74. Hook EW, Handsfield HH. Gonococcal infections in adults. In: Holmes KK, Sparling PF, Mardh P-A, et al, eds. Sexually Transmitted Diseases, 3rd edn. New York: McGraw-Hill, 1999: 451–66.
75. Eschenbach DA. Epidemiology and diagnosis of acute pelvic inflammatory disease. Obstet Gynecol 1980;55:142(S).
76. Cunningham FG, Hauth JC, Gilstrap LC, et al. The bacterial pathogenesis of acute pelvic inflammatory disease. Obstet Gynecol 1978;152:161.
77. Holtz F. Klinische studien uber die nicht tuberkulose salpingoophoritis. Acta Obstet Gynecol 1930;10(S):5.
78. Falk V. Treatment of acute nontuberculous salpingitis with antibiotics alone and in combination with glucocorticoids. Acta Obstet Gynecol Scand 1965;44(S-16):65.
79. Hundley JM, Diehl WK, Baggott JW. Bacteriologic studies in salpingitis with special reference to gonococcal viability. Am J Obstet Gynecol 1950;60:97.
80. Jacobson L, Westrom L. Objectivized diagnosis of acute pelvic inflammatory disease. Am J Obstet Gynecol 1969;105:1088.
81. Lip J, Burgoyne X. Cervical and peritoneal bacterial flora associated with salpingitis. Obstet Gynecol 1966;28:561.
82. Sweet RL, Mills J, Hadley WK, et al. Use of laparoscopy to determine the microbiologic etiology of acute salpingitis. Am J Obstet Gynecol 1979;134:68–74.
83. Thompson SE, Hager WD, Wong KH, et al. The microbiology and therapy of acute pelvic inflammatory disease in hospitalized patients. Am J Obstet Gynecol 1980;136:179.
84. Rendtorff RC, Curran JC, Chandler RW, et al. Economic consequences of gonorrhea in women. J Am Vener Dis Assoc 1974;1:40.
85. Westrom L. Decrease in the incidence of women treated in hospital for acute salpingitis in Sweden. Genitourin Med 1988;64:59.
86. Ness RB, Soper DE, Holley RL, et al. Effectiveness of inpatient and outpatient treatment strategies for women with pelvic inflammatory disease. Results from the Pelvic Inflammatory Disease Evaluation and Clinical Health (PEACH) Randomized Trial. Am J Obstet Gynecol 2002;186:929–37.
87. Rabe LK, Hillier SL, Wiesenfeld HC, et al. Endometrial microbiology in women with pelvic inflammatory disease. Abstract 182 International Society Sexually Transmitted Diseases Research. July 11–14, 1999, Denver, CO.
88. Bukusi EA, Cohen CR, Stevens CE, et al. Effects of human immunodeficiency virus I infection on microbial origins of pelvic

inflammatory disease and on efficacy of ambulatory oral therapy. Am J Obstet Gynecol 1999;181:1374–81.
89. Eckert LO, Hawes SE, Wolner-Hanssen PK, et al. Endometritis: The clinical–pathologic syndrome. Am J Obstet Gynecol 2002;186:690–5.
90. Wiesenfeld HC, Sweet RL, Ness RJ, et al. Comparison of acute and subclinical pelvic inflammatory disease. Sex Transm Dis 2005;32:400–5.
91. Toth A, O'Leary WM, Ledger WJ. Evidence for microbial transfer by spermatozoa. Obstet Gynecol 1982;59:556–9.
92. Nowicki S, Nowicki B, Martens M. Host factors in the attachment of gonococcal cells to pelvic tissue. In: Ades EW, Rest RF, Morse SA, eds. Microbial Pathogenesis and Immune Response. New York: New York Academy of Sciences, 1994: 292–4.
93. Nowicki S, Martens M, Kaul A, Nowicki B. Gonococcal attachment to human ovarian tissue. In: Conde-Glez CJ, Morse S, Rice P, et al., eds. Pathobiology and Immunobiology of Neisseriaceae. Cuernavaca, Mexico 1994: 730–4.
94. Nowicki S, Ram P, Pham T, et al. Pelvic inflammatory disease isolates of Neisseria gonorrhoeae are distinguished by Ciq-dependent virulence for newborn rats and by the sac-4 region. Infect Immun 1997;65:2094–9.
95. Mardh P-A. An overview of infectious agents of salpingitis, their biology, and recent advances in detection. Am J Obstet Gynecol 1980;138:933–51.
96. Sweet RL, Draper D, Hadley WK. Etiology of acute salpingitis: influence of episode number and duration of symptoms. Obstet Gynecol 1981;58:62.
97. Soper DE, Brockwell NJ, Dalton HP. Microbial etiology of urban emergency department acute salpingitis: treatment with olfoxacin. Am J Obstet Gynecol 1992;167:653–60.
98. Carney FE, Taylor-Robinson D. Growth and effect of *Neisseria gonorrhoeae* in organ cultures. Br J Vener Dis 1973;49:435.
99. McGee ZA, Johnson AP, Taylor-Robinson D. Pathogenic mechanisms of *Neisseria gonorrhoeae*. Observations on damage to human fallopian tubes in organ culture by gonococci of colony type 1 or type 4. J Infect Dis 1981;143:413–22.
100. Melly MA, Gregg CR, McGee ZA. Studies of toxicity of *Neisseria gonorrhoeae* for human fallopian tube mucosa. J Infect Dis 1981;143:423–31.
101. Gregg CR, Melly MA, McGee ZA. Gonococcal lipopolysaccharide: a toxin for human fallopian tube mucosa. Am J Obstet Gynecol 1980;138:981.
102. Melly MA, McGee ZA, Rosenthal RS. Ability of monomeric peptidoglycan fragments from *Neisseria gonorrhoeae* to damage human fallopian tube mucosa. J Infect Dis 1984;149:378–86.
103. Mulks MH, Plaut AG. IgA protease production as a characteristic distinguishing pathogenic from harmless Neisseria. N Engl J Med 1978;299:973–6.
104. Grifo JA, Jeremias J, Ledger WE, et al. Interferon-gamma in the diagnosis and pathogenesis of pelvic inflammatory disease. Am J Obstet Gynecol 1989;160:26–30.
105. Draper DL, James JF, Brooks GF, Sweet RL. Comparison of virulence markers of peritoneal and fallopian tube isolates with endocervical *Neisseria gonorrhoeae* isolates from women with acute salpingitis. Infect Immun 1980;27:882–8.
106. Draper DL, James JF, Hadley WK, Sweet RL. Auxotypes and antibiotic susceptibilities of *Neisseria gonorrhoeae* from women with acute salpingitis. Comparison with gonococci causing uncomplicated genital tract infections in women. Sex Transm Dis 1981;8:43–50.
107. Draper DL, Donegan EA, James JF, et al. Scanning electron microscopy of attachment of *Neisseria gonorrhoeae* colony phenotypes to surfaces of human genital epithelia. Am J Obstet Gynecol 1980;138:818–26.
108. Sparling PF. Biology of Neisseria gonorrhoeae. In: Holmes KK, Sparling PF, Mardh P-A, et al, eds. Sexually Transmitted Diseases, 3rd edn. New York: McGraw-Hill, 1999: 433–49.
109. Meyer TF. Pathogenic Neisseriae: complexity of pathogen–host cell interplay. Clin Infect Dis 1999;28:433–41.
110. Kellogg DS Jr, Peacock WL Jr, Deacon WE, et al. *Neisseria gonorrhoeae*. I. Virulence genetically linked to clonal variation. J Bacteriol 1963;85:1274–9.
111. Ward ME, Watt DJ, Robertson JN. The human fallopian tube: a laboratory model for gonococcal infection. J Infect Dis 1974;129:650–9.
112. Pierce WA, Buchanan TM. Attachment role of gonococcal pili: optimum conditions and quantification of adherence of isolated pili to human cells in vitro. J Clin Invest 1978;61:931.
113. James JF, Swanson J. Studies on gonococcus infection. XIII. Occurrence of color/opacity colonial variant in clinical cultures. Infect Immun 1978;19:332–40.
114. Kupsch E-M, Knepper B, Kuroti T, et al. Variable opacity (Opa) outer membrane proteins account for the cell tropism displayed by *Neisseria gonorrhoeae* for human leukocytes and epithelial cells. EMBO J 1993;12:641–50.
115. Rice PA. Serum resistance of *Neisseria gonorrhoeae*. Does it thwart the inflammatory response and facilitate the transmission of infection? Ann NY Acad Sci 1994;730:7–14.
116. Buchanan TM, Eschenbach DA, Knapp JS, Holmes KK. Gonococcal salpingitis is less likely to recur with *Neisseria gonorrhoeae* of the same principal outer membrane protein antigen type. Am J Obstet Gynecol 1981;138:978–80.
117. Centers for Disease Control and Prevention. *Chlamydia trachomatis* genital infections – United States, 1995. MMWR 1997;46:193–8.
118. Mangione-Smith R, O'Leary J, McGlynn EA. Health and cost-benefits of chlamydia screening in young women. Sex Transm Dis 1999;26:309–16.
119. Sweet RL, Gibbs RS. Chlamydial infection. In: Infectious Diseases of the Female Genital Tract, 4th edn. Philadelphia: Lippincott, Williams & Wilkins, 2002: 57–100.
120. Schachter J. Infection and disease epidemiology. In Stephens RS, ed. Chlamydia: Intracellular Biology, Pathogenesis and Immunity. Washington, DC: American Society for Microbiology; 1999, 139–69.
121. Schachter J. Biology of *Chlamydia trachomatis*. In: Holmes KK, Sparling PF, Mardh P-A, et al, eds. Sexually Transmitted Diseases, 3rd edn. New York: McGraw-Hill, 1999: 391–405.
122. Byrne GI, Moulder JW. Parasite-specified phagocytosis of *Chlamydia psittaci* and *Chlamydia trachomatis* by L and HeLa cells. Infect Immun 1978;19:598.
123. Hodinka RL, Wyrick PB. Ultrastructural study of mode of entry of *Chlamydia psittaci* into L-929 cells. Infect Immun 1986;54:855–63.
124. Barbour AG, Amano KI, Hackstadt T, et al. *Chlamydia trachomatis* has penicillin-binding proteins but not detectable muramic acid. J Bacteriol 1982;151:420–8.
125. Newhall WJ, Jones RB. Disulfide-linked oligomers of the major outer membrane protein of chlamydiae. J. Bacteriol 1983;154:998–1001.
126. Newhall WJ. Biosynthesis and disulfide cross-linking of outer membrane components during the growth cycle of *Chlamydia trachomatis*. Infect Immun 1987;55:162–8.
127. Bavoil PA, Ohlin A, Schachter J. Role of disulfide bonding in outer membrane structure and permeability in *Chlamydia trachomatis*. Infect Immun 1984;44:479–85.
128. Nurminen M, Leinonen M, Saikku P, Makela PH. The genus-specific antigen of chlamydia: resemblance to the lipopolysaccharide of enteric bacteria. Science 1983;220:1279–81.
129. Sellors JW, Mahoney J, Chernesky M, et al. *Chlamydia trachomatis* in fertile and infertile Canadian women. In: Chlamydia Infections,

Sixth International Symposium Proceedings, June 1986. Cambridge: Cambridge University Press, 1986: 233.
130. Mardh P-A, Moller BR, Paavonen J. Chlamydial infection of the female genital tract with emphasis on pelvic inflammatory disease. A review of Scandinavian studies. Sex Transm Dis 1981;8(S):140–55.
131. Ripa KR, Moller BR, Mardh P-A, et al. Experimental acute salpingitis in grivet monkeys provoked by *Chlamydia trachomatis*. Acta Pathol Microbiol Scand 1979;87:65.
132. Eilard ET, Brorsson J-E, Hanmark B, Forssman L. Isolation of chlamydia in acute salpingitis. Scand J Infect Dis 1976;9(S):82–4.
133. Mardh P-A, Ripa T, Svensson L, et al. *Chlamydia trachomatis* infection in patients with acute salpingitis. N Engl J Med 1977;298:1377.
134. Gjonnaess H, Dalaker K, Anestad G, et al. Pelvic inflammatory disease: etiological studies with emphasis on chlamydial infection. Obstet Gynecol 1982;59:550–5.
135. Treharne JD, Ripa KT, Mardh P-A, et al. Antibodies to *Chlamydia trachomatis* in acute salpingitis. Br J Vener Dis 1979;5:26.
136. Paavonen J, Saikku P, Vesterinen E, Ako K. *Chlamydia trachomatis* in acute salpingitis. Br J Vener Dis 1979;55:203–6.
137. Paavonen J. *Chlamydia trachomatis* in acute salpingitis. Am J Obstet Gynecol 1980;138:957–9.
138. Mardh P-A, Lind I, Svensson L, et al. Antibodies to *Chlamydia trachomatis*, *Mycoplasma hominis* and *Neisseria gonorrhoeae* in serum from patients with acute salpingitis. Br J Vener Dis 1981;57:125–9.
139. Ripa KT, Svensson L, Treharne JD, et al. *Chlamydia trachomatis* infection in patients with laparoscopically verified acute salpingitis. Results of isolation and antibody determinations. Am J Obstet Gynecol 1980;138:960–4.
140. Moller BR, Mardh P-A, Ahrons S, Nussler E. Infection with *Chlamydia trachomatis*, *Mycoplasma hominis*, and *Neisseria gonorrhoeae* in patients with acute pelvic inflammatory disease. Sex Transm Dis 1981;8:198–202.
141. Osser S, Persson K. Epidemiology and serodiagnostic aspects of chlamydial salpingitis. Obstet Gynecol 1982;59:206–9.
142. Svensson L, Westrom L, Ripa KT, et al. Differences in some clinical laboratory parameters in acute salpingitis related to culture and serologic findings. Am J Obstet Gynecol 1980;138:1017–21.
143. Kiviat NB, Wolner-Hanssen P, Peterson M, et al. Localization of *Chlamydia trachomatis* infection by direct immunofluorescence and culture in pelvic inflammatory disease. Am J Obstet Gynecol 1986;154:865–73.
144. Kiviat NB, Wolner-Hansses P, Eschenbach DA, et al. Endometrial histopathology in patients with culture-proved upper genital tract infection and laparoscopically diagnosed acute salpingitis. Am J Surgical Pathol 1990;14:167–75.
145. Livengood CH 3rd, Hill GB, Addison WA. Pelvic inflammatory disease: findings during inpatient treatment of clinically severe, laparoscopy-documented disease. Am J Obstet Gynecol 1992;166:519–24.
146. Bevan CD, Johal BJ, Mumtaz G, et al. Clinical, laparoscopic and microbiologic findings in acute salpingitis: report on United Kingdom cohort. Br J Obstet Gynecol 1995;102:407–14.
147. Monif GRG, Welkos SL, Baer H, Thompson RJ. Cul-de-sac isolates from patients with endometritis, salpingitis, peritonitis, and gonococcal endocervicitis. Am J Obstet Gynecol 1976;126:158–61.
148. Cunningham FG, Hauth JC, Strong JD, et al. Evaluation of tetracycline or penicillin and ampicillin for the treatment of acute pelvic inflammatory disease. N Engl J Med 1977;296:1380–3.
149. Henry-Suchet J, Loffredo V, Sarfaty D. *Chlamydia trachomatis* and mycoplasma research by laparoscopy in cases of pelvic inflammatory disease and in cases of tubal obstruction. Am J Obstet Gynecol 1980;138:1022.
150. Soper DE, Brockwell NJ, Dalton HP. Microbial etiology of urban emergency department acute salpingitis: treatment with ofloxacin. Am J Obstet Gynecol 1992;167:653–60.
151. Punnonen R, Terho P, Nikkanen V, Meurman O. Chlamydial serology in infertile women by immunofluorescence. Fertil Steril 1979;31:656–9.
152. Jones RB, Ardery BR, Hui SL, Cleary RE. Correlation between serum antichlamydial antibodies and tubal factor as a cause of infertility. Fertil Steril 1982;38:553–8.
153. Moore DE, Foy HM, Dalin JR, et al. Increased frequency of serum antibodies to *Chlamydia trachomatis* in infertility due to tubal disease. Lancet 1982;2:574.
154. Gump DW, Gibson M, Ashikaga T. Evidence of prior pelvic inflammatory disease and its relationship to *C. trachomatis* antibody and intrauterine contraceptive device use in infertile women. Am J Obstet Gynecol 1983;146:153–9.
155. Cevanini R, Possati G, LaPlaca M. *Chlamydia trachomatis* infection in infertile women. In: Mardh P-A, Holmes KK, Oriel JD, Piot P, Schachter J, eds. Chlamydial Infections. Amsterdam: Elsevier Biomedical Press, 1982: 182–92.
156. Gibson M, Gump D, Ashikaga T, Hall B. Patterns of adnexal inflammatory damage: chlamydia, the intrauterine device, and history of pelvic inflammatory disease. Fertil Steril 1984;41:47–51.
157. Conway D, Glazener CM, Caul EO, et al. Chlamydial serology in fertile and infertile women. Lancet 1984;i:191–3.
158. Kane JL, Woodland RM, Forsey T, et al. Evidence of chlamydial infection in infertile women with and without fallopian tube obstruction. Fertil Steril 1984;42:843–8.
159. Brunham RS, MacLean IW, Binns B, Peeling RW. *Chlamydia trachomatis*: its role in tubal infertility. J Infect Dis 1985;152:1275–82.
160. Chow JM, Yonekura L, Richard GA, et al. The association between *Chlamydia trachomatis* and ectopic pregnancy: a matched-pair, case–control study. JAMA 1990;263:3164–7.
161. Brunham RS, Binns B, McDowell J, Paraskeras M. *Chlamydia trachomatis* infection in women with ectopic pregnancy. Obstet Gynecol 1986;67:722–6.
162. Svensson L, Mardh P-A, Ahlgren M, Nordenskjold F. Ectopic pregnancy and antibiotics to *Chlamydia trachomatis*. Fertil Steril 1985;44:313–17.
163. Hartford SL, Silva PD, diZerega GS, Yonekura ML. Serologic evidence of prior chlamydial infection in patients with tubal ectopic pregnancy and contralateral tubal disease. Fertil Steril 1987;47:118–21.
164. Morrison RP, Belland RJ, Lyngk, Caldwell HD. Chlamydial disease pathogenesis. The 57-kD hypersensivitity antigen in a stress response protein. J Exp Med 1989;170:1271–83.
165. Witkin SS, Jeremias J, Toth M, Ledger WL. Cell-mediated immune response to the recombinant 57-kDa heat-shock protein of *Chlamydia trachomatis* in women with salpingitis. J Infect Dis 1993;167;1379–83.
166. Morrison RP, Manning DS, Caldwell HD. Immunology of *Chlamydia trachomatis* infections: immunoprotective and immunopathogenic responses. In: Gallin JI, Fauci AS, Quinn TC, eds. Advances in Host Defense Mechanisms. Vol 8: Sexually Transmitted Diseases. New York: Raven Press, 1992: 57–84.
167. Patton DL, Cosgrove Sweeney YT, Kuo C-C. Demonstration of delayed hypersensitivity in *Chlamydia trachomatis* salpingitis in monkeys. A pathogenic mechanism of tubal damage. J Infect Dis 1994;169:680–3.
168. Brunham RC, Peeling RW. *Chlamydia trachomatis* antigens: role in immunity and pathogenesis. Infect Agents Dis 1994;3:218–33.
169. Peeling RW, Kimani J, Plummer F, et al. Antibody to chlamydial hsp 60 predicts an increased risk for chlamydial pelvic inflammatory disease. J Infect Dis 1997;175:1153–8.

170. Eckert LO, Hawes SE, Wolner-Hanssen P, et al. Prevalence and correlates of antibody to chlamydial heat shock protein in women attending sexually transmitted diseases clinic and women with confirmed pelvic inflammatory disease. J Infect Dis 1997;175:1453–8.
171. Morrison RP, Lyng K, Caldwell HD. Chlamydial disease pathogenesis: ocular hypersensitivity elicited by a genus-specific 57-kD protein. J Exp Med 1989;169:663–75.
172. Hutchinson GR, Taylor-Robinson D, Dourmashkin RR. Growth and effect of chlamydia in human and bovine oviduct cultures. Br J Vener Dis 1979;55:194–202.
173. White HJ, Rank RG, Soloff BL, Barron AL. Experimental chlamydial salpingitis in immunosuppressed guinea pigs infected in the genital tract with agent of guinea pig inclusion conjunctivitis. Infect Immun 1979;26:573.
174. Sweet RL, Banks J, Sung M, et al. Experimental chlamydial salpingitis in the guinea pig. Am J Obstet Gynecol 1980;138:952.
175. Swenson CE, Donegan E, Schachter J. *Chlamydia trachomatis-induced* salpingitis in mice. J Infect Dis 1983;148:1101–7.
176. Swenson CE, Schachter J. Infertility as a consequence of chlamydial infection of the upper genital tract in female mice. Sex Transm Dis 1984;11:64–7.
177. Patton DL, Halbert SA, Kuo CC, et al. Host response to primary *Chlamydia trachomatis* infection of the fallopian tube in pig-tailed monkeys. Fertil Steril 1983;40:829–40.
178. Patton DL, Kuo CC, Wang SP, Halbert SA. Distal obstruction induced by repeated *Chlamydia trachomatis* salpingeal infection in pig-tailed mocaques. J Infect Dis 1987;155:1292–9.
179. Cooper MD, Jeffery C. Scanning and transmission electron microscopy of bacterial attachment to mucosal surfaces with particular reference to human fallopian tube. Scan Electron Microsc 1985;3:1183–90.
180. Cooper MD, Rapp J, Jeffery-Wiseman C, et al. *Chlamydia trachomatis* infection of human fallopian tube organ cultures. J Gen Microbiol 1990;136:1109–15.
181. Phillips DM, Svenson CE, Schachter J. Ultrastructure of *Chlamydia trachomatis* infection of the mouse oviduct. J Ultrastruc Res 1984;88:244–56.
182. Patton DL, Swenson CE, Schachter J. Immunopathology and histopathology of experimental chlamydial salpingitis. Rev Infect Dis 1982;7:746–51.
183. Grayston JT, Wang SP, Yeh L-J, Kuo CC. Importance of reinfection in the pathogenesis of trachoma. Rev Infect Dis 1985;7:717–25.
184. Moller BR, Westrom L, Ahrons S, et al. *Chlamydia trachomatis* infection of the fallopian tubes: histological findings in two patients. Br J Vener Dis 1979;55:422–8.
185. Wagar EA, Schachter J, Bavoil P, Stephens RS. Differential human serologic response to two 60,000 molecular weight *Chlamydia trachomatis* antigens. J Infect Dis 1990;162:922–7.
186. Brunham RC, Peeling R, Maclean I, et al. Postabortal *Chlamydia trachomatis* salpingitis: correlating risk with antigenic-specific serological responses and with neutralization. J Infect Dis 1987;155:749–55.
187. Ward ME. Mechanisms of chlamydia-induced disease. In: Stephens RS, ed. Chlamydia: Intracellular Biology, Pathogenesis and Immunity. Washington DC: American Society for Microbiology, 1999: 171–210.
188. Byrne GL, Grubbs B, Marshall JJ, et al. Gamma interferon-mediated cytotoxicity related to murine *Chlamydia trachomatis* infection. Infect Immun 1988;56:2023–7.
189. Williams DM, Bonewald LF, Roodman GD, et al. Tumor necrosis factor as a cytotoxin induced by murine *Chlamydia trachomatis* infection. Infect Immun 1989;57:1351–5.
190. Rothermel CD, Schachter J, Lavrich P, et al. *Chlamydia trachomatis*-induced production of interleukin-1 by human monocytes. Infect Immun 1989;57:2705–11.
191. Rasmussen SJ, Eckmann L, Quayle AJ, et al. Secretion of proinflammatory cytokines by epithelial cells in response to chlamydia infection suggests a central role for epithelial cells in chlamydial pathogenesis. J Clin Invest 1997;99:77–87.
192. Fitzpatrick DR, Wie J, Webb D, et al. Preferential binding of *Chlamydia trachomatis* to subsets of human-lymphocytes and induction of interluekin-6 and interferon-gamma. Immunol Cell Biol 1991;69:337–48.
193. Morrison RP, Belland RJ, Lyngk, Caldwell HD. Chlamydial disease pathogenesis. The 57-KD hypersensitivity antigen in a stress response protein. J Exp Med 1989;170:1271–83.
194. Coehn CR, Brunham RC. Pathogenesis of chlamydia induced pelvic inflammatory disease. Sex Transm Inf 1999;75:21–4.
195. Beatty WL, Belanger TA, Desai AA, et al. Tryptophan depletion as a mechanism of gamma interferon-mediated chlamydial persistence. Infect Immun 1994;62:3705–11.
196. Witkin S, Toth M, Jeremias J, Ledger WJ. Increased inducibility of inflammatory mediators from peripheral blood mononuclear cells in women with salpingitis. Am J Obstet Gynecol 1991;165:719–23.
197. Arno JN, Ricker VA, Batteiger BE, et al. Interferon-gamma in endocervical secretions of women infected with *Chlamydia trachomatis.* J Infect Dis 1990;162:1385–9.
198. Mabey DC, Bailey RL, Dunn D, et al. Expression of MHC class II antigens by conjunctival epithelial cells in trachoma: Implications concerning the pathogenesis of blinding disease. J Clin Opthalmol 1991;44:285–9.
199. Peeling RW, Kimani J, Plummer F, et al. Antibody to chlamydial hsp 60 predicts an increased risk for chlamydial pelvic inflammatory disease. J Infect Dis 1997;175:1153–8.
200. Eckert LO, Hawes SE, Wolner-Hansses P, et al. Prevalence and correlates of antibody to chlamydial heat shock protein in women attending sexually transmitted diseases clinic and women with confirmed pelvic inflammatory disease. J Infect Dis 1997;175:1453–8.
201. Brunham RC, Peeling R, MacLean I, et al. *Chlamydia trachomatis* - associated ectopic pregnancy: serologic and histologic correlates. J Infect Dis 1992;165:1076–81.
202. Toye B, Laferriere C, Claman P, et al. Association between antibody to the chlamydial heat-shock protein and tubal infertility. J Infect Dis 1993;168:1236–40.
203. Arno JN, Yuan Y, Cleary RE, Morrison RP. Serologic responses of infertile women to the 60-kd chlamydial heat shock protein (Hsp 60). Fertil Steril 1995;64:730–5.
204. Money DM, Hawes SE, Eschenbach DA, et al. Antibodies to the chlamydial 60kd heat-shock protein are associated with laparoscopically confirmed perihepatitis. Am J Obstet Gynecol 1997;176:870–7.
205. Domeika M, Domeika K, Paavonen J, et al. Humoral immune response to conserved epitopes of *Chlamydia trachomatis* and human 60-kDa heat-shock protein in women with pelvic inflammatory disease. J Infect Dis 1998;177:714–19.
206. Witkin SS, Jeremais J, Toth M, Ledger WL. Cell-mediated immune response to the recombinant 57-KD heat-shock protein of *Chlamydia trachomatis* in women with salpingitis. J Infect Dis 1993;167:1379–83.
207. Witkin SS, Askienazy-Elbhar M, Henry-Suchet J, et al. Circulating antibodies to a conserved epitope of the *Chlamydia trachomatis* 60kDa heat shock protein (hsp 60) in infertile couples and its relationship to antibodies to *C. trachomatis* surface antigens and the *Escherichia coli* and human HSP60. Hum Reprod 1998;13:1175–9.
208. Kimani J, Maclean IW, Bwayo JJ, et al. Risk factors for *Chlamydia trachomatis* pelvic inflammatory disease among sex workers in Nairobi, Kenya. J Infect Dis 1996;173:1437–44.

209. Cohen CR, Sinei SS, Bukusi EA, et al. Human leukocyte antigen class II DQ alleles associated with *Chlamydia trachomatis* tubal infertility. Obstet Gynecol 2000;95:72–7.
210. Chow AW, Malkasian KL, Marshall JR, Guze LB. The bacteriology of acute pelvic inflammatory disease. Am J Obstet Gynecol 1975;122:876–9.
211. McCormack WM, Nowroozi K, Alpert S, et al. Acute pelvic inflammatory disease: characteristics of patients with gonococcal infection and evaluation of their response to treatment with aqueous procaine penicillin G and spectinomycin hydrochloride. Sex Transm Dis 1977;4:125–31.
212. Soper DE, Brockwell NJ, Dalton HP. False-positive cultures of the cul-de-sac associated with culdocentesis in patients undergoing laparoscopy. Obstet Gynecol 1991;77;134–8.
213. Eckert LO, Thwin SS, Hillier SL, et al. The antimicrobial treatment of subacute endometritis: a proof of concept study. Am J Obstet Gynecol 2004;190:305–13.
214. Paavonen J, Valtonen VV, Kasper DL, et al. Serological evidence for the role of *Bacteroides fragilis* and enterobacteriaceae in the pathogenesis of acute pelvic inflammatory disease. Lancet 1981;1:293–5.
215. Pheifer TA, Forsyth PS, Durfee MA, et al. Nonspecific vaginitis: role of *Haemophilus vaginalis* and treatment with metronidazole. N Engl J Med 1978;298:1429–34.
216. Holmes KK, Spiegel C, Amsel R, et al. Nonspecific vaginosis. Scand J Infect Dis 1981;26:110–14.
217. Spiegel CA, Amsel R, Eschenbach DA, et al. Anaerobic bacteria in nonspecific vaginitis. N Engl J Med 1980;303:601–7.
218. Taylor E, Barlow D, Blackwell AL, Phillips I. *Gardnerella vaginalis*, anaerobes and vaginal discharge. Lancet 1982;i:1376–9.
219. Spiegel CA, Eschenbach DA, Amsel R, Holmes KK. Curved anaerobic bacteria in bacterial (nonspecific) vaginosis and their response to therapy. J Infect Dis 1983;148:817–22.
220. Klebanoff SJ, Hillier SL, Eschenbach DA, Waltersdorph AM. Control of the microbial flora of the vagina by H_2O_2-generating lactobacilli. J Infect Dis 1991;164:94–100.
221. Hawes SE, Hillier SL, Benedetti J, et al. Hydrogen peroxide-producing lactobacilli and acquisition of vaginal infections. J Infect Dis 1996; 174:1058–63.
222. Eschenbach DA, Davick PR, William BL, et al. Prevalence of hydrogen peroxide-producing *Lactobacillus* species in normal women and women with bacterial vaginosis. J Clin Microbiol 1989;17:251–56.
223. Schwebke JR. Gynecologic consequences of bacterial vaginosis. Obstet Gynecol Clin North Am 2003;30:685–94.
224. Hillier SL. Bacterial vaginosis. In: Holmes KK, Sparling PF, Mardh PA et al, eds. Sexually Transmitted Diseases, 3rd edn. New York: McGraw-Hill, 1999:563–86.
225. Eschenbach DA, Hillier S, Critchlow C, et al. Diagnosis and clinical manifestations of bacterial vaginosis. Am J Obstet Gynecol 1988;158:819–28.
226. Korn AP, Bolan G, Padian N, et al. Plasma cell endometritis in women with symptomatic bacterial vaginosis. Obstet Gynecol 1995;85:387–90.
227. Sweet RL. Role of bacterial vaginosis in pelvic inflammatory disease. Clin Infect Dis 1995;20(Suppl 2):S276–85.
228. Ness RB, Hillier SL, Kip KE, et al. Bacterial vaginosis and risk of pelvic inflammatory disease. Obstet Gynecol 2004;104:761–9.
229. Goldacre MJ, Watt B, London N, et al. Vaginal microbial flora in normal young women. BMJ 1979;i:1450–3.
230. Eschenbach DA. Acute pelvic inflammatory disease. Urol Clin North Am 1984;11:65–81.
231. Sweet RL. Microbial etiology of pelvic inflammatory disease. In: Landers DV, Sweet RL, eds. Pelvic Inflammatory Disease. New York: Springer-Verlag, 1997: 30–59.
232. Centers for Disease Control and Prevention. Sexually Transmitted Disease Treatment Guidelines 2002. MMWR 2002.
233. Bartlett JG, Onderdonk AB, Drude E, et al. Quantitative bacteriology of the vaginal flora. J Infect Dis 1977;126:271–7.
234. Westrom L, Wolner-Hanssen P. Pathogenesis of pelvic inflammatory disease. Genitourin Med 1993;69:9–17.
235. Walker CK, Workowski KA, Washington AE, et al. Anaerobes in pelvic inflammatory disease: implications for the Centers for Disease Control and Prevention's guidelines for treatment of sexually transmitted diseases. Clin Infect Dis 1999;28(Suppl 1):S29–36.
236. Lemcke R, Csonka GW. Antibodies against pleuropneumonia-like organisms in patients with salpingitis. Br J Vener Dis 1962;38:212–17.
237. Mardh P-A, Westrom L. Tubal and cervical cultures in acute salpingitis with special reference to *Mycoplasma hominis* and T-strain mycoplasmas. Br J Vener Dis 1970;46:179–86.
238. Møller BR. The role of mycoplasmas in the upper genital tract of women. Sex Transm Dis 1983;10(S):281–4.
239. Mardh P-A, Lind I, Svensson L, et al. Antibodies to *Chlamydia trachomatis*, *Mycoplasma hominis* and *Neisseria gonorrhoeae* in serum from patients with acute salpingitis. Br J Vener Dis 1981;57:125–9.
240. Taylor-Robinson D, Carney FE. Growth and effect of mycoplasmas in fallopian tube organ cultures. Br J Vener Dis 1974;50:212–16.
241. Henry-Suchet J, Loffredo V, Sarfaty D. *Chlamydia trachomatis* and mycoplasma research by laparoscopy in cases of pelvic inflammatory disease and in cases of tubal obstruction. Am J Obstet Gynecol 1980;138:1022–5.
242. Hare MJ, Barnes CFJ. Fallopian tube organ culture in the investigation of *Bacteroides* as a cause of pelvic inflammatory disease. In: Philips I, Collier J, eds. Metronidazole: Royal Society of Medicine International Congress and Symposium Series No. 18. London: Academic Press, 1979.
243. Møller BR, Freundt EA, Black FT, Frederiksen P. Experimental infection of the genital tract of female grivet monkeys for *Mycoplasma hominis*. Infect Immun 1978;20:248–57.
244. Mardh P-A, Westrom L, van Mecklenberg C, Hammar E. Studies on ciliated epithelia of the human genital tract. I. Swelling of the cilia of fallopian tube epithelium in organ cultures infected with *Mycoplasma hominis*. Br J Vener Dis 1976;52:52–7.
245. Moller BR, Freundt EA. Monkey animal model for study of mycoplasmal infections of the urogenital tract. Sex Transm Dis 1983;10:359–62.
246. Palmer HM, Gilroy CB, Claydon EJ, Taylor-Robinson D. Detection of *Mycoplasma genitalium* in the genitourinary tract of women by the polymerase chain reaction. Int J STD AIDS 1991;2:261–3.
247. Taylor-Robinson D. The history of *Mycoplasma genitalium* in sexually transmitted diseases. Genitourin Med 1995;71:1–8.
248. Taylor-Robinson D, Furr PM, Tully JG, et al. Animal models of *Mycoplasma genitalium* urogenital infections. Isr J Med Sci 1987;23:561–4.
249. Paavonen J, Teisala K, Heinonen PK, et al. Endometritis and acute salpingitis associated with *Chlamydia trachomatis* and herpes simplex virus type two. Obstet Gynecol 1985;65:288–91.
250. Lehtinen M, Rantala I, Teisala K, et al. Detection of herpes simplex virus in women with acute pelvic inflammatory disease. J Infect Dis 1985;152:78–82.
251. Clarke LM, Duerr A, Yeung KH, et al. Recovery of cytomegalovirus and herpes simplex virus from upper and lower genital tract specimens obtained from women with pelvic inflammatory disease. J Infect Dis 1997; 176:286–8.

252. Clarke LM, Duerr A, Feldman J, et al. Factors associated with cytomegalovirus infection among human immunodeficiency virus type 1-seronegative and -seropositive women from an urban minority community. J Infect Dis 1996; 173:77–82.

253. Moodley P, Wilkinson D, Connolly C, et al. *Trichomonas vaginalis* is associated with pelvic inflammatory disease in women infected with human immunodeficiency virus. Clin Infect Dis 2002; 34:519–22.

3. Pathogenesis

Harold C. Wiesenfeld

Pelvic inflammatory disease (PID) results from ascension of microorganisms from the cervix and/or vagina to the upper genital tract. During the ascent, these organisms overcome barriers along the path to infect the endometrial cavity, fallopian tubes, and the abdominopelvic peritoneal cavity. Spermatozoa, talc, and dyes can be found in the peritoneal cavity, indicating that the upper genital tract is not impenetrable. It has become evident that ascent of microorganisms can occur in the absence of establishment of infection. Once in the upper genital tract, one of three events can occur:

- first, the host may clear the microbial invaders and prevent the establishment of infection
- secondly, pelvic infection can be manifested in either the endometrium, fallopian tubes or both, as well as the associated pelvic structures (e.g., tubo-ovarian abscess)
- a third scenario is the establishment of subclinical and ongoing infection in the uterus and/or fallopian tubes.

The mechanisms of each of these possible scenarios remain to be determined.

CERVICAL FACTORS

Ascension of microorganisms requires traversing through the cervical canal into the endometrium and other upper genital tract structures. Toth et al have postulated that spermatozoa facilitate ascension of microorganisms to the upper genital tract.[1] Whether these postulations reflect an actual pathogenic mechanism remains to be determined, as there are no confirmatory in-vivo studies and many cases of PID are not temporally related to recent coitus. Cervical mucus has long been believed to have an important role in the natural host defense against ascending infections. Several investigators have studied the antibacterial properties of cervical mucus. Zuckerman et al demonstrated that human cervical mucus inhibited growth of several microorganisms, including *Micrococcus lysodeikticus*, *Staphylococcus* and *Streptococcus* species, and *Escherichia coli*.[2] Using a modified agar diffusion assay, Eggert-Kruse and colleagues tested antimicrobial activity of cervical mucus from 122 women undergoing infertility evaluation.[3] All samples inhibited growth of *M. lysodeikticus*. Interestingly, antibacterial activity was greater for cervical mucus samples that were obtained from women who had recent intercourse (within 12 hours) and contained spermatozoa, compared with cervical mucus samples obtained from women after sexual abstinence. This finding may reflect leukocyte-derived antimicrobial peptides arising from seminal fluid or as a response to coitus, or perhaps due to other antimicrobial agents. Further, the antibacterial activity of cervical mucus that was colonized with potentially pathogenic bacteria was lower than the activity of sterile cervical mucus. Cervical mucus in pregnancy has also been examined for its antibacterial properties. Complete or partial inhibition of growth has been demonstrated for several bacterial species including *E. coli*, *Pseudomonas aeruginosa*, *Staphylococcus aureus*, *Streptococcus agalactiae*, *Streptococcus pyogenes*, and *Enterococcus faecium*.[4]

How the cervical mucus provides a line of defense against ascension of organisms is not well understood. Some have proposed that the cervical mucus acts as a physical barrier to prevent access of microbes to the upper genital tract.[5,6] Perhaps more likely is that cervical secretions contain antimicrobial products that aid in the control of infection and ascent of microorganisms. Possible contributors to the local defense include secretory leukocyte protease inhibitor (SLPI), lysozyme, lactoferrin, and defensins. SLPI is a component of the innate immunity and is produced from a number of different cells, including neutrophils, macrophages, and epithelial cells lining mucus membranes.[7] SLPI has been detected in the female lower genital tract, and high levels of vaginal SLPI levels have been associated with lower vertical HIV (human immunodeficiency virus) transmission rate.[8] Further, current research suggests that SLPI possesses bactericidal properties. SLPI production from uterine epithelial cells is associated with antibacterial activity.[9] Levels of SLPI in vaginal fluid are lower in women with a sexually transmitted infection, supporting evidence that SLPI is an integral component of innate immunity regarding sexually transmitted diseases (STDs) in women. Interestingly, expression of SLPI in the cervical mucus varies during the menstrual cycle.[10] Endometrial production of SLPI is greater in the late secretory phase than in the proliferative phase of the menstrual cycle.[11] This differential SLPI production may, in part, explain the findings of some investigators that PID more commonly manifests during the proliferative phase of the menstrual cycle.

Defensins are antimicrobial peptides that are integral components of innate immunity, probably acting by disrupting the outer membrane of microbes and other target cells. Human beta-defensin-1 has been found at high levels in endocervical tissue.[12] In a cohort of women at-risk for subclinical PID, we have demonstrated a strong association between vaginal levels of neutrophil defensins and STDs, including *Neisseria gonorrhoeae, Chlamydia trachomatis*, and *Trichomonas vaginalis*.[13] Moreover, elevated human defensin levels were highly correlated with endometritis, suggesting that defensins are important in the host–pathogen interaction in the female reproductive tract. Defensins, in addition to other antimicrobial peptides located at the cervical level, probably play key roles in host defense against ascending pelvic infection.

HORMONAL FACTORS INFLUENCING ASCENDING INFECTION

Many lines of evidence point to the influential role of endogenous and exogenous hormones in the pathogenesis of PID. Symptoms of acute PID often start during or shortly following menses. Further, diagnosis of gonococcal cervicitis is more common in the follicular phase than in the luteal phase. A number of events are linked to the menstrual cycle, and may explain this timely relationship. Menstrual blood is rich in iron, and iron acquisition is important for bacterial pathogenesis, including *Neisseria* species.[14] In addition, menstrual blood may contain other nutrients that promote growth of *N. gonorrhoeae*. Retrograde menstruation may also facilitate microbial ascension to the upper genital tract.

Further support for the influence of hormones on the pathogenesis of PID are a number of studies demonstrating that women using oral contraceptives are at lower risk of symptomatic PID than women who do not use oral contraceptives or who use other methods. Nearly three decades ago, reports began to suggest that oral contraceptive use may have a protective effect against acute PID.[15,16] In a case–control study comparing 648 women hospitalized with acute PID and 2516 hospitalized control subjects, Rubin et al demonstrated that the risk of acute PID for women using oral contraceptives was 0.5 (95% confidence limits (CI) 0.4, 0.6).[17] The protective effect of oral contraceptives could not be explained by demographic characteristics or sexual practices. A case–control study of women hospitalized with a first diagnosis of acute PID demonstrated that the risk of PID was reduced 60–80% among women using oral contraceptives for at least 1 year.[18] Further analysis showed a non-statistically significant protective effect when examining solely low-dose oral contraceptives containing less than 50 μg of estrogen. In a prospective study of Kenyan commercial sex workers, depot medroxyprogesterone acetate (DMPA) was associated with a 60% reduction in incident PID, whereas oral contraceptive use demonstrated a reduced risk that was not statistically significant: hazard ratio (HR) = 0.7; 95% CI 0.3, 1.4.[19] Wolner-Hanssen and colleagues examined whether the relationship of oral contraceptives and acute PID is influenced by specific pathogens.[20] In women with PID who were infected with *C. trachomatis*, oral contraceptive use was negatively associated with PID: odds ratio (OR) = 0.22; 95% CI 0.08, 0.64. In contrast, no such protection was observed among women with PID who were infected with *N. gonorrhoeae*: OR = 0.92; 95% CI 0.31, 2.63. In the Swedish cohort of women with laparoscopy-confirmed acute PID, oral contraceptive use was associated with a dramatic reduction in the risk of acute PID: relative risk (RR) 0.24, 95% CI 0.15, 0.28.[21] Thus, there have been a number of studies suggesting that oral contraceptive use may be associated with a lower risk of acute symptomatic PID.

In contrast to the negative association between oral contraceptives and acute PID, oral contraceptive use is associated with an increased risk of chlamydial cervicitis. As *C. trachomatis* is one of the major etiologic agents of acute PID, how can the contrasting findings of oral contraceptive use be reconciled? Over two decades ago, leading experts expressed concern about concluding that oral contraceptives protect against PID.[22] One hypothesis was that oral contraceptives alter the host immune response to infection and perhaps reduce the inflammatory response in the upper genital tract. This concept is supported by the findings in the Swedish cohort of women with laparoscopically confirmed acute PID, as women using oral contraceptives had visually less severe inflammatory changes compared with women using other contraceptive methods.[23] Ness et al further attempted to explain these paradoxical findings in a comparative analysis of women with subclinical PID and women with acute PID.[24] Oral contraceptive use was more common in women with subclinical PID than in women with acute PID, suggesting that oral contraceptive use is associated with either subtler, milder, or subclinical disease. If in fact oral contraceptives increase the risk for subclinical PID, a condition that may be responsible for the majority of cases of infection-mediated tubal factor infertility, these findings could have major implications in the reproductive choices and subsequent outcomes of women.

Gonadal hormones may directly influence growth of microorganisms, thereby influencing the pathogenesis of PID. Over 5 decades ago, Koch demonstrated that progesterone is bactericidal against *N. gonorrhoeae*, findings confirmed by Morse and Fitzgerald 20 years later.[25,26] Animal studies have demonstrated that exogenous estrogen may enhance genital chlamydial infection.[27] Moreover, estrogen or oral contraceptive therapy promotes ascending chlamydial infection in a number of experiments using guinea pigs.[27–29] One of potential mechanisms by which estrogen promotes chlamydial infection is by enhancing attachment to endometrial gland epithelial cells.[30] On the other hand, Kleinman et al investigated the susceptibility of cultured endometrial cells and did not demonstrate an impact on chlamydial infection by estrogen or progestins.[31] To further complicate the issue, Kaushic and colleagues examined the influence of estradiol and progesterone on intrauterine chlamydial infection in a rat model. These investigations revealed that progesterone increases, and estradiol decreases, susceptibility to intrauterine chlamydial infection.[32] Further, Patton and colleagues studied the influence of oral contraceptives on the clinical course of chlamydial salpingitis using a monkey model in which subcutaneous salpingeal pockets were inoculated with *C. trachomatis*.[33] The administration of oral contraceptive agents did not influence the duration of shedding of chlamydial organisms or the histopathology of acute chlamydial infection. At present, the precise delineation of the hormonal influence on the pathogenesis of PID is lacking. As large proportions of reproductive-aged women use hormonal contraception, further studies examining the influence of sex steroids on the virulence of microbial pathogens, host defenses, and the pathogenesis of PID are greatly needed.

INFECTION AND INFLAMMATION OF THE FALLOPIAN TUBES

Ascension of microbes to the upper genital tract, particularly *N. gonorrhoeae* and *C. trachomatis*, is frequently the initial step of a complex process of microbe-induced inflammation and damage, and subsequent humoral and cellular immune host defense. A description of how *N. gonorrhoeae* and *C. trachomatis* establish infection in the human genital tract and the various strategies to evade human host defense is beyond the scope of this text, but the reader is referred to in-depth reviews on these topics.[34–36] This discussion focuses on gonococcal and chlamydial infections of the upper genital tract.

NEISSERIA GONORRHOEAE

Elegant experiments using organ cultures of human fallopian tubes have demonstrated that *N. gonorrhoeae* attaches primarily to non-ciliated mucosal cells.[37] After increasing the number of organisms within these cells, the gonococci then proceed to invade the subepithelial tissues. Interestingly, although attachment and entry occur foremost on non-ciliated cells, the ciliated cells bear the brunt of gonococcal-induced damage. Mucosal damage characteristic of gonococcal tubal infection is sloughing of the ciliated mucosal cells. This damage is believed to be mediated through toxic factors resulting from gonococcal infection. Sterilized supernatant from gonococcus-infected organ cultures produced similar damage to fallopian tube organ cultures directly infected with *N. gonorrhoeae*, indicating that toxins, perhaps expressed by the gonococcus, can directly cause epithelial damage.[38] Candidates for such toxins to the fallopian tube include lipopolysaccharide (LPS) and peptidoglycan.[39,40]

The release of proinflammatory mediators is essential to gonococcal infection of the upper genital tract. The biochemical mediators LPS and peptidoglycan may increase the production of the proinflammatory cytokine tumor necrosis factor-alpha (TNF-α).[41] Macrophages exposed to *N. gonorrhoeae* secrete high levels of proinflammatory cytokines, including TNF-α and interleukin-6 (IL-6).[42] The mucosal tissue concentration of TNF-α, in turn, is highly correlated with the degree of loss of mucosal ciliated cells.[43] Further, high levels of TNF-α in peritoneal fluid correlate with tubal occlusion.[44] IL-6 may be involved in fibrosis and tubal scarring. Together, these data indicate that proinflammatory cytokines, particularly TNF-α, play critical roles in the pathogenesis of gonococcal PID.

Much work has focused on the attachment of *N. gonorrhoeae* to the epithelia of the upper genital tract in an effort to delineate the access to the endometrial and fallopian tube tissues and thereby to understand the early stages of the pathogenesis of PID. Lutropin receptor (LHr) has been postulated to be a receptor for gonococcal invasion of the endometrial and fallopian tube mucosa.[45] LHr is up-regulated during menses, which correlates chronologically with the initiation of many cases of PID. Further, expression of this receptor increases from the endometrium to the fallopian tube. The endometrium expresses a number of other receptors for *N. gonorrhoeae* in addition to LHr, including CEACAM, CR3, asialoglycoprotein receptor (ASGP-R), and TLR-4.[46] CEACAM is a receptor molecule of the carcinoembryonic antigen (CEA) family. CEACAM binds to several Opa protein outer membrane proteins of *N. gonorrhoeae*. CEACAM is not essential for initiation and establishment of infection, but *N. gonorrhoeae* will exploit this receptor, if present, for mucosal adherence and invasion.[47] Recently, Boulton and Gray-Owen studied the interaction between gonococci and CEACAM1.[48] They demonstrated that the binding of *N. gonorrhoeae* to CEACAM1 on $CD4^+$ cells suppressed the activation and proliferation of these lymphocytes. Their work suggests that one mechanism of immune evasion and propagation of infection is due to the gonococcus itself, by suppressing the immune response that results from binding to CEACAM1. In summary, the pathogenesis of PID and the immunologic mechanism of disease due to *N. gonorrhoeae* are highly complex and poorly understood, with much work needed to elucidate the various mechanisms of initiation and propagation of infection of the upper genital tract.

Additional inherent properties of *N. gonorrhoeae* may facilitate infection. Mucosal immunoglobulin A (IgA) is an important component of the host defense against infection, by preventing adherence of the microorganism to the mucosal surface. The interaction between the gonococcus and secretory IgA may represent an additional pathogenic mechanism of this organism. *N. gonorrhoeae* produces IgA proteases that are capable of breaking down secretory IgA, thereby facilitating mucosal adherence and inactivating host mucosal defense.[49] Gonococcal IgA proteases are probably key to the early stages of gonococcal infections of the lower genital tract, facilitating the establishment of infection. Whether gonococcal IgA protease assists in the pathogenesis of salpingitis is not currently known. *N. gonorrhoeae* also produces additional compounds that have been postulated to be involved in the pathogenesis of disease. For example, lipopolysaccharide (LPS) is expressed on the surface of gonococci. Gonococcal LPS may be directly toxic to epithelial cells, as noted above.[39] Whether this virulence factor is important in the establishment of salpingitis is currently unknown.

Draper et al studied virulence factors of paired *N. gonorrhoeae* strains isolated from lower and upper genital tract sites in women with acute PID.[50,51] The colony phenotype of *N. gonorrhoeae* differed according to disease severity. Organisms isolated from the fallopian tubes from women with acute PID tended to be of the transparent colony phenotype, unlike the opaque strains found at the cervix. These investigators further studied the pathogenic nature of the transparent strains of *N. gonorrhoeae*.[52] A study using explant systems comprising human fallopian tube and cervical tissue demonstrated that transparent colony phenotype of *N. gonorrhoeae* attaches more avidly to fallopian tube mucosa than opaque colonies. Other studies indicate that PID is more common with certain serotypes of *N. gonorrhoeae*.[53] Other potential gonococcal virulence factors include iron-repressible proteins, opacity (Opa) proteins, and porin protein. Further information is needed to help understand the pathogenic role of *N. gonorrhoeae* in salpingitis.

CHLAMYDIA TRACHOMATIS

The host inflammatory response to chlamydial antigens may determine the pathogenesis of PID due to *C. trachomatis*. Much attention has been focused lately on the role of the chlamydial 60 kDa heat shock protein (Hsp 60) in chlamydial pelvic inflammatory disease and infertility. Antibodies to chlamydial Hsp 60 correlate with acute PID.[54,55] Moreover, antibodies to chlamydial Hsp 60 are associated with more severe infection and tissue damage.[56] In a study of women with laparoscopically-confirmed PID, high levels of chlamydial Hsp 60 antibody were identified in 80% of women with tubal occlusion compared with 19% of women with patent tubes.[55] Higher titres of chlamydial Hsp 60 antibody are also seen in women with PID who have perihepatitis and severe pelvic adhesions.[57] There is considerable homology between chlamydial Hsp 60 and human Hsp 60. Consequently, fallopian tube infection with *C. trachomatis* may lead to production of antibodies to chlamydial Hsp 60. By virtue of the close amino acid sequence homology to human Hsp 60, chlamydial Hsp 60 antibodies create an autoimmune response, cross-reacting and targeting fallopian tube mucosa, and causing subsequent damage and scarring.[58]

The host inflammatory response, mediated through cytokine production is believed to be a critical pathogenic mechanism of PID. The T-helper (Th1) response, primarily interferon-γ (IFN-γ) , is a critical component of the host defense against chlamydial infection. The Th1 response in the fallopian tubes infected with *C. trachomatis* is considerable, and this immune response contributes to subsequent tubal scarring and damage.[59,60] Employing an animal model using subcutaneous pockets containing autologous salpingeal tissue in *Macaca nemestrina*, Van Voorhis and colleagues demonstrated that the inflammatory response following inoculation with *C. trachomatis* consisted primarily of $CD8^+$ T-cell lymphocytes with a Th1-like cytokine response. The Th1 cytokines can promote killing of intracellular pathogens. In particular, IFN-γ has demonstrated chlamydial killing and clearance in both in-vitro and animal experiments.[61,62] On the contrary, IFN-γ can promote tissue fibrosis.[63] Further confusing the picture is that moderate IFN-γ levels (in contrast to high levels) may actually promote ongoing chlamydial infection.[61] The Th1 cytokine response in chlamydial infections has been associated with inflammatory changes that lead to progression of fibrosis.[60] A Th2 cytokine response is also witnessed during chlamydial infection. Whereas the Th2 cytokines may down-regulate the Th1 response, this immunomodulatory effect may paradoxically promote tissue damage by enabling ongoing and persistent chlamydial infection. IL-10 secretion from peripheral blood mononuclear cells (PBMCs) that were stimulated with chlamydial Hsp 60 was greater from cells obtained from women with tubal factor infertility than from women with other types of infertility.[64] These findings suggest that anti-inflammatory cytokines may suppress the host immune response to chlamydial infections and enable persistence of *C. trachomatis*.

Delayed-type hypersensitivity responses may play critical roles in the pathogenesis of chlamydial PID. In monkeys previously infected with *C. trachomatis*, recombinant chlamydial Hsp 60 elicited an inflammatory response similar to that seen in women with chlamydial PID.[65] In a cohort of Kenyan commercial sex workers, Peeling and colleagues demonstrated that women with pre-existing chlamydial Hsp 60 antibodies were at significant increased risk for developing acute PID during a new chlamydial infection compared with those women without pre-existing chlamydial Hsp 60 antibody.[66] These data suggest that prior sensitization by chlamydia followed by a subsequent chlamydial infection can lead to a more robust inflammatory response and greater damage to the fallopian tubes.

Repeated infections are associated with far greater tubal damage and infertility, suggesting the importance of immunologic mediation of tubal damage due to *C. trachomatis*. An early report on the pathogenesis of trachoma suggests that more severe scarring occurs after reinfection with *C. trachomatis*.[67] A similar relationship has been observed in PID. Westrom et al examined the risk of infertility in women with laparoscopy-confirmed acute PID.[68] The rate of infertility doubled after each repeated episode of PID. The rate of infertility following a single episode of acute PID was 8%, and this rate rose to 19.5% and 40% after a second and third episode of PID, respectively. The exponential increase in infertility highlights the relationship between repeat infections and tubal scarring. The adverse impact of repeated chlamydial infections has been best studied in an animal model using pig-tailed macaques. Patton et al demonstrated that a single inoculation with *C. trachomatis* caused a self-limited infection of the lower genital tract, whereas repeated inoculation caused fallopian tube obstruction.[69] A subsequent study in the same monkey model evaluated fallopian tube damage from tubal chlamydia inoculation in animals with multiple cervical infections.[70] Following a series of cervical chlamydial infections occurring at no less than weekly intervals, the fallopian tubes were inoculated with *C. trachomatis*. All animals that received five cervical inoculations with *C. trachomatis* developed peritubal adhesions, whereas no adhesions developed in the animals receiving three or fewer cervical inoculations. As noted above, Van Voorhis et al used the subcutaneous salpingeal pocket model in macaques to demonstrate that repeated chlamydial infections of the fallopian tube caused an infiltrate primarily of $CD8^+$ T cells and a Th1-like cytokine response that was associated with subsequent fibrosis.[60] Thus, animal and human data indicate that, compared with a single infection, repeated chlamydial infections cause far greater fallopian tube damage. Either repeat infections or untreated chronic infections may perpetuate the host inflammatory responses and result in tubal damage.

NONGONOCOCCAL, NONCHLAMYDIAL PELVIC INFLAMMATORY DISEASE

As outlined in Chapter 2, salpingitis is a polymicrobial infection. Aerobic and anaerobic organisms are frequently isolated from the upper genital tract of women with acute PID. Although we know that the lower genital tract (i.e. vagina and cervix) in women is typically heavily colonized with aerobic and anaerobic organisms, little is known on how these organisms ascend to the endometrium and fallopian tubes. One theory is that a critical number of organisms are needed to overcome the local host defense. Evidence is mounting that bacterial vaginosis (BV)-related microorganisms play a critical role in the pathogenesis of PID. In studies employing microbiologic evaluation of the endometrium and/or fallopian tubes, BV-associated organisms have often been isolated from the upper genital tract of women with acute PID.[71–73] In addition to the association with acute PID, we have demonstrated that women with BV are at increased likelihood for concomitant subclinical PID.[74] A prospective observational study of a cohort of women at high risk for STDs by Ness et al did not identify an increased risk of incident PID among women with BV.[75] However, further analysis of this same cohort demonstrated that incident PID was associated with heavy growth of BV-associated organisms (particularly *Gardnerella vaginalis, Mycoplasma hominis*, and anaerobic Gram-negative rods).[76] Further, those women with heavy growth of these organisms and who had a new sexual partner were at greatest risk for PID. The findings of this study suggest that because women with BV have far greater vaginal concentrations of potentially pathogenic bacteria compared with women with normal vaginal flora, it is possible that the numbers of pathogenic bacteria simply overcome cervical barriers to ascent. Moreover, the relationship between BV, a new sexual partner, and PID suggests that sexually activity or a sexually transmitted cofactor enhances the risk of PID in women with BV. This does not explain why only a limited number of women with BV develop PID. Potentially pathogenic bacteria in the vagina may excrete products that alter the integrity of the cervical barrier. Hydrogen peroxide (H_2O_2)-producing lactobacilli, typically absent in women with BV, have the capability to inhibit the growth of *N. gonorrhoeae* in vitro.[77] Perhaps the absence of H_2O_2-producing lactobacilli enables enhanced growth of *N. gonorrhoeae* and facilitates access to the upper genital tract. An abnormal vaginal microenvironment, mediated by microbial products, may also alter the host susceptibility to infection. Succinate, produced by anaerobic Gram-negative rods commonly associated with BV, alters leukocyte function and may compromise host defenses.[78] Vaginal fluid of women with BV contains sialidase and other glycosides that affect vaginal fluid viscosity and may facilitate ascending infection. However, the fact that the great majority of women with BV do not develop acute or subclinical PID highlights the limited current understanding in the pathogenesis of nongonococcal, nonchlamydial acute PID.

HUMAN LEUKOCYTE ANTIGEN AND PELVIC INFLAMMATORY DISEASE

As the host immune response is critical to the development of PID and its sequelae, work has begun to explore the role of the host's innate response to chlamydial and gonococcal infection. The initial stages of infection involve the host's presentation of peptides to $CD4^+$ T cells. Recognition of peptide requires that major histocompatibility complex (MHC) molecules bind intracellular antigen and deliver it to the cell surface. These MHC molecules are coded by human leukocyte antigen (HLA) genes. To explore the immunogenetic response to *C. trachomatis* infection, Cohen et al studied HLA alleles in a cohort of Kenyan women with suspected tubal factor infertility.[79,80] Possession of HLA DQA*0101 and DQB*0501 alleles was associated with tubal factor infertility due to *C. trachomatis*, whereas the detection of two Class II alleles, HLA-DR1*1503 and DRB5*0101, was less frequent among infertile women seropositive for *C. trachomatis* than among women without the *C. trachomatis* antibodies. Among women with clinically suspected acute PID, HLA DQA*0301 was associated with endometritis and infertility.[81] These works suggest that some women have the innate capability to modify the pathogenic response to *C. trachomatis* infection and its associated fallopian tube damage.

SUMMARY

It is evident that the pathogenesis of PID is complex and our current understanding is limited. Many microbial virulence factors, particularly for *N. gonorrhoeae*, have been identified and yet there have been few correlates between pathogen-derived virulence factors and PID. Moreover, work exploring the interactions between *N. gonorrhoeae, C. trachomatis*, the BV-associated organisms, and the host innate immune response is only in its infancy. The individual's immunologic responses at the mucosal, local, and systemic levels are critical in determining whether the PID-associated pathogens gain access to the upper genital tract, establish infection in the endometrium and fallopian tubes, and cause fallopian tube scarring and infertility. Despite the great advances in our knowledge of the pathogenesis of PID, there remains much work to accurately characterize the pathogenic mechanisms of the disease.

REFERENCES

1. Toth A, O'Leary WM, Ledger WJ. Evidence for microbial transfer by spermatozoa. Obstet Gynecol 1982;59:556–9.
2. Zuckerman H, Kahana, A, Carmel S. Antibacterial activity of human cervical mucus. Gynecol Invest 1975;6:265–71.
3. Eggert-Kruse W, Botz I, Pohl S, et al. Antimicrobial activity of human cervical mucus. Human Reprod 2000;15:778–84.
4. Hein M, Helmig RB. Schonheyder HC, et al. An in vitro study of antibacterial properties of the cervical mucus plug in pregnancy. Am J Obstet Gynecol 2001; 185:586–92.
5. Odeblad E. The functional structure of human cervical mucus. Acta Obstet Gynecol Scand 1986;47(Suppl 1):59–79.
6. Chretien FC. Ultrastructure and variations of human cervical mucus during pregnancy and the menopause. Acta Obstet Gynecol Scand 1978;57:337–48.
7. Doumas S. Kolokotronis A, Stefanopoulos P. Anti-inflammatory and antimicrobial roles of secretory leukocyte protease inhibitor. Infect Immun 2005;73:1271–4.
8. Pillay K, Coutsoudis A, Agadzi-Naqvi AK, et al. Secretory leukocyte protease inhibitor in vaginal fluids and perinatal human immunodeficiency virus type-1 transmission. J Infect Dis 2001;183:653–6.
9. Fahey JV, Wira CR. Effect of menstrual status on antibacterial activity and secretory leukocyte protease inhibitor production by human uterine epithelial cells in culture. J Infect Dis 2002;185:1606–13.
10. Moriyama A, Shimoya K, Ogata I, et al. Secretory leukocyte protease inhibitor (SLPI) concentrations in cervical mucus of women with normal menstrual cycle. Mol Human Reprod 1999;5:656–61.
11. King AE, Critchley HOD, Kelly RW. Presence of secretory leukocyte protease inhibitor in human endometrium and first trimester decidua suggests an antibacterial protective role. Mol Human Reprod 2000;6:191–6.
12. Valore EV, Park CH, Quayle AJ, et al. Human beta-defensin-1: an antimicrobial peptide of urogenital tissues. J Clin Invest 1998;101(8):1633–42.
13. Wiesenfeld HC, Heine RP, Krohn MS, et al. Association between elevated neutrophil defensins and endometritis. J Infect Dis 2002;186:792–7.
14. Litwin CM, Calderwood SB. Role of iron in regulation of virulence genes. Clin Microbiol Rev 1993;6:137–49.
15. Eschenbach DA, Harnisch JP, Holmes KK. Pathogenesis of acute pelvic inflammatory disease: role of contraception and other risk factors. Am J Obstet Gynecol 1977;128:838–50.
16. Senanayake P, Kramer DG. Contraception and the etiology of pelvic inflammatory disease: new perspectives. Am J Obstet Gynecol 1980;138:852–60.
17. Rubin GL, Ory HW, Layde PM. Oral contraceptives and pelvic inflammatory disease. Am J Obstet Gynecol 1982;144:630–5.
18. Panser LA, Phipps WR. Type of oral contraceptive in relation to acute, initial episodes of pelvic inflammatory disease. Contraception 1991;43:91–9.
19. Baeten JM, Nyange PM, Richardson BA, et al. Hormonal contraception and risk of sexually transmitted disease acquisition: results from a prospective study. Am J Obstet Gynecol 2001;185:380–5.
20. Wolner-Hanssen P, Eschenbach DA, Paavonen J, et al. Decreased risk of symptomatic chlamydial pelvic inflammatory disease associated with oral contraceptive use. JAMA 1990;263(1):54–9.
21. Wolner-Hanssen PK, Svensson L, Mardh PA, Westrom L. Laparoscopic findings and contraceptive use in women with signs and symptoms suggestive of acute salpingitis. Obstet Gynecol 1985;66:233–8.
22. Washington AE, Gove S, Schachter J, Sweet RL. Oral contraceptives, *Chlamydia trachomatis* infection, and pelvic inflammatory disease. A word of caution about protection. JAMA 1985;253(15):2246–50.
23. Svensson L, Westrom L, Mardh PA. Contraceptives and acute salpingitis. JAMA 1984;251:2553–5.
24. Ness RB, Keder LM, Soper DE, et al. Oral contraception and the recognition of endometritis. Am Obstet Gynecol 1997;176(3):580–5.
25. Koch ML. The bactericidal action of beta progesterone. Am J Obstet Gynecol 1950;59:168–71.
26. Morse SA, Fitzgerald TJ. Effect of progesterone on *Neisseria gonorrhoeae*. Infect Immun 1974;10:1370–7.
27. Rank RG, White HJ, Hough AJ Jr, et al. Effect of estradiol on chlamydial genital infection of female guinea pigs. Infect immun 1982;38:699–705.
28. Pasley JN, Rank RG, Hough AJ Jr, et al. Effects of various doses of estradiol on chlamydial genital infection in overiectomized guinea pigs. Sex Transm Dis 1985;12:8–13.
29. Barron AL, Pasley JN, Rank RG, et al. Chlamydial salpingitis in female guinea pigs receiving oral contraceptives. Sex Transm Dis 1988;15:169–73.
30. Maslow AS, Davis CH, Choong J, Wyrick PB. Estrogen enhances attachment of *Chlamydia trachomatis* to human endometrial epithelial cells in vitro. Am J Obstet Gynecol 1988;159:1006–14.
31. Kleinman D, Sarov B, Insler V. The effects of contraceptive hormones on the replication of *Chlamydia trachomatis* in human endometrial cells. Contraception 1987;35:533–42.
32. Kaushic C, Zhou F, Murdin AD, Wira CR. Effects of estradiol and progesterone on susceptibility and early immune responses to *Chlamydia trachomatis* infection in the female reproductive tract. Infect Immun 2000;68:4207–16.
33. Patton DL, Sweeney YT, Kuo CC. Oral conceptives do not alter the course of experimentally induced chlamydial salpingitis in monkeys. Sex Transm Dis 1994;21:89–92.
34. Brunham RC, Rey-Ladino J. Immunology of chlamydia infection: implications for a *Chlamydia trachomatis* vaccine. Nat Rev Immunol 2005;5:149–61.
35. Cohen MS, Sparling PF. Mucosal infection with *Neisseria gonorrhoeae*. J Clin Invest 1992;89:1699–705.
36. Edwards JL, Apicella MA. The molecular mechanisms used by *Neisseria gonorrhoeae* to initiate infection differ between men and women. Clin Microbiol Rev 2004; 17:965–81.
37. McGee ZA, Johnson AP, Taylor-Robinson D. Pathogenic mechanisms of *Neisseria gonorrhoeae*: observations on damage to human fallopian tubes in organ culture by gonococci of colony type 1 or type 4. J Infect Dis 1981;143:413–22.
38. Melly MA, Gregg CR, McGee ZA. Studies of toxicity of *Neisseria gonorrhoeae* for human fallopian tube mucosa. J Infect Dis 1981;143:423–31.
39. Gregg CR, Melly MA, McGee ZA. Gonococcal lipopolysaccharide: a toxin for human fallopian tube mucosa. Am J Obstet Gynecol 1980;138:981–4.
40. Melly MA, McGee ZA, Rosenthal RS. Ability of monomeric peptidoglycan fragments from *Neisseria gonorrhoeae* to damage human fallopian-tube mucosa. J Infect Dis 1984; 149:378–86.
41. McGee ZA, Clemens CM, Jensen RL, et al. Local induction of tumor necrosis factor as a molecular mechanism of mucosal damage by gonococci. Microb Pathog 1992;12:333–41.

42. Makepeace BL, Watt PJ, Heckels J, Christodoulides M. Interactions of *Neisseria gonorrhoeae* with mature human macrophage opacity proteins influence production of proinflammatory cytokines. Infect Immun 2001;69:1909–13.
43. McGee ZA, Jensen RL, Clemens CM, et al. Gonococcal infection of human fallopian tube mucosa in organ culture: relationship of mucosal tissue TNF-alpha concentration to sloughing of ciliated cells. Sex Transm Dis 1999;26:160–5.
44. Guerra-Infante FM, Flores-Medina S, Lopez-Hurtado M, et al. Tumor necrosis factor in peritoneal fluid from asymptomatic infertile women. Arch Med Res 1999;30:138–43.
45. Spence JM, Chen JCR, Clark VL. A proposed role for the lutropin receptor in contact-inducible gonococcal invasion of Hec1B cells. Infect Immunol 1997;65:3736–42.
46. Timmerman MM, Shao JQ, Apicella MA. Ultrastructural analysis of the pathogenesis of *Neisseria gonorrhoeae* endometrial infection. Cell Microbiol 2005;7:627–36.
47. Swanson KV, Jarvis GA, Brooks GF. CEACAM is not necessary for *Neisseria gonorrhoeae* to adhere to and invade female genital epithelial cells. Cell Microbiol 2001;3:681–91.
48. Boulton IC, Gray-Owen SD. Neisserial binding to CEACAM1 arrests the activation and proliferation of CD4$^+$ T lymphocytes. Nat Immunol 2002;3:229–36.
49. Mulks MH, Plaut AG, IgA protease production as a characteristic distinguishing pathogenic from harmless Neisseria. N Engl J Med 1978;1978:973–6.
50. Draper DL, James JF, Brooks GF, Sweet RL. Comparison of virulence markers of peritoneal and fallopian tube isolates with endocervical *Neisseria gonorrhoeae* isolates from women with acute salpingitis. Infect Immun 1980;27(3):882–8.
51. Draper DL, James JF, Hadley WK, Sweet RL. Auxotypes and antibiotic susceptibilities of *Neisseria gonorrhoeae* from women with acute salpingitis. Comparison with gonococci causing uncomplicated genital tract infections in women. Sex Transm Dis 1981;8(2):43–50.
52. Draper DL, Donegan EA, James JF, et al. Scanning electron microscopy of attachment of *Neisseria gonorrhoeae* colony phenotype to surfaces of human genital epithelia. Am J Obstet Gynecol 1980;138:818–26.
53. Buchanan TM, Eschenbach DA, Knapp JS, et al. Gonococcal salpingitis is less likely to recur with *Neisseria gonorrhoeae* of the same principal outer membrane protein antigen type. Obstet Gynecol 1981;138:978–80.
54. Witkin SS, Jeremias J, Toth M, Ledger WJ. Cell-medicated immune response to the recombinant 57-kDa heat-shock protein of *Chlamydia trachomatis* in women with salpingitis. J Infect Dis 1993;167(6):1379–83.
55. Eckert LO, Hawes SE, Wolner-Hanssen P, et al. Prevalence and correlates of antibody to chlamydial heat shock protein in women attending sexually transmitted disease clinics and women with confirmed pelvic inflammatory disease. J Infect Dis 1997;175(6):1453–8.
56. Dieterle S, Wollenhaupt J. Humoral immune response to the chlamydial heat shock proteins hsp60 and hsp70 in chlamydia-associated chronic salpingitis with tubal occlusion. Hum Reprod 1996;11:1352–6.
57. Money DM, Hawes SE, Eschenbach DA, et al. Antibodies to the chlamydial 60 kd heat-shock protein are associated with laparoscopically confirmed perihepatitis. Am J Obstet Gynecol 1997;176(4):870–7.
58. Domeika M, Domeika K, Paavonen J, et al. Humoral immune response to conserved epitopes of *Chlamydia trachomatis* and human 60-kDa heat-shock protein in women with pelvic inflammatory disease. J Infect Dis 1998;177(3):714–19.
59. Rank RG, Bowlin AK, Kelly KA. Characterization of lymphocyte response in the female genital tract during ascending chlamydial infection in the guinea pig model. Infect Immun 2000;68:5293–8.
60. van Voorhis WC, Barrett LK, Sweeney YT, et al. Repeated *Chlamydia trachomatis* infection of *Macaca nemestrina* fallopian tubes produces a Th1-like cytokine response associated with fibrosis and scarring. Infect Immun 1997;65:2175–82.
61. Beatty WL, Byrne GI, Morrison RP. Morphologic and antigenic characterization of interferon gamma-mediated persistent *Chlamydia trachomatis* infection in vitro. Proc Natl Acad Sci USA 1993;90:3998–4002.
62. Rank RG, Ramsey KH, Pack EA, Williams DM. Effect of gamma interferon on resolution of murine chlamydial genital infection. Infect immun 1992;60:4427–9.
63. Kovacs EJ. Fibrogenic cytokines: the role of immune mediators in the development of scar tissue. Immunol Today 1991;12:17–23.
64. Kinnunen A, Surcel HM, Halttunen M, et al. *Chlamydia trachomatis* heat shock protein-60 induced interferon-gamma and interleukin-10 production in infertile women. Clin Exp Immunol 2003;131:299–303.
65. Patton DL, Sweeney YT, Kuo CC. Demonstration of delayed hypersensitivity in *Chlamydia trachomatis* salpingitis in monkeys: a pathogenic mechanism of tubal damage. J Infect Dis 1994;169(3):680–3.
66. Peeling RW, Kimani J, Plummer F, et al. Antibody to chlamydial hsp60 predicts an increased risk for chlamydial pelvic inflammatory disease. J Infect Dis 1997;175(5):1153–8.
67. Grayston JT, Wang SP, Yeh LJ, Kuo CC. Importance of reinfection in the pathogenesis of trachoma. Rev Infect Dis 1985;7:717–25.
68. Westrom L, Joesoef R, Reynolds G, et al. Pelvic inflammatory disease and fertility. A cohort study of 1844 women with laparoscopically verified disease and 657 control women with normal laparoscopic results. Sex Transm Dis 1992;19:185–92.
69. Patton DL, Kuo CC, Wang SP, Halbert SA. Distal tubal obstruction induced by repeated *Chlamydia trachomatis* salpingeal infections in pig-tailed macaques. J Infect Dis 1987;155:1292–9.
70. Patton DL, Wolner-Hanssen P, Cosgrove SJ, Holmes KK. The effects of *Chlamydia trachomatis* on the female reproductive tract of the *Macaca nemestrina* after a single tubal challenge following repeated cervical inoculations. Obstet Gynecol 1990;76:643–50.
71. Jossens MO, Schachter J, Sweet RL. Risk factors associated with pelvic inflammatory disease of differing microbial etiologies. Obstet Gynecol 1994;83(6):989–97.
72. Soper DE, Brockwell NJ, Dalton HP, Johnston D. Observations concerning the microbial etiology of acute salpingitis. Am J Obstet Gynecol 1994;170(4):1008–14.
73. Hillier SL, Kiviat NB, Hawes SE, et al. Role of bacterial vaginosis-associated microorganisms in endometritis. Am J Obstet Gynecol 1996;175(2):435–41.
74. Wiesenfeld HC, Hillier SL, Krohn MA, et al. Lower genital tract infection and endometritis: insight into subclinical pelvic inflammatory disease. Obstet Gynecol 2002;100(3):456–63.
75. Ness RB, Hillier SL, Kip KE, et al. Bacterial vaginosis and risk of pelvic inflammatory disease. Obstet Gynecol 2004;104:761–9.
76. Ness RB, Kip KE, Hillier SL, et al. A cluseter analysis of bacterial vaginosis-associated microflora and pelvic inflammatory disease. Am J Epidemiol 2005;162(6):1–6.
77. Zheng H, Alcorn TM, Cohen MS. Effects of H_2O_2-producing lactobacilli on *Neisseria gonorrhoeae* growth and catalase activity. J Infect Dis 1994;170:1209–15.
78. Rotstein OD, Pruett TL, Fiegel VD, et al. Succinic acid, a metabolic by-product of *Bacteroides* species, inhibits polymorphonuclear leukocyte function. Infect Immunol 1985;48:402–5.

79. Cohen CR, Sinei SS, Bukusi EA, et al. Human leukocyte antigen class II DQ alleles associated with *Chlamydia trachomatis* tubal infertility. Obstet Gynecol 2000;95:72–7.
80. Cohen CR, Gichui J, Rukaria R, et al. Immunogenetic correlates for *Chlamydia trachomatis*-associated tubal infertility. Obstet Gynecol 2003;101:438–44.
81. Ness RB, Brunham RC, Shen C, Bass DC. Associations among human leukocyte antigen (HLA) class II DQ variants, bacterial sexually transmitted diseases, endometritis, and fertility among women with clinical pelvic inflammatory disease. Sex Transm Dis 2004;31:301–4.

4. Pathology

Dorothy L. Patton and Anne B. Lichtenwalner

INTRODUCTION

Chlamydia trachomatis infections are still the most frequently reported bacterial sexually transmitted disease (STD) in the United States, with 834 555 infections reported to the Centers for Disease Control and Prevention (CDC) in 2002. An estimated 3 million new cases occur in the US yearly.[1] Pelvic inflammatory disease (PID) due to *C. trachomatis* genital tract infections in women remains significant in the United States, with estimates that approximately 1 million cases of PID were treated yearly in the 1980s, and perhaps 780 000 cases per year more recently.[2,3] A recent study of young adults reported a chlamydial genital infection prevalence in women of 4.74%.[4] In a large study of female army recruits, overall prevalence of *C. trachomatis* detection using ligase chain reaction was 9.5%, but a significant and progressive increase from 8.5% to 9.9% occurred over the 4-year course of study.[5] Animal studies indicate that the substantial inflammation caused by chlamydial upper genital tract infection is a delayed-type hypersensitivity response, occurring as a result of repeated exposures to *C. trachomatis*. A recent clinical study established that the reinfection rate among over 32 000 women successfully treated for initial chlamydial genital tract infections over a 3–4-year period was 15%.[6] Based on these reports, chlamydial PID will continue to impact US health care in the near future.

HUMAN STUDIES

The clinical presentation of chlamydial PID varies, but lower abdominal tenderness, adnexal tenderness, and cervical motion tenderness, combined with fever and a high white blood cell count, are considered to be relatively sensitive and specific markers for the syndrome, whereas imaging with power Doppler transvaginal ultrasound can be effective in detecting fallopian tube inflammation.[7] Laparoscopic examination of women with chlamydial PID often reveals pelvic adhesions and tubal occlusion.[8] In women, *C. trachomatis* PID is thought to arise from an initial cervical infection that extends into the upper reproductive tract, affecting the uterus, fallopian tubes, and occasionally the peritoneum. In one study, only 17% of women with suspect PID (based on lower abdominal pain of greater than 3 weeks' duration and abnormal adnexal tenderness on pelvic examination) had endometritis alone. In contrast, 55% of the women studied had salpingitis, and 85% of these women had both endometritis and salpingitis.[9] Chlamydial PID may culminate in tubal factor infertility, painful abdominal adhesions, and fibrinopurulent perihepatitis (Fitz-Hugh–Curtis syndrome).[10]

Whereas the reproductive pathology associated with acute PID (Figure 4.3) includes extensive intraperitoneal inflammation, pathology associated with chronic PID (Figure 4.4) is linked to loss of reproductive function. In early studies of women with tubal factor infertility (TFI), greater than 50% of those with overt or silent salpingitis were serologically positive for *C. trachomatis* (vs 0% of controls). Laparoscopy revealed intra-abdominal adhesions and uni- or bilateral hydrosalpinges (See Figure 4.5b, as compared to the normal fallopian tube shown in Figure 4.1b). Gross histologic and electron microscopic studies showed that tubal tissues from women with overt or silent salpingitis had dilated lumina characterized by flattened epithelial cells with an absence of cilia. In contrast, the lumina of normal fallopian tube tissues have closely packed mucosal folds that are lined with secretory and ciliated epithelial cells as shown in

Figure 4.2. In women with TFI, tubal ciliary activity was significantly impaired.[11] This impairment of fallopian tube ciliary activity may affect transport of sperm and ova and contribute to the infertility that commonly follows chronic chlamydial salpingitis. Tubal tissues of women with acute chlamydial salpingitis (Figure 4.3) showed both epithelial damage and marked inflammatory cell infiltration of the submucosal layers with polymorphonuclear leukocytes (PMNs) and lymphocytes.[12]

These inflammatory changes are also seen in endometrial tissue during chlamydial infection. Polymorphonuclear cell shedding, detected in vaginal smears, is significantly correlated with histologic endometritis in *C. trachomatis*-infected women.[13] Inflammatory changes may be associated with severe abdominal pain, which is significantly associated with the presence of plasma cell endometritis. With the development of upper tract infection, tubal and endometrial inflammation is primarily lymphocytic (Figure 4.4). In a study of women that coupled laparoscopic visual assessment with endometrial biopsy and multisite cultures for *C. trachomatis*, *Neisseria gonorrhoeae*, and other STDs, endometrial plasma cell (activated B-lymphocyte) inflammation and lymphoid follicle formation were positively correlated with salpingitis and with the presence of either *C. trachomatis* or *N. gonorrhoeae*.[14]

The time course of histologic and immunologic responses to chlamydial infection is difficult to characterize in clinical studies. In a small study of serologically chlamydia-positive women, endometrial plasma cells were characterized as producing immunoglobulins IgG, IgA, and IgM, suggesting that the principal local response is humoral. Indeed, in the patients with large aggregations of endometrial plasma cells (lymphoid follicles) in this study, IgA-producing plasma cells were in the majority.[15] However, in women with either tubal factor infertility or PID, tissue-derived T-lymphocyte lines reacted with chlamydial antigens,

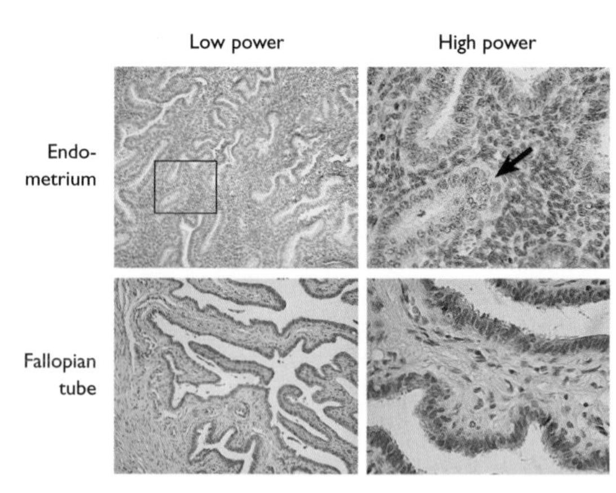

Figure 4.2 Normal histology (human). The endometrium (proliferative phase) consists of elongated glands (low power) lined by a pseudostratified epithelial cells (arrow) and a supportive cellular stroma (high power). The ampulla of the fallopian tube consists of delicate mucosal folds lined by simple columnar epithelial cells supported by a loose connective tissue, the submucosa, resting on the muscularis (low power). Both ciliated and secretory epithelial cells form the tubal epithelium (high power).

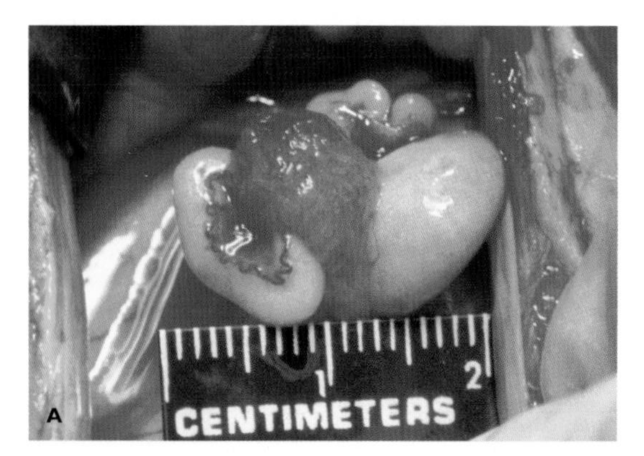

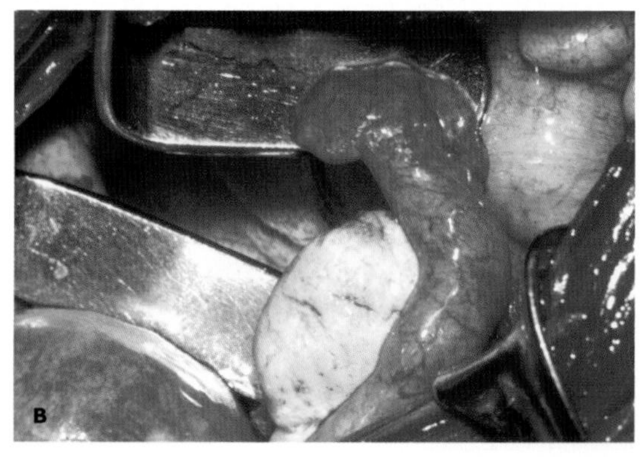

Figure 4.1 Normal pelvic anatomy of upper reproductive tract tissues of (A) *Macaca nemestrina* (monkey) and (B) human. The fallopian tube, fimbria, and ovary of the monkey are smaller than in the human but similar in gross anatomic structure.

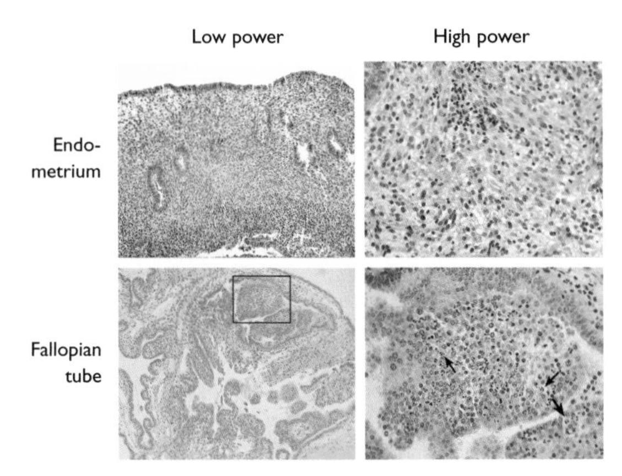

Figure 4.3 Acute pelvic inflammatory disease (human). Endometrial stroma contains an inflammatory infiltrate that consists primarily of polymorphonuclear leukocytes (PMNs) (low and high power). The superficial layer (low power) of the endometrium and the stroma are permeated by numerous PMNs (high power). The fallopian tube mucosal folds are characterized by a PMN infiltrate (low and high power, arrows) within the submucosa consistent with acute salpingitis/PID.

Low power High power

Endo-
metrium

Fallopian
tube

Figure 4.4 Chronic pelvic inflammatory disease (human). The endometrial stroma contains a mixed inflammatory infiltrate consisting of lymphocytes (low power) and plasma cells (high power). The submucosa of the fallopian tube contains a widespread lymphocytic infiltrate (low power) and numerous plasma cells (high power). The lymphocytes appear to form small clusters or foci near capillaries (high power, arrows).

characterized by Th-1 activity,[16] suggesting an important role for cell-mediated immunity. Recent studies of genetic predisposition to PID,[17–19] of the persistence of chlamydial DNA or antigens following antimicrobial treatment of infection,[20,21] and of variations in serologic responses to chlamydial antigens[16,22] suggest that host factors influencing immunologic responses to chlamydial antigens in the reproductive tract tissues of susceptible individuals may exacerbate the pathology of PID.

ANIMAL STUDIES

In animal studies, we attempt to test hypotheses that are suggested by clinical studies in humans. However, the more complex the model (i.e. the

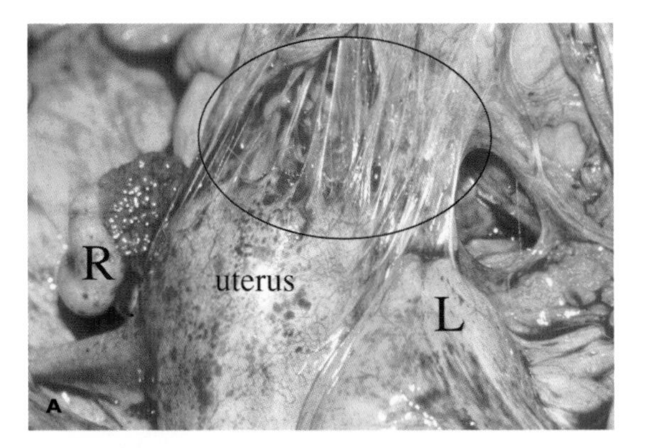

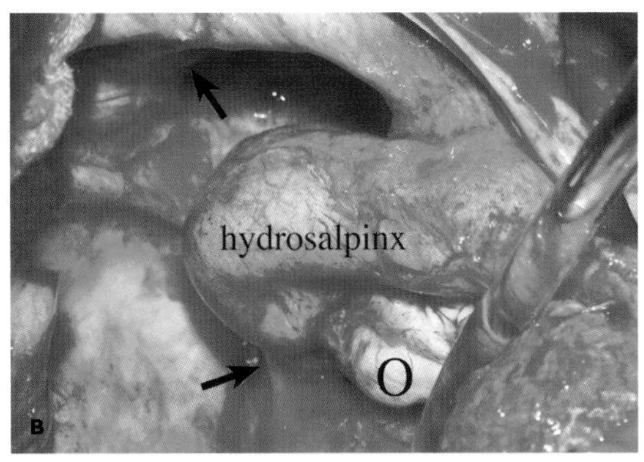

Figure 4.5 *Chlamydia trachomatis* pelvic inflammatory disease (PID). Laparatomy views: experimentally induced chlamydial PID in *Macaca nemestrina* and a clinical case of human disease. (A) In the monkey, extensive adhesion formation (ellipse) occurred between the fundus of the uterus (uterus) and the greater omentum. The left fallopian tube (L) is occluded, whereas the right tube (R) is both erythematous and edematous. (B) In the human, a large right hydrosalpinx (hydrosalpinx) is shown, tucked around the ovary (O). Numerous pelvic adhesions are present (arrows).

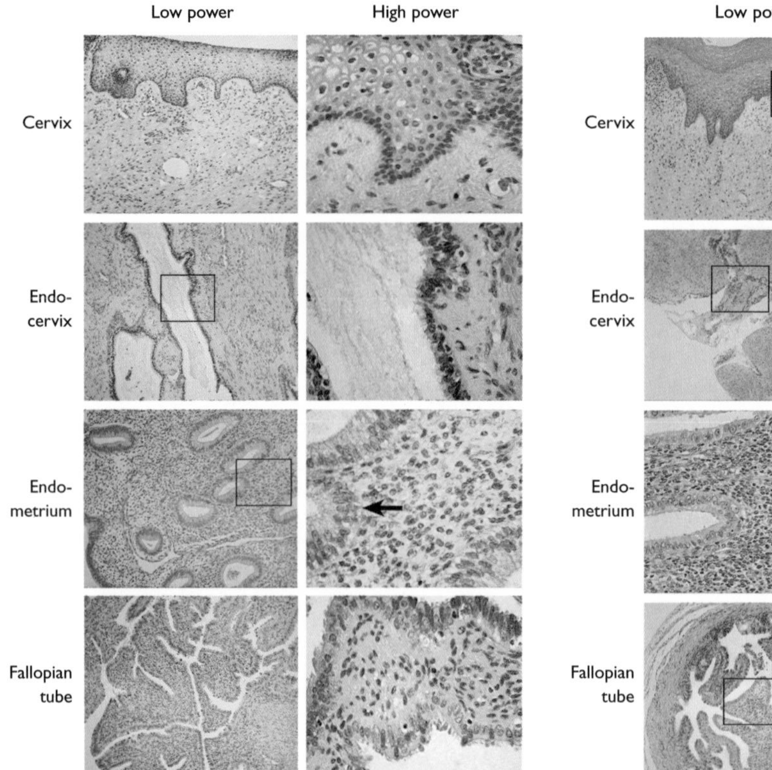

Figure 4.6 Normal histology of the reproductive tract from *Macaca nemestrina*. The cervical mucosa is composed of simple stratified squamous epithelium covering a cellular submucosa rich in capillaries. The endocervical canal has an irregular appearance of invagination of the epithelial lining, consisting of a simple columnar epithelium. Cervical mucus is present in the endocervical canal. The endometrium (proliferative phase) is typical, with simple glands lined by pseudostratified columnar epithelium surrounded by a cellular stroma (high power, arrow). The fallopian tube contains delicate mucosal folds that fill the luminal space of the tube itself. Ciliated and secretory epithelial cells form the simple columnar epithelium of the mucosal fold. The center of the mucosal fold consists of loose connective tissue, the submucosa.

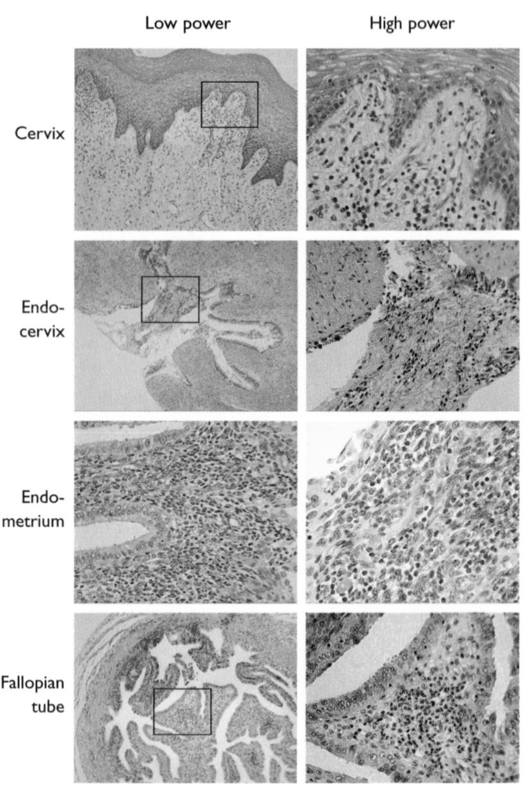

Figure 4.7 Acute pelvic inflammatory disease in *Macaca nemestrina*. By contrast to the normal histology, the cervical tissues contain a mixed inflammatory infiltrate of PMNs and lymphocytes in the submucosa (low and high power). Areas of the epithelial lining of the endocervix have been sloughed (low and high power) and the cervical mucus contains large numbers of PMNs (high power). The endometrium, as well, shows a moderate infiltration of PMNs and lymphocytes within the stroma (low and high power). The mucosal folds of the fallopian tube are characterized by an extravasation of red blood cells into the tissues (low power) and an increased presence of PMNs in the mucosa and submucosal tissues (high power).

closer to the human subject), the more ethical, financial, and practical constraints pertain. Additionally, mammalian model systems require strictly regulated housing, nutrition, and behavioral conditions, none more so than the non-human primate.

Because numerous species of animals act as natural host to chlamydial infections, various animal models have been used to study the course of chlamydial disease in humans. Cats, rabbits, guinea pigs, rats, grivet monkeys, and non-human primates have been used in earlier studies of chlamydial genital infection.[23–27] Current models range from macaques, in which the course of chlamydial disease and its sequelae most closely mimic human disease (Figures 4.5a, 4.7, 4.8), to mice, which act as important and relatively easily manipulated models of immunologic factors.

As early as the mid-1960s, the organism causing guinea pig inclusion conjunctivitis (GPIC) was found to be related to the organisms causing psittacosis, lymphogranuloma, and trachoma in

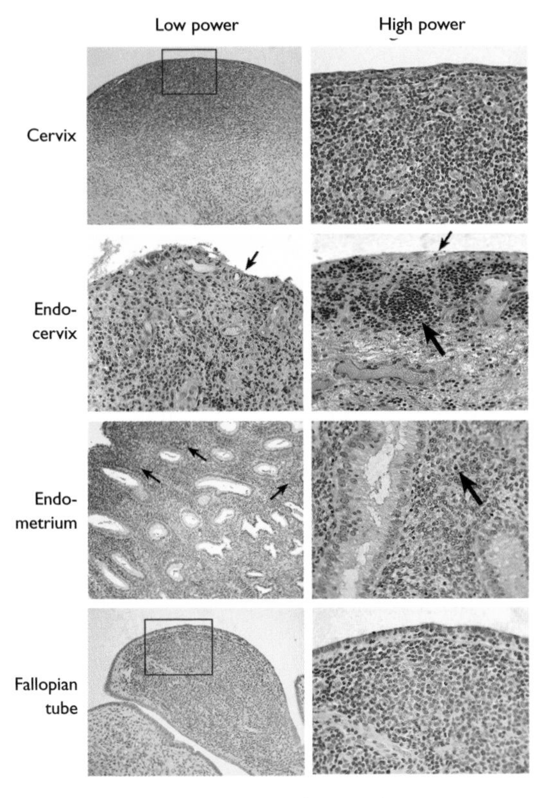

Figure 4.8 Chronic pelvic inflammatory disease in the *Macaca nemestrina*. The submucosa of the cervix is engorged with an extensive lymphocytic infiltrate (low and high power). Thinning of the epithelium is common (low and high power). Large numbers of plasma cells accompany the lymphocytic response (high power). The endocervical epithelium continues to show evidence of sloughing of the cells (low and high power, small arrows) and lymphocytes permeate the tissues (high power, large arrow). Plasma cells (high power, large arrow) and lymphocytes (low power, small arrows) are present within the endometrial stroma. The mucosal folds of the fallopian tube, like cervical tissue, are engorged with an extensive invasion of lymphocytes.

humans, and the guinea pig came to be utilized as an animal model of human chlamydial genital tract infection.[27] Vaginal inoculation of GPIC resulted in a self-limited cervicitis, characterized by a transient migration of PMNs into the endocervical epithelium by day 5 post-infection, followed by mononuclear (primarily lymphocytic) infiltration by day 10.[28] Infection of the upper genital tract could be produced following vaginal inoculation in a subset of animals, although immunosuppression with cyclophosphamide, estradiol pretreatment, or direct intrauterine inoculation increased the development of salpingitis. After immunosuppression, approximately 25% of animals developed histologic upper tract disease. Estradiol treatment for 2 weeks prior to and during infection with GPIC substantially increased inflammation and chlamydial shedding in the upper genital tract vs infected controls.[29] The guinea pig model demonstrated a bimodal inflammatory response to chlamydial infection, suggested that the local immune response reduced the chance of developing upper tract disease, and also suggested that endogenous hormones might play a role in developing upper tract disease.

Both the guinea pig model and the cat model utilize *Chlamydia psittaci*, a natural pathogen of each animal that causes conjunctivitis. In cats, direct fimbrial inoculation with *C. psittaci* using laparoscopy resulted in tubal scarring and/or adhesions by 6 weeks post-inoculation. Cytology samples revealed polymorphonuclear inflammation for up to 7 weeks; however, this model did not show the marked lymphocytic inflammation seen in human chlamydial salpingitis and PID.[24] Studies of the effects of endogenous hormones on chlamydial infection are not appropriate in cats, which are induced ovulators, and so do not experience regular cyclic hormonal effects.

Rabbits have been used as a model of chlamydial salpingitis, developing acute salpingitis characterized by a neutrophilic inflammatory response after direct inoculation with *C. trachomatis* D or F. Inflammatory changes were self-limited; however, a rechallenge inoculation did result in recrudescence of inflammation.[26] Like cats, rabbits are induced ovulators and experience prolonged periods of estrogen dominance.

Mouse studies originally used a strain of chlamydia known to induce pneumonitis in that host (MoPn, current taxonomy *Chlamydia muridarum*). Ascending chlamydial infection could be induced in this model by intravaginal inoculation with MoPn, which resulted in cervicitis of 2–3 weeks' duration.[30–31] Later studies utilized either MoPn or *C. trachomatis* human biovars. Possibly due to the rapid (4–5 day) murine estrus cycle, infection was dependent upon either progesterone pretreatment or cycle stage at inoculation.[32,33] Mice developed both neutrophilic and lymphocytic salpingeal inflammation, consisting of both plasma cell (B) and T lymphocytes.[34] Although this study indicated that mice would be a relevant model for the human histologic response to *C. trachomatis*, dependence upon exogenous hormone stimulation for development of upper tract disease suggested that conclusions drawn from this model might be limited. However, the great strength of the mouse model lies in the relative ease of genetic manipulation of the model, which can thus be utilized to test hypotheses regarding pathogenesis.

Non-human primates, in contrast to other models, can be infected genitally with human strains of *C. trachomatis*, and develop PID without hormonal manipulation (Figures 4.5a, 4.7, 4.8).

In early experimental work using a small number of grivet monkeys, cervical or uterine inoculation with *C. trachomatis* type K resulted in lymphocytic salpingitis, tubal adhesions, and persistent tubal occlusion. In this study, multiple laparotomies and tubal biopsies were conducted in each subject, a technique that might be expected to induce some inflammatory changes, but detailed control animal data were not reported. Although current animal-use protocols would be unlikely to allow this experimental design, the study answered, and raised, worthwhile questions. Several animals were assigned to cervical or uterine chlamydial inoculation, while two were assigned to infection following tubal ligation and endometrial curettage. In theory, tubal ligation would prevent intraluminal spread of the organism, and curettage would promote vascular and/or lymphatic spread. By day 14 post-inoculation, these two animals had elevated white blood cell counts and prolonged erythrocyte sedimentation rates; both were positive for *C. trachomatis* by culture. One of the two ligation/curettage subjects died and was found on postmortem to have severe perihepatitis, splenic distention and inflammation, subserosal salpingeal inflammation, and vascular inflammatory cell cuffing. The other animal showed mild salpingeal subserosal inflammation that resolved by 14 days post-inoculation. In contrast, no salpingeal intraluminal inflammation was seen in cervically or transcervically infected animals. Although the experiment was supportive of the conclusion that chlamydial salpingitis occurs via epithelial spread from cervical exposure, it suggested that marked serosal and peritoneal changes, such as are seen in PID in women, may occur by a different mechanism. The small number of animals used precluded an adequate control of the curettage portion of the experiment.[35]

Marmosets were studied as a model for ascending chlamydial infection; whereas intravaginal inoculation resulted in cervicitis, only one of five animals showed upper tract inflammation at necropsy.[36]

Pigtailed macaques were first used in the early 1980s as a model for chlamydial genital disease. The advantages of this primate model include the animal's size, relatively quiet temperament, and well-characterized menstrual cycle. Additionally, cyclic changes in salpingeal ciliary and epithelial activity have been defined for this species.[25] The normal anatomy and histology of the macaque reproductive tract are depicted in Figures 4.1a and 4.6. Using this model, direct cervical inoculation with human serovars of *C. trachomatis* caused cervicitis and chlamydial cervical shedding for a mean of 9 weeks. Cervical immunity apparently occurs, because if rechallenged once culture-negative, most animals were resistant to reinfection. However, weekly repeated cervical inoculations resulted in upper tract disease.[37]

Direct intratubal inoculation with *C. trachomatis* serovar E or F resulted in both cervicitis and salpingitis, and invoked both a humoral and a cellular immune response. In this study, predominantly B and T lymphocytes invaded salpingeal tissues by days 7–14. Extensive deciliation and rupture of secretory cells accompanied increasing submucosal inflammation by day 14. Although inflammation decreased by days 21–35, deciliation and mucosal cellular disruption persisted. Interestingly, a neutrophilic early response to direct intratubal infection was not detected in this study.[25] Repeated salpingeal inoculations using this model caused more extensive PID, with peritubal adhesions in 3 of 3 experimental monkeys Figure 4.5a, but not in the sham-inoculated control.[38]

Using repeated cervical inoculations caused salpingitis and peritubal adhesions, although following repeated cervical inoculations with a direct intratubal challenge increased the incidence of severe upper tract disease.[39]

In order to further define the salpingeal response to chlamydial infection over time, an autotransplant ("pocket") model was derived.[40–42] Using this model, in which up to 20 fimbrial autotransplants can be established in the subcutis of the abdomen, both local sIgA responses (in the fluid surrounding the transplanted tissue) and circulating antibody to the infecting strain can be detected. Serum IgM was detectable by day 7, then tended to decrease by day 14, whereas IgG persisted up to 42 days.[40] By day 2 post-inoculation, a neutrophilic response was seen in tubal autograft tissues, followed on days 3–7 by an increasing mononuclear cell inflammatory response, including plasma cells. This response was reduced by days 21–28.

Repeating the *C. trachomatis* inoculation in previously inoculated pockets resulted in a robust, primarily mononuclear response by days 2 and 3. Lymphoid follicles, consisting primarily of plasma cells with a T-lymphocyte cap, were seen in the submucosa. Mononuclear cell infiltration was reduced by day 10, but epithelial disruption persisted in infected tissues.[42] This increased pathologic response to repeated infection, seen in both the in-situ and the autograft models, suggested that the salpingeal response to chlamydial infection might be a delayed-type hypersensitivity (DTH) response to repeated presentation of certain chlamydial antigens.

Following reports that, as in women, macaques with PID had intense and long-lasting immune responses to chlamydial 60 kDa heat shock protein (Hsp 60),[43] and that the corneal scarring seen in experimental trachoma could be induced by chlamydial Hsp 60, chlamydial Hsp 60 was used in the autograft model and found to be capable of inducing severe lymphoid follicle formation in pocket tissues. Animals were exposed to *C. trachomatis* by direct inoculation into two-thirds of the pockets; one-third of the pockets were inoculated with a control vehicle. Infected pockets had a self-limiting inflammatory response, as previously seen using this model. Repeat inoculation of both infected and uninfected pockets at day 21, using only purified chlamydial Hsp 60, caused a strong mononuclear response within 48 hours. In contrast, only slight inflammation occurred in infected pockets that were challenged with vehicle control. Thus, in this model, the systemic immune system controlled the response to a specific antigen eliciting a localized DTH response.[44] Experimentally, chlamydial Hsp 60 appears to be a more effective inducer of the DTH response than other chlamydial antigens.[45]

As in women, some genetic predisposition towards severity of upper tract disease exists in macaques. In macaques, expression of major histocompatibility complex (MHC) Class I alleles has been found to be correlated with the severity of experimental chlamydial PID. MHC Class II alleles were not available for macaque evaluation at the time of the study. In women, MHC Class II-associated susceptibility to upper tract disease has been supported in clinical studies.[19,46]

The predominant lymphocytic response in chlamydia-infected macaque salpingeal tissues using the autograft model was activated $CD8^+$ lymphocytes, although both $CD4^+$ and B cells were also recruited. The $CD4^+$ response was characterized by Th1-type cytokines.[47] Similar responses were obtained using the in-situ model, although in this study $CD8^+$ cell activation could not be assessed due to high background levels of perforin in control, uninfected tubal tissues.[48]

RESPONSE TO TREATMENT

Meta-analysis of studies in women suggests that the best intervention to prevent PID is to screen for early chlamydial infection, in the hope of providing early antibiotic therapy.[49] In women treated with doxycycline and metronidazole, the main predictor of fecundity following treatment was the severity of salpingitis at the time of treatment.[50]

Treatment of mice with doxycycline prevented infertility associated with the MoPn biovar of chlamydia, as long as treatment was begun within a week of infection.[51] Roxithromycin treatment was also effective in *C. trachomatis*-infected mice, but protection was associated with higher (100 vs 50 mg/kg) doses given earlier in infection (7 vs 10 days).[52] Azithromycin was not effective in preventing upper tract disease in a mouse model unless administered at the time of chlamydial inoculation.[53]

In macaques, doxycycline alone was curative, but adding nonsteroidal anti-inflammatory treatment increased the likelihood of persistent chlamydial antigen detection in a macaque model of chlamydial PID.[54] Experimental quinolone treatment effectively killed chlamydia in the macaque model, although chlamydial antigens and DNA persisted in both treated and untreated monkeys for up to 1 month following quinolone or control treatment.[55] Recent studies reveal that, in contrast to murine models, the macaque model responded well to azithromycin administered after chlamydial infection was established by repeated weekly cervical inoculations. Azithromycin treatment of both uncomplicated chlamydial cervicitis (14 mg/kg single dose) and chlamydial PID (14 mg/kg/day for 1 week) resulted in clearance of chlamydial antigens, and significantly reduced the inflammatory response in the macaque model when compared with untreated or doxycycline-treated controls.[56,57]

CONCLUSION

Chlamydial PID apparently arises from a complex host response to a sophisticated pathogen. *C. trachomatis* appears to be capable of modulating the local and systemic immune response to the eventual detriment of the host. The use of animal models has led to a better understanding of the immunopathology of the organism, and most recently to cogent evidence for changing recommendations for treatment of clinical PID.

ACKNOWLEDGMENTS

Non-human primate research was supported in part by NIH Grants AI 40307 and AI 022082 of the National Institute of Allergy and Infectious Diseases and RR00166 of the Washington National Primate Research Center.

REFERENCES

1. Centers for Disease Control and Prevention. Sexually transmitted diseases treatment guidelines 2002. MMWR Morb Mortal Wkly Rep 2002;51:1–77.
2. Beigi RH, Wiesenfeld HC. Pelvic inflammatory disease: new diagnostic criteria and treatment. Obstet Gynecol Clin North Am 2003;30:777–93.
3. Rein DB, Kassler WJ, Irwin KL, et al. Direct medical cost of pelvic inflammatory disease and its sequelae: decreasing but still substantial. Obstet Gynecol 2000;95:397–402.
4. Miller WC, Ford CA, Morris M, et al. Prevalence of chlamydial and gonococcal infections among young adults in the United States. JAMA 2004;291(18):2229–36.
5. Gaydos CA, Howell MR, Quinn TC, et al. Sustained high prevalence of *Chlamydia trachomatis* infections in female army recruits. Sex Transm Dis 2003;30(7):539–44.
6. Xu F, Schillinger JA, Markowitz LE, et al. Repeat *Chlamydia trachomatis* infection in women: analysis through a surveillance case registry in Washington State, 1993–1998. Am J Epidemiol 2000;152(12):1164–70.
7. Ross JD. An update on pelvic inflammatory disease. Sex Transm Infect 2002;78:18–19.
8. Bevan CD, Johal BJ, Mumtaz G, et al. Clinical, laparoscopic and microbiological findings in acute salpingitis: report on a United Kingdom cohort. Br J Obstet Gynaecol 1995;102(5):407–14.
9. Eckert LO, Hawes SE, Wolner-Hanssen PK, et al. Endometritis: the clinical–pathologic syndrome. Am J Obstet Gynecol 2002;186(4):690–5.
10. Eschenbach D. Fitz-Hugh–Curtis syndrome. In: Holmes KK, Mardh P-A, Sparling PF, Weisner PJ, eds. Sexually Transmitted Diseases. New York: McGraw-Hill, 1984: 633–8.
11. Patton DL, Moore DE, Spadoni LR, et al. A comparison of the fallopian tube's response to overt and silent salpingitis. Obstet Gynecol 1989;73:622–30.
12. Patton DL. Microbiology and pathology of pelvic inflammatory disease. In: Berger GS, Weström LV, eds. Pelvic Inflammatory Disease. New York: Raven Press, 1992.
13. Yudin MH, Hillier SL, Wiesenfeld HC, et al. Vaginal polymorphonuclear leukocytes and bacterial vaginosis as markers for histologic endometritis among women without symptoms of pelvic inflammatory disease. Am J Obstet Gynecol 2003;188:318–23.
14. Paavonen J, Teisala K, Heinonen PK, et al. Microbiological and histopathological findings in acute pelvic inflammatory disease. Br J Obstet Gynaecol 1987;94(5):454–60.
15. Lehtinen M, Rantala I, Aine R, et al. B cell response in *Chlamydia trachomatis* endometritis. Eur J Clin Microbiol 1986;5:596–8.
16. Kinnunen A, Molander P, Laurila A, et al. *Chlamydia trachomatis* reactive T lymphocytes from upper genital tract tissue specimens. Hum Reprod 2000;15(7):1484–9.
17. Kimani J, Maclean IW, Bwayo JJ, et al. Risk factors for *Chlamydia trachomatis* pelvic inflammatory disease among sex workers in Nairobi, Kenya. J Infect Dis 1996;173:1437–44.
18. Gaur LK, Peeling RW, Cheang M, et al. Association of *Chlamydia trachomatis* heat-shock protein 60 antibody and HLA class II DQ alleles. J Infect Dis 1999:180:234–7.
19. Cohen CR, Sinei SS, Bukusi EA, et al. Human leukocyte antigen class II DQ alleles associated with *Chlamydia trachomatis* tubal infertility. Obstet Gynecol 2000;95:72–7.
20. Patton DL, Askienazy-Elbhar M, Henry-Suchet J, et al. Detection of *Chlamydia trachomatis* in fallopian tube tissue in women with postinfectious tubal infertility. Am J Obstet Gynecol 1994;171:95–101.
21. Beatty WL, Morrison RP, Byrne GI. Persistent chlamydiae: from cell culture to a paradigm for chlamydial pathogenesis. Microbiol Rev 1994;58:686–99.
22. Peeling RW, Kimani J, Plummer F, et al. Antibody to chlamydial HSP60 predicts an increased risk of pelvic inflammatory disease. J Infect Dis 1997;175:1153–8.

23. Moller BR, Mardh PA. Animal models for the study of chlamydial infections of the urogenital tract. Scand J Infect Dis Suppl 1982;32:103–8.
24. Kane JL, Woodland RM, Elder MG, et al. Chlamydial pelvic infection in cats: a model for the study of human pelvic inflammatory disease. Genitourin Med 1985;61(5):311–18.
25. Patton DL, Halbert SA, Kuo C-C, et al. Host response to primary *Chlamydia trachomatis* infection of the fallopian tube in pig-tailed monkeys. Fertil Steril 1983;40:829–40.
26. Patton DL, Halbert SA, Wang SP. Experimental salpingitis in rabbits provoked by *Chlamydia trachomatis*. Fertil Steril 1982;37(5):691–700.
27. Howard LV, O'Leary MP, Nichols RL. Animal model studies of genital chlamydial infections. Immunity to re-infection with guinea-pig inclusion conjunctivitis agent in the urethra and eye of male guinea-pigs. Br J Vener Dis 1976;52(4):261–5.
28. Barron AL, White HJ, Rank RG, et al. Target tissues associated with genital infection of female guinea pigs by the chlamydial agent of guinea pig inclusion conjunctivitis. J Infect Dis 1979;139:60–68.
29. White HJ, Rank RG, Soloff BL, Barron AL. Experimental chlamydial salpingitis in immunosuppressed guinea pigs infected in the genital tract with the agent of guinea pig inclusion conjunctivitis. Infect Immun 1979;26:729–35.
30. Barron AL, White HJ, Rank RG, et al. A new animal model for the study of *Chlamydia trachomatis* genital infections: infection of mice with the agent of mouse pneumonitis. J Infect Dis 1979;26:573–9.
31. Barron AL, Rank RG, Moses EB. Immune response in mice infected in the genital tract with mouse pneumonitis agent (*Chlamydia trachomatis* biovar). Infect Immun 1984;44:82–5.
32. Tuffrey M, Falder P, Taylor-Robinson D. Genital tract infection and disease in nude and immunologically competent mice after inoculation of a human strain of *Chlamydia trachomatis*. Br J Exp Pathol 1982;63:539–46.
33. Tuffrey M, Falder P, Gale J, et al. Salpingitis in mice induced by human strains of *Chlamydia trachomatis*. Br J Exp Pathol 1986;67:605–16.
34. Patton DL, Landers DV, Schachter J. Experimental *Chlamydia trachomatis* salpingitis in mice: initial studies on the characterization of the leukocyte response to chlamydial infection. J Infect Dis 1989;159(6):1105–10.
35. Møller BR, Mårdh P-A. Experimental salpingitis in grivet monkeys by *Chlamydia trachomatis*. Acta Path Microbiol Scand B 1980;88:107–14.
36. Johnson AP, Hare MJ, Wilbanks GD, et al. A colposcopic and histological study of experimental chlamydial cervicitis in marmosets. Br J Exp Pathol 1984;65(1):59–65.
37. Patton DL. Immune responses to *C. trachomatis* infections in a non-human primate model. Infect Dis Obstet Gynecol 1996;4:159–62.
38. Patton DL, Kuo CC, Wang SP, Halbert SA. Distal tubal obstruction induced by repeated *Chlamydia trachomatis* salpingeal infections in pig-tailed macaques. J Infect Dis 1987;155:1292–9.
39. Patton DL, Wølner-Hanssen P, Cosgrove SJ, et al. The effects of *Chlamydia trachomatis* on the female reproductive tract of the *Macaca nemestrina* after a single tubal challenge following repeated cervical inoculations. Obstet Gynecol 1990;76:643–50.
40. Patton DL, Kuo CC, Wang SP, et al. Chlamydial infection of subcutaneous fimbrial transplants in cynomolgus and rhesus monkeys. J Infect Dis 1987;155:229–35.
41. Patton DL, Kuo CC, Brenner RM. Chlamydia trachomatis oculogenital infection in the subcutaneous autotransplant model of conjunctiva, salpinx and endometrium. Br J Exp Pathol 1989;70:357–67.
42. Patton DL, Kuo CC. Histopathology of *Chlamydia trachomatis* salpingitis after primary and repeated reinfections in the monkey subcutaneous pocket model. J Reprod Fertil 1989;85:647–56.
43. Peeling RW, Patton DL, Cosgrove Sweeney YT, et al. Antibody response to the chlamydial heat-shock protein 60 in an experimental model of chronic pelvic inflammatory disease in monkeys (*Macaca nemestrina*). J Infect Dis 1999;180:774–9.
44. Patton DL, Sweeney YT, Kuo CC. Demonstration of delayed hypersensitivity in *Chlamydia trachomatis* salpingitis in monkeys: a pathogenic mechanism of tubal damage. J Infect Dis 1994;169:680–3.
45. Lichtenwalner AB, Patton DL, Van Voorhis WC, et al. Heat shock protein 60 is the major antigen which stimulates delayed-type hupersensitivity reaction in the macaque model of *Chlamydia trachomatis* salpingitis. Infect Immun 2004;72:1159–61.
46. Lichtenwalner AB, Patton DL, Cosgrove Sweeney YT, et al. Evidence of genetic susceptibility to *Chlamydia trachomatis-induced* pelvic inflammatory disease in the pig-tailed macaque. Infect Immun 1997;65:2250–3.
47. Van Voorhis WC, Barrett LK, Sweeney YT, et al. Analysis of lymphocyte phenotype and cytokine activity in the inflammatory infiltrates of the upper genital tract of female macaques infected with *Chlamydia trachomatis*. J Infect Dis 1996;174(3):647–50.
48. Van Voorhis WC, Barrett LK, Sweeney YT, et al. Repeated *Chlamydia trachomatis* infection of *Macaca nemestrina* fallopian tubes produces a Th1-like cytokine response associated with fibrosis and scarring. Infect Immun 1997;65:2175–82.
49. Honey E, Templeton A. Prevention of pelvic inflammatory disease by the control of *C. trachomatis* infection. Int J Gynecol Obstet 2002;78:257–61.
50. Heinonen PK, Leinonen M. Fecundity and morbidity following acute pelvic inflammatory disease treated with doxycycline and metronidazole. Arch Gynecol Obstet 2003; 268(4):284–8.
51. Swenson CE, Sung ML, Schachter J. The effect of tetracycline treatment on chlamydial salpingitis and subsequent fertility in the mouse. Sex Transm Dis 1986;13(1):40–4.
52. Zana J, Muffat-Joly M, Thomas D, et al. Roxithromycin treatment of mouse chlamydial salpingitis and protective effect on fertility. Antimicrob Agents Chemother 1991;35(3):430–5.
53. Tuffrey M, Woods C, Taylor-Robinson D. The effect of a single oral dose of azithromycin on chlamydial salpingitis in mice. J Antimicrob Chemother 1991;28(5):741–6.
54. Patton DL, Sweeney YC, Bohannon NJ, et al. Effects of doxycycline and antiinflammatory agents on experimentally induced chlamydial upper genital tract infection in female macaques. J Infect Dis 1997;175(3):648–54.
55. Patton DL, Cosgrove YT, Kuo CC, et al. Effects of quinolone analog CI-960 in a monkey model of *Chlamydia trachomatis* salpingitis. Antimicrob Agents Chemother 1993;37(1):8–13.
56. Patton DL, Cosgrove Sweeney YT, Stamm WE. Azithromycin vs doxycycline vs placebo for resolution of chlamydial infection and associated inflammation in the pig-tailed macaque model. In: Schachter J, Christiansen G, Clarke IN, et al, eds. Chlamydial Infections. Antalya: Basin Yeri, 2002: 365–8.
57. Patton DL, Sweeney YT, Stamm WE. Significant reduction in inflammatory response in the macaque model of chlamydial pelvic inflammatory disease with azithromycin. J. Infect Dis 2005;192:129–35.

5. Sequelae

Andrea Ries Thurman and David E. Soper

BACKGROUND

Each year in the United States, more than 1 million women experience an episode of pelvic inflammatory disease (PID).[1] Silent salpingitis is under-diagnosed, under-reported, and under-treated. In general, after one episode of PID, one in four women will develop potentially irreversible or life-threatening complications, such as infertility, ectopic pregnancy, and chronic pelvic pain (CPP).[2] After recurrent episodes of salpingitis, almost one in two women will develop serious sequelae.[2] Direct medical expenditures for treatment of acute PID and sequelae within 1 year of diagnosis in the United States were 2 billion dollars.[3] This amount actually represents a decrease in projections from the 1990s, with savings from increased availability of directly observed, single-dose treatment of sexually transmitted infections (STIs), improved screening techniques, and education regarding prevention strategies.[3,4] When economic projections extend to 5 years after diagnosis, the average per-person lifetime cost of PID ranges from $1060 to $3180, making screening and prevention strategies cost-effective.[5] These economic data do not encompass the emotional toll, loss of productivity, and quality of life problems that women experience when facing infertility, ectopic pregnancy, or CPP.

When considering the following data regarding the sequelae of PID, it is important to note whether the patient population was diagnosed clinically or surgically. In older studies, ultrasound and microbiologic testing was not as advanced; therefore, laparoscopy was used to confirm the diagnosis. Now, less-invasive, and therefore less-accurate, clinical diagnostic criteria are used.

In a review of the signs and symptoms of PID, Eschenbach et al concluded that clinical and laboratory criteria used traditionally to judge the clinical severity of acute PID only partially predict the degree of tubal or other pelvic damage on laparoscopy and are not reliable in assessing an individual patient's future risk of adverse sequelae.[6] In women whose fallopian tubes are damaged by a previous infection, endogenous organisms from the vagina can cause a primary infection or reactivation of a latent tubal infection.[7] This statement is supported by observations that repeated episodes of PID tend to be less often STI-associated.[7] After an initial infection of the upper genital tract (UGT), tubal damage can occur, causing subsequent absolute infertility, relative infertility leading to ectopic pregnancy, and/or CPP.[8]

INFERTILITY

Several studies have examined infertility after PID. Common themes suggest that the severity of PID, recurrent infections, and delay in care exceeding 3 days are poor prognostic factors for future fertility. Antichlamydial antibodies are common among women with tubal factor infertility (TFI), with and without a history of PID, suggesting a role of "silent salpingitis". Finally, modern treatment studies have shown that PID causes comparable adverse fertility outcomes, whether treatment is rendered in the outpatient or inpatient setting.

LUND, SWEDEN COHORT

The world's largest and longest prospective cohort study of women with acute PID was conducted in Lund, Sweden, over a 24-year period.[9–15] In 1974, Westrom followed 415 women with surgically verified PID for 9.5 years.[9] After the index PID episode, 21.2% of patients were infertile compared with 3% of control patients, who had normal pelvic anatomy verified at laparoscopy.[9] Tubal obstruction was the cause of infertility in 82% of the infertile couples. Reinfection was the factor most predictive of subsequent TFI: 12.8% after one PID episode, 35.5% after two PID episodes, and 75% of patients had occluded tubes after three or more episodes of PID.[9] Infertility rates were also correlated with the severity of the index PID case, with rates of 2.6%, 13.1%, and 28.6% with mild, moderate, and severe PID, respectively. Westrom evaluated a subset of women with only one PID episode, based on the causative agent. In 6/99 (6%) of women who had *Neisseria gonorrhoeae* (GC) PID and 26/150 (17%) who had non-GC PID, the tubes were occluded, although the severity of tubal changes in this cohort did not differ significantly with the causative organism. From this, they concluded that fertility is more preserved after GC PID as opposed to *Chlamydia trachomatis* (CT)-associated PID. This is probably because GC-associated PID has overt symptoms and is therefore detected and treated earlier than the silent salpingitis of CT-associated PID. However, these findings must be interpreted with caution, as the antibiotic regimens used during this study, which mainly targeted GC, were different from those used today.

In an interim report on 1204 salpingitis patients from the Lund, Sweden cohort, Westrom reemphasized that the most important factor in post-PID TFI was the number of PID infections, with each new PID episode approximately doubling the rate of TFI.[13] At this point in the study, CT was not recognized as a major contributor to PID.[13]

Once CT was recognized as a major contributor to PID, Svensson et al reported a subset of the Lund, Sweden cohort ($n = 299$), with special reference to CT- vs GC-associated PID.[14] They found that after one episode of laparoscopically verified PID, patients with an index diagnosis of CT, GC, both, or neither in the cervix had similarly poor fertility prognoses. Of patients with PID, 23% were infertile. Rather than the etiology of PID, post-PID infertility was again correlated with reinfection rates, erythrocyte sedimentation rate (ESR) at admission, and the severity of the inflammatory reactions of the tubes.[14]

Due to the poor fertility outcomes in the 1983 subset described by Svensson et al,[14] different inpatient antibiotic regimens were attempted, which provided more potent coverage of CT, in hopes of improving fertility outcomes in these patients.[15] In this subset of the Lund, Sweden cohort, 608 women with a first case of laparoscopically verified PID were divided into 4 treatment groups, one of which consisted of doxycycline. They hypothesized that patients receiving doxycycline would have improved outcomes. However, after 17 years of follow-up, no differences were found in fertility between the different antibiotic regimens after controlling for the age of the women, etiology of PID, and severity of PID.

The most recent findings regarding fertility prognosis of the Lund, Sweden cohort were reported between 1991 and 1997 by Westrom and coworkers.[10–12] Beginning in 1960, patients suspected of having acute PID ($n = 2501$) underwent laparoscopy: 1844 patients had abnormal pelvic findings and 657 patients who had a normal pelvis were used as controls.[11,12] A subset of 1309 patients with PID and 451 controls, who attempted to conceive, were available for follow-up and are summarized in Table 5.I.

Of the 1309 infertile patients, 47 had incomplete fertility evaluations and 21 had reasons for infertility other than TFI, leaving a subset of 1241 patients with PID for further evaluation. This group's fertility prognosis, based on age, number of PID episodes, and severity of the index case is illustrated in Table 5.2.

Table 5.1 Lund, Sweden cohort fertility prognosis

Category	PID patients *n/N* (%)	Control patients *n/N* (%)
Attempting pregnancy	1309	451
Pregnant	1100/1309 (84.0)	439/451 (96.1)
First pregnancy ectopic	100/1100 (9.1)	6/439 (1.4)
Not pregnant	209/1309 (16.0)	12/451 (2.7)
Infertility evaluation	162	3
Proven TFI	141/162 (87.0)	0/3 (0.0)
Other cause	21/162 (13.0)	3/3 (100.0)
Incomplete infertility evaluation	47	9

Table 5.2 Lund, Sweden Cohort fertility prognosis based on age and disease

Number of PID episodes	< 25 years old		> 25 years old		Total	
	Percent	n/N	Percent	n/N	Percent	n/N
One	7.7	59/771	9.1	20/220	8.0	79/991
Mild	0.8	2/241	0.0	0/71	0.6	2/312
Moderate	6.4	23/361	5.6	5/89	6.2	28/452
Severe	20.1	34/169	25.0	15/60	21.4	49/229
Two	18.4	29/158	25.9	7/27	19.5	36/185
Three or more	37.7	23/61	75.0	3/4	40.0	26/65
Total	11.2	111/990	12.0	30/251	11.4	141/1241

In a subset analysis of the recent Lund, Sweden data, Lepine and coworkers found that women with an index case of severe PID disease and recurrent PID were eight times more likely to fail to conceive compared with women with a single episode of mild PID.[10] In addition, women with severe index disease and no recurrences were 1.7 times more likely to be infertile than women with a single episode of mild PID and no subsequent PID.[10] The occurrence of subsequent PID in women with mild index PID did not diminish their long-term probability of live birth, whereas it significantly lowered the probability of live birth in women with severe PID during the index case.[10]

Initially, Westrom reported that age at the time of the index PID case was correlated with impaired future fertility, occurring in 26% of those over 25 years old and 14% of patients younger than age 25.[12] However, when examining the reasons for impaired fertility, there was no difference in the proportions of women with TFI (7.7% vs 9.1%).[12] This suggests that impaired fertility in older patients with PID is also related to decreased fecundity of age. Also, after more than one infection, no age difference in the infertility rates was observed, which suggests that longer duration of risky behavior will predispose to recurrent infections, and increasing levels of tubal damage, regardless of age.[2]

Delay in seeking care for PID was also found to be an important prognostic factor for future infertility.[16] Hillis and coworkers found that women who delay seeking care for PID were three times more likely to experience infertility or ectopic pregnancy than women who sought care promptly, after adjustment for age, organism, year of diagnosis, type of contraception, and history of recent gynecologic events.[16] Delay in care was defined as seeking care after 3 or more days of symptoms. Approximately 20% of those who delayed care suffered later infertility or ectopic pregnancy, compared with 8.3% of those who sought care within 3 days. The longer a patient delayed care (linear trend analysis), the higher the chance of adverse sequelae.[16] When the analysis was stratified according to organism, a positive association was found between delayed care and impaired fertility among women infected with CT, GC, or both. The effect of delay was strongest for women with chlamydia.

FERTILITY PROGNOSIS OF CHLAMYDIAL PELVIC INFLAMMATORY DISEASE

McCormack et al found that women with GC PID were more likely to become ill during the first 10 days of the menstrual cycle, presented to care sooner, had higher admission white blood cell (WBC) counts, and were more severely ill than patients with non-GC PID.[17] The diagnosis of PID was based on clinical criteria, and GC PID patients were more likely to be treated as inpatients compared with non-GC PID patients.[17] During an average of 17 months follow-up, 29% of women with GC PID were infertile vs 71% of women with non-GC PID.

Svensson et al compared women with laparoscopically confirmed PID caused by CT vs GC vs neither.[18] They found that women with GC PID were more acutely ill on presentation and sought medical attention earlier than other patients. Tubal damage at the time of laparoscopy was generally more severe than expected from the patient's clinical symptoms in the CT PID group.

"Silent salpingitis" is thought to be as destructive as clinically overt PID. Patton and coworkers compared the fallopian tubes of women with a history of overt PID vs those with distal tubal obstruction, and found similar antichlamydial antibody levels and tubal damage in both groups.[19] There was no difference in the American Fertility Society classification scores for pelvic adhesions between women with overt PID and those with silent PID.

ANTIBODY TESTING AND FERTILITY

As the diagnosis of PID becomes less invasive, laparoscopic verification of PID will be less common in patients presenting for fertility evaluation. In this case, antichlamydial antibodies can be used to make some conclusions regarding fertility. Antichlamydial antibodies are present in the serum of almost all CT-infected individuals shortly after acquisition of infection, and may persist for years, even following curative therapy.[20] Several studies have found that women with TFI have higher rates and higher titers of anticlamydial antibodies than controls.[21–23]

Brunham et al found that seropositivity with antichlamydial antibodies and TFI is independent of number of sexual partners.[24]

Moore and coworkers compared factors that predict tubal disease: abnormal hysterosalpingogram (HSG), CT antibody, history of PID, history of intrauterine device (IUD) use, and history of pregnancy, and found that CT antibody was most predictive.[25] CT serology predicted 72% of tubal disease, abnormal HSG 76%, and abnormal HSG + CT antibodies 84%. Based on this data, they concluded that the presence or absence of antibodies to CT was as discriminatory in the detection of TFI as HSG, and the serologic test should become a routine part of the infertility investigation.[25]

Authors have also been able to isolate CT antigen from the fallopian tubes of women with TFI, antichlamydial antibodies, and absence of active endocervical CT infection.[20,23,26] This suggests that women exposed to CT can possess a chronic, relapsing infection of the fallopian tubes.

MODERN FINDINGS OF PELVIC INFLAMMATORY DISEASE AND INFERTILITY

A more recent follow-up study of patients diagnosed with PID by laparoscopy was conducted by Bernstine and coworkers in 1987.[27] Like the Lund, Sweden cohort, they found that the incidence of infertility increased as the patient's PID progressed in severity. TFI was present in 21%, 45%, and 67% of women with mild, moderate, and severe PID, respectively. These numbers are much higher than that found by Jacobseon and Westrom, which may reflect new etiologies of PID, particularly CT.[9,11]

In the Swedish studies, tubal occlusion was diagnosed after PID with HSG; however, a more accurate diagnosis of post-PID tubal disease is provided by second-look laparoscopy. In 1996, Gerber and Krause reported on 158 women who underwent second-look laparoscopy, an average 10 weeks after surgically proven PID.[28] Similar to the 1974 Westrom study, second-look laparoscopy revealed bilateral tubal occlusion in 21.7% of patients.[1–9] Also, tubal damage was associated with the severity of the index PID case: 9.5% after mild PID, 20% after moderate PID, and 32% after severe PID. The rate of infertility during follow-up was 9.5% for patients with mild PID, 35% for patients with moderate PID, and 40% for patients with severe PID.[28]

The largest, most recent study to follow women diagnosed with PID in the United States is the PEACH study.[29] This study is comparable to the manner in which PID is often diagnosed today, i.e. clinically, and used recent antibiotic regimens. In contrast to the findings of Westrom and coworkers, who found that the severity of PID was an independent risk factor for TFI, Haggerty and coworkers, looking at a cohort of the PEACH study, found that endometritis and/or UGT infection with GC or CT, as diagnosed by endometrial biopsy, were not independent risk factors for subsequent infertility, reduced pregnancy rates, recurrent PID, or CPP.[30] Neither chronic nor acute endometritis was associated with infertility, recurrent PID, or CPP.

Their findings suggest that endometritis is not associated with reduced pregnancy rates in women with mild-to-moderate PID. These findings are not intuitive, as endometritis has been associated with salpingitis, and salpingitis has been strongly associated with these reproductive morbidities. However, this study supports the assumption that endometritis is not a precise marker for future tubal disease and morbidity. Endometritis is a spotty disease of the endometrium and endometrial pipelle may miss a focus of endometritis. Also, salpingitis may not be associated with endometritis in women with mild-to-moderate disease.

A small, recent study in 2003 in Finland may provide good prognostic information for fertility after PID.[31] Heinonen and Leinonen followed 39 women with a first episode of PID (20 with mild PID and 19 with severe PID); the grade and etiology were classified using laparoscopy, endometrial biopsy, and cervical and fallopian tube cultures for a mean of 125 months.[31] In addition, 51% of the women had laparotomy or second laparoscopy during the 125 months of follow-up. Of the women who attempted pregnancy, 11% were infertile after the index PID. The conception rate was not influenced by etiology or severity of the PID, although women with CT were more likely to have severe PID as compared with those without an STI. The weakness of the study is the small number of patients, but the treatment regimen of doxycycline and metronidazole is used for PID today, and may guide prognosis.

FERTILITY SUCCESS AFTER TUBAL REPAIR

Ries, in 1909, proposed a theory as to the mechanism of hydrosalpinx formation.[32] Ries differentiated fallopian tube damage into perimetric vs salpingitic.[32] In perimetric closure, the parametrium is inflamed and these inflammatory mediators encircle the tube, collapsing it, with the fimbriae pointed outward.[32] In salpingitic closure, the ostium is occluded by changes within the walls of the tube that cause them to swell; the fimbriae become little plicae, and the walls bulge and close in over the fimbriae, which point inward into the hydrosalpinx.[32]

Prior to in-vitro fertilization, attempts were made to repair damaged tubes, to improve fertility. The success of microsurgical repair of damaged tubes depends on the extent of tubal damage prior to repair.[33] One series reported that pregnancy rates after repair of mild, moderate, and severely damaged tubes were 80%, 31%, and 16% respectively.[33] Patton and coworkers found that women with distal tubal damage had reduced ciliary beat frequency throughout the endosalpinx.[19] Salpingitis caused not only deciliation but also persistent ciliary dyskinesia.[19] This inherent tubal dysfunction probably contributes to persistent infertility and ectopic pregnancy risk even after successful reestablishment of a patent tubal lumen.

PREVENTION OF PELVIC INFLAMMATORY DISEASE

In 1997, the incidence of CT in the United States was 207 cases per 100 000 people, a rate that exceeds all other reportable infectious diseases.[34] However, many women at risk for PID are unaware of their risk. It is important for healthcare providers to educate the public on prevention techniques.

The largest study in the United States to experimentally verify that routine screening for STIs is effective in preventing PID was carried out by Scholes and coworkers.[35] They identified women at risk for chlamydial infection and randomized them to routine chlamydia screening vs usual care.[35] In the screening group, 7% tested positive for chlamydia and were treated.[35] At the end of 1-year follow-up there were 9 verified cases of PID among women in the screening group and 33 cases among women receiving the usual care.[35] Screening for lower genital tract infection is probably one of the most important prevention strategies for UGT infection.[35]

ORAL CONTRACEPTIVE PILLS AND PREVENTION OF PELVIC INFLAMMATORY DISEASE

Using oral contraceptive pills (OCPs) was thought to decrease an ascending cervicitis. OCP users have decreased myometrial activity, which may decrease propulsion of microorganisms to the UGT.[36] By decreasing menstrual blood flow, OCPs may reduce ascending infection, as menstrual fluid provides a medium favorable for bacterial growth.[37,38] The progesterone component of OCPs may make the cervical mucus more impermeable to bacteria.[38,39] However, the hormonal effect of OCPs may be more complicated than providing a barrier to ascent of infection. Maslow et al found that adding estrogen to endometrial gland epithelial cells, in vitro, enhanced CT serovar E attachment.[40] However, adding progesterone in combination with estrogen reduced attachment in a dose-dependent fashion.[40] With scanning electron microscopy, Maslow and colleagues showed that the endometrial cavity and fallopian tube had marked degeneration of epithelial microvilli during the secretory phase of the menstrual cycle. CT is an obligate intracellular parasite and must attach to these villi to enter cells to initiate the infectious process. The protective effect of OCPs may also be related to bias. OCP users may be more familiar with the healthcare system.[38,40] Finally, contraception use and age are often collinear.

EVIDENCE SUPPORTING A PROTECTIVE EFFECT OF ORAL CONTRACEPTIVE PILLS

The first study to report that OCP use was less common in patients with laparoscopically diagnosed PID was done in 1976 by Westrom and colleagues.[39] They compared women with acute PID diagnosed by laparoscopy with controls matched for sexual activity, age, and socioeconomic status. Cases were significantly less likely to use OCPs than controls, but they did not comment on duration of use or dose of the OCPs.

In a follow-up study of the Lund, Sweden cohort, in 1984, Svensson et al found that OCP use diminished the grade of laparoscopically verified PID.[39] Age, which could reflect past history of PID, did not explain the differences observed.[39]

In 1986, Wolner-Hanssen described a subset of the Lund, Sweden cohort: 94 women with acute salpingitis at laparoscopy compared with 12 women with salpingitis and perihepatitis.[41] All patients were infected with chlamydia. None of the patients with perihepatitis, a marker of more severe PID, used OCPs.[41] Of the patients with acute salpingitis, 40% used OCPs.[41] The geometric mean titer of serum immunoglobulin G (IgG) antibody to CT was lower in OCP users than in OCP non-users.[41]

In the most recent summary of the Lund, Sweden PID cohort ($n = 1844$) in 1992, Westrom et al again confirmed that women who were using OCPs at the time of their index PID episode had a less severe infection than women using other methods of contraception.[11] Importantly, over a 24-year follow-up period, the relative risk of TFI was significantly lower in PID patients using OCPs at the time of diagnosis than users of other methods or no contraception.

Rubin and colleagues interviewed 648 women hospitalized with an initial episode of PID and 2516 hospitalized control subjects.[37] The relative risk of PID is summarized in Table 5.3.

This association was not explained by differences between case subjects and control subjects in age (over or under age 24), education, race, gravidity, number of sexual partners, gynecologic history, or medical history. Importantly, the protective effect of OCPs was restricted to women using OCPs for more than 12 months. Based on the data from this large multicenter case–control study, conducted in 1982, it was concluded that, annually, an estimated 50 000 initial cases of PID and 12 500 hospitalizations are prevented by OCP use.

In a review of 11 published studies on contra-

Table 5.3 Risk of pelvic inflammatory disease (PID) controlling for oral contraceptive pill (OCP) use

OCP use	Comparison group	Relative risk of PID (CI)
Ever used OCP	Never OCP	0.8 (0.6–1.0)
Past OCP	Never OCP	0.9 (0.7–1.1)
Current OCP	Never OCP	0.7 (0.5–0.9)
Current OCP	Current other contraception	0.5 (0.4–0.6)
Current long-term OCP use (13–24 months)	No contraception	0.3 (0.2–0.4)
Current short-term OCP use (1–12 months)	No contraception	1.1 (0.8–1.5)

ception and PID from 1980, Senanayake and Kramer reported on the relative risk of developing PID for OCP users or OCP users vs OCP non-users.[42] With one exception (where PID was defined very loosely), these studies show a relative risk of PID of 0.3–0.9 for OCP users compared with non-users of contraceptives.

ORAL CONTRACEPTIVE PILLS AND PREVENTION OF CHLAMYDIA-ASSOCIATED PELVIC INFLAMMATORY DISEASE

There is controversy over whether OCPs protect against both CT and GC PID. Of concern, in vitro, progesterone depresses the growth of GC, but estrogen may slightly increase the growth of this organism.[43] Women who use OCPs are at an increased risk for developing cervical infection with CT, compared with women with a comparable number of sexual partners who do not use OCPs. Of concern clinically is the possibility that OCP use may mask signs and symptoms of ascending infection, resulting in a greater proportion of untreated, silent PID.

In 1990, Wolner-Hanssen and coworkers compared 141 women with PID, verified by endometrial biopsy or laparoscopy, with 739 sexually active women with no clinical evidence of disease.[38] Case and control subjects were stratified on the basis of infection with CT, GC, or neither organism. Women with CT-associated PID were less likely to use OCPs than controls infected with CT. This association was significant when OCP use was compared with all other types of contraception and with non-use of contraception. Among cases and controls infected with GC, OCPs were not protective. Among women infected with both CT and GC, OCP use provided a mild, but not statistically significant, protective effect, compared with non-use of contraception. After adjusting for age, race, parity, years of formal education, current smoking, age at coitarche, frequency of intercourse, douching during the preceding 2 months, and history of CT, GC, and/or PID, OCP use remained negatively associated with PID compared with non-use of OCPs and with use of no method of birth control. It was concluded that OCP use protects against symptomatic PID among women infected with CT but not among those infected with GC.

EVIDENCE SUPPORTING A PROTECTIVE EFFECT OF ORAL CONTRACEPTIVE PILLS ON NEISSERIA GONORRHOEAE-ASSOCIATED PELVIC INFLAMMATORY DISEASE

Ryden et al studied 87 patients with GC-associated PID, confirmed by laparoscopy, and compared them with 174 women with uncomplicated GC cervicitis. OCP users had an 8.8% rate of PID compared with a 23.5% rate in IUD users and a 15.5% rate in non-users of contraception.[44] However, this study, conducted in Sweden in 1979, may not be comparable to OCP formulations and antibiotic regimens used today.

Eschenbach et al found that OCP use was protective against GC PID, but was not protective against nongonococcal PID.[45] They compared 204 patients with clinically diagnosed PID, 45% of whom had GC, with 707 sexually active women attending a contraception clinic, without gynaecologic complaints. PID patients were more likely to use IUDs and no contraception. Patients with GC-associated PID were less likely to use OCPs than patients with nongonococcal PID. Having a tubal ligation was protective against PID.

EVIDENCE REFUTING A PROTECTIVE EFFECT OF ORAL CONTRACEPTIVE PILLS

In 1985, Washington and coworkers cautioned physicians regarding the protective effect of OCPs on PID.[46] They noted that many of the articles that supported the protective effect of OCPs were limited to hospitalized women, who represent less than 25% of all PID cases and are likely to have relatively severe forms of the disease. Also, as CT began to be recognized as a major contributor to PID, the authors were concerned that many studies on OCPs and PID did not distinguish between gonococcal and nongonococcal PID. They were concerned that OCPs may protect against clinically apparent PID but not against the long-term damage after PID. Also, studies did not elaborate on the duration or dose of OCPs, and did not differentiate between recurrent and initial episodes of PID. They pointed out that women using OCPs have higher rates of CT cervicitis, and may have higher rates of silent PID, than GC-associated PID. The increased cervical ectropion exposed on the vaginal aspect of the cervix may lead to a greater chance that infection will be acquired after sexual contact with an infected partner due to a greater number of susceptible columnar cells.

Targum and Wright found no protective effect of OCP use, when comparing women with a first episode of PID with matched controls.[47] PID was diagnosed in this 1974 study by a fever of over 99.8°F (37.7°C), and two clinical symptoms. Of cases, 22% were using OCPs compared with 33% of controls ($p > 0.1$). The organism causing the PID was not determined.

In a follow-up of the PEACH study, the investigators compared OCP users with barrier contraception users for evidence of UGT infection, as diagnosed by endometrial biopsy cultures.[48] As expected, inconsistent condom use was significantly and independently associated with a 2.3 times elevated risk for UGT infection. OCPs did reduce clinical severity of PID, as OCP users had less tenderness on clinical examination. However, UGT infection was not significantly associated with use of OCPs, depot medroxyprogesterone, consistent condom use, or other barrier methods. It was concluded that no hormonal or barrier contraceptive method was related to a reduction in upper genital tract disease among women with clinically diagnosed PID. This study differs from conclusions of the Lund, Sweden cohort studies on the protective effect of OCPs.[11,39,41] However, in the Lund, Sweden cohort studies, PID was diagnosed by laparoscopy instead of clinically. Also, the Lund, Sweden cohort was collected between 1960 and 1984, when higher-dose OCP formulations were used, and there were different rates of GC- and CT-associated PID. The PEACH investigators suggest that the difference in their findings with older studies may be based on the different formulations of modern day OCPs. Another discrepancy may be explained by the fact that the PEACH investigators classified OCP use as use within 4 weeks of index PID episode. Recall that Rubin and associates found that only long-term OCP use, over 12 months, was protective against PID.[37] Based on this data, the PEACH investigators posed the question of whether OCP use masks the clinical symptoms of PID.

To address this question, Ness and coworkers, in continuing follow-up of the PEACH cohort, studied women with unrecognized endometritis vs those with symptomatic endometritis.[49] Asymptomatic endometritis patients ($n = 43$) were ascertained by contact tracing of partners with STIs or patients with asymptomatic cervical STIs. Comparison was made with women with clinical symptoms of PID ($n = 111$) with biopsy-proven endometritis. Women with unrecognized endometritis were 4.3 times more likely than women with recognized endometritis to use OCPs. It was hypothesized that OCP use might reduce the inflammatory reaction associated with UGT infection or reduce the bacterial inoculum by increasing the viscosity of the cervical mucus. Importantly, OCP use was associated with asymptomatic, unrecognized disease, but was highly associated with silent endometritis.

Although the Lund, Sweden cohort studies were extensive, when deciding whether OCPs exert protection against PID, the recent PEACH studies are probably the most applicable to modern-day medicine, and physicians should encourage consistent condom use and frequent STI screening to prevent PID. Studies are needed to address the implications to public health messages of using OCPs to protect against PID.

NONSTEROIDAL ANTI-INFLAMMATORY DRUGS AND PREVENTION OF PELVIC INFLAMMATORY DISEASE

Another possible frontier in prevention of the sequelae of PID is using nonsteroidal anti-inflammatory drugs (NSAIDs) in conjunction with antibiotics. Since much of the tubal damage from chlamydia is thought to be secondary to hypersensitivity or immune-mediated reactions rather than direct infectious damage, NSAIDs may reduce this inflammation and improve fertility. Infection of human monocyte-derived macrophages with CT induces production of prostaglandin E_2.[50] In guinea pig models, treatment with physiologic doses of estradiol results in an increase in the output of uterine prostaglandin $F_{2\alpha}$. Treatment of these guinea pigs with the prostaglandin inhibitors indomethacin and ibuprofen results in decreased effect of estradiol-enhanced genital chlamydia infection.[51] In mice, Landers and coworkers found that adding ibuprofen to tetracycline therapy for chlamydia did not alter the inflammatory response, or improve subsequent fertility or ectopic pregnancy rates.[52] However, the addition of an NSAID did decrease immune response, as measured by antichlamydial antibody IgM.[53] Blanco and colleagues performed a similar study, and found that adding ibuprofen to clindamycin in chlamydia-infected mice did not effect inflammatory damage to the pelvis.[53] Of note, inflammatory changes were similar in mice treated with clindamycin alone, ibuprofen alone, and combination of the two.[53] These studies may not reflect the effectiveness of adding an NSAID to newer antibiotic regimens for PID, and it is unclear how early NSAID therapy must be initiated to achieve clinical effect. More research needs to be done to determine if inexpensive, over-the-counter NSAIDs can decrease the costly, long-term sequelae of PID.

ECTOPIC PREGNANCY

The tubal damage resulting from PID may be absolute, causing tubal factor infertility, or relative, causing damage that is not enough to impede pregnancy but is sufficient to cause abnormal ectopic gestations. The incidence of ectopic pregnancy has increased since 1970.[54] In 1992, CDC reported there were 20 ectopic gestations per 1000 pregnancies, accounting for 9% of pregnancy-related deaths.[54]

To establish general risk factors for ectopic pregnancy, Marchbanks and coworkers conducted a population-based, case–control study in Minnesota in 1988.[55] Twenty-two potential risk factors for ectopic pregnancy were assessed in 274 women with ectopic pregnancies and 548 matched controls.[55] Current IUD use, a history of infertility or PID, and prior tubal surgery remained independent risk factors for ectopic pregnancy.

In 1981, Westrom's group examined 30 822 intrauterine and 249 ectopic pregnancies from the Lund, Sweden birth registry.[56] They found that the incidence of ectopic pregnancy increases with age: 4.1 ectopic pregnancies per 100 woman-years in teenagers and 12.9 ectopic pregnancies per 100 woman-years in 30–39-year-old women.[56] This may be explained by the likelihood that the older a woman is, the higher the chance of being exposed to risks for ectopic pregnancy, namely PID. The relationship between PID, IUD use, and ectopic pregnancy was also examined and it was found that in women aged 20–29 years, the total ectopic pregnancy rate per 100 woman-years of IUD use was 0.4, which was similar to the rate of ectopic pregnancies in women with no history of PID or IUD use, 0.3 per 100 woman-years. The rate of ectopic pregnancy in women with a history of PID, but no history of IUD use, was 1.9 ectopics per 100 woman-years. It was concluded that the incidence of ectopic pregnancy among women who have never had salpingitis is the same in women not using contraceptives as in those using non-medicated or copper-medicated IUDs. A history of laparoscopically verified salpingitis, not the history of IUD use, elevates the risk of ectopic pregnancy seven-fold.

In 1985, Westrom reported on the association of ectopic pregnancy in 1204 patients with laparoscopically verified PID, compared with 150 women with surgically verified normal pelvis.[13] In control patients, 75% became pregnant, with 1 of 112 pregnancies being ectopic. Of PID patients, 62% subsequently became pregnant, with 1 of 16 pregnancies being ectopic, a seven-fold increase.

When different antibiotic regimens for PID were compared in a subset of the Lund, Sweden cohort ($n = 608$), there were no differences in the ratios of ectopic to intrauterine pregnancy (IUP) between the different treatment regimens used.[15] However, the rate of ectopic pregnancy was significantly lower after GC PID than after non-GC PID.

In 1991, Joesoef et al found that once a woman has PID, her risk of a subsequent ectopic pregnancy remains elevated, even if she achieves an IUP.[57] Joesoef and colleagues performed laparoscopy on 2501 women with PID and graded the pelvis as normal (score = 0), mild (score = 1), moderate (score = 2), or severe (score = 3) PID. Of the 2899 pregnancies that occurred during more than 20 years of follow-up after index laparoscopy, 193 (6.7%) were ectopic. Among first-order pregnancies after the index PID episode, 6.8% were ectopic. Among second-order or higher pregnancies after surgically confirmed PID, women with a prior IUP still had a 5.6% rate of ectopic pregnancy, whereas those with a prior ectopic had a 21.7% rate of repeat ectopic.[58] This group also reemphasized that risk of an ectopic pregnancy was directly related to age at pregnancy, severity of the index PID episode, and prior adnexal operations, as shown in Table 5.4.

A study in the United States, by Bernstine and coworkers followed 187 women with an initial episode of PID, verified by laparoscopy.[27] They found the rates of ectopic pregnancy also increased based on the severity of the index case: 14%, 11%, and 42% after mild, moderate, or severe PID respectively.[27] The increased rates seen in this study, versus the Lund Sweden cohort, may be due to different etiologies of PID and different treatment regimens in the 1960s vs the 1980s.

Table 5.4 Risk factors for ectopic pregnancy after laparoscopically verified pelvic inflammatory disease (PID)

Risk factor	Percent ectopic rate after index PID
Age at pregnancy (years):	
<25	3.6[a]
26–30	8.5
>30	8.7
Prior adnexal operations:	
0	5.8[a]
1	18.4
>1	25.7
Prior salpingitis:	
0	2.2[a]
1	8.0
2	11.0
>2	15.4
Index salpingitis score:	
0	2.2[a]
1–2	6.0
3	13.5
>3	18.1

[a]$p < 0.01$ for linear trend.

In a study by Chaparro and coworkers, 223 women with suspected PID underwent laparoscopy: 46% had PID, 31% had other serious conditions, and 23% had a normal pelvis.[58] Like the Swedish studies, the PID was surgically graded as mild, moderate, or severe. The number of patients is smaller than in the Joesoef group's study (103 vs 2501), but when the diagnosis of PID is based on objective surgical visualization, the ectopic pregnancy rate after PID was similar in these studies: 2.7% after mild PID and 6.5% after moderate PID. There were no pregnancies, ectopic or intrauterine, in the patients with severe PID.

Gerber and Krause followed women for an average of 76 months after laparoscopically verified PID and found ectopic pregnancies in 7.3% of patients.[28] In addition, second-look laparoscopy was performed, on average 10 weeks after initial diagnosis. For the patients with ectopic pregnancies, four of five had at least one tube patent at second-look laparoscopy, indicating that a patent tube is not necessarily functioning correctly.

When the diagnosis of PID is not confirmed by laparoscopy, other diseases, such as endometriosis or ovarian cysts, may be present, driving down the rate of ectopic pregnancy in the future. For example, Safrin and coworkers followed a small ($n = 55$) cohort of women released from the hospital with a discharge diagnosis of PID, based on clinical, not surgical, criteria.[59] At a mean of 37 months follow-up, 2.4% had experienced an ectopic pregnancy and 48% had an intrauterine pregnancy.[59] These rates of ectopic pregnancy differ from those found by Joesoef and Chaparro, as the diagnosis of PID was made differently in these three studies.

Further support for the role of STIs in ectopic pregnancy is that women experiencing ectopic pregnancies, like infertile women, have higher rates and titers of antichlamydial antibody than women with intrauterine pregnancies.[60,61] Interestingly, among women with tubal pregnancies, higher titers of antichlamydial antibody have been correlated with higher grades of inflammatory tubal mucosal damage.[61,62]

Chow and coworkers compared patients with ectopic gestations with those with IUPs, and found that, even after controlling for factors known to be associated with ectopic pregnancy – including age at coitarche, total lifetime partners, douching, previous infertility, and parity – elevated antichlamydial IgG titers conferred a 2.4 relative risk of ectopic pregnancy.[63]

Hartford and coworkers examined 24 patients undergoing exploratory laparotomy and salpingectomy for ruptured ectopic pregnancy and divided them into two groups, based on the presence or absence of gross abnormalities in the fallopian tube contralateral to the ectopic gestation.[64] Antichlamydial IgG was significantly higher in patients with ectopic pregnancies and evidence of contralateral chronic salpingitis than in patients with ectopic pregnancies but otherwise normal contralateral tubal anatomy. This study is interesting because it compared ectopic gestations with ectopic gestations.

As the diagnosis of PID turns to less-invasive methods, the findings of the studies regarding antichlamydial antibody titers may provide patients with PID prognostic information on their risk for subsequent tubal damage.

CHRONIC PELVIC PAIN

CPP refers to menstrual or non-menstrual pain of at least 6 months' duration that occurs below the umbilicus and is severe enough to cause functional disability or require treatment. Patients diagnosed with PID are at an increased risk of CPP. The incidence of CPP may be higher in women with more severe PID, as diagnosed by laparoscopy,[27,58] although some authors have found that any pelvic damage is associated with CPP, regardless of severity.[28] The cause of post-PID CPP is not known but may be related to increased intraovarian pressure induced by menstrual cycle-related volume changes, which are restricted by adhesions surrounding the ovaries.[65]

Buchan and coworkers found that patients with PID were 10 times more likely to be readmitted to hospital for abdominal pain, 4 times more likely to be readmitted for gynecologic pain, 6 times more likely to be readmitted for endometriosis, and 8 times more likely to have a hysterectomy than hospitalized controls.[66]

Safrin and coworkers followed 51 women admitted for the treatment of PID for 37 months.[59] CPP occurred in 24% of the women after the index hospitalization, and was more common in women with a history of PID prior to the index admission, which may reflect more severe, recurrent disease.[59]

A more global picture of the consequences of post-PID pelvic pain was obtained by Adler and coworkers, who followed 78 patients admitted with PID vs 77 controls for up to 21 months. They recorded all complaints of abdominal pain, not just complaints severe enough to result in hospitalization. In general, 75% of the PID patients reported abdominal pain other than dysmenorrhea, compared with 25% of controls. Due to pelvic pain, the PID patients were significantly more likely to alter their daily routine, take time off work, present as outpatients, experience dyspareunia, and be admitted and undergo abdominal operations than controls.[67] Pelvic pain has often been associated with psychological stress and somatic complaints. The Adler et al study was unique because patients were also questioned regarding attitude/interpersonal relationships, sexual function, and work adjustment at each follow-up. The cases did not differ significantly from the controls on the psychological parameters, suggesting that cases were experiencing altered social and work functioning due to physical and not somatic pain.[67]

In the early years of the Lund, Sweden cohort, Westrom described 415 women with laparoscopically verified PID.[2] At 9.5 years of follow-up, CPP was reported by 18.1% of the PID patients vs 5% of controls.[2]

The above studies followed women with severe enough PID to be admitted to the hospital. A better sense of a woman's risk of CPP may be offered by the PEACH study, since it included women more representative of the general PID population, namely those with mild and moderate PID. At a mean of 35 months follow-up, 36% of patients in the PEACH study experienced CPP.[68] Factors associated with CPP after PID included previous episodes of PID, previous pelvic surgery, less than a high school education, non-black race, smoking, being married, and douching. Not intuitively, women with GC, CT, or an elevated WBC count during the index PID episode had a lower risk of post-PID CPP.[68] However, recall that patients in the PEACH study were diagnosed by clinical rather than surgical criteria. Some patients included in the PEACH cohort may have had other causes of acute pelvic pain such as endometriosis. Positive cervical cultures or leukocytosis are markers for "curable" pelvic infection. This may indicate that patients without objective evidence of infection should undergo laparoscopy to detect other causes of acute pelvic pain. Non-black patients enrolled in the PEACH study may have represented a larger cohort of patients with endometriosis or other non-PID conditions, increasing their risk of CPP. It is unclear why being married was found to be a stronger predictor of subsequent CPP than age. Douching, which disrupts normal vaginal flora and may facilitate repeated, subclinical PID infections, was a risk factor for CPP. Smoking may be a coping mechanism for the chronic stress of pelvic pain.

Similar to the Adler et al study, Haggerty et al provided detailed information on the effect CPP had on the lives of a cohort of the PEACH study patients.[69] They showed that individual physical function, bodily pain, general health, vitality, social function, and mental health scores, measured by Mean Medical Outcomes Study Short Form, were progressively lower among women with increasing grades of CPP.

In summary, evidence shows that women with either laparoscopically or clinically diagnosed PID are at higher risk of post-PID CPP. Furthermore, the risk for debilitating pain applies to women with mild-to-severe PID and those treated as inpatients or outpatients. Finally, the pain puts the woman at increased risk for several medical interventions and decreased psychological and social functioning, leading to a high societal cost of PID.

RECURRENT PELVIC INFLAMMATORY DISEASE

When considering prevention strategies, prevention of recurrent PID is an important goal, as it has been shown that the sequelae of PID worsen with repeated episodes of PID.

In the large Lund, Sweden cohort, Westrom found that the frequency of reinfection after index PID episode depended on age.[9] For women under age 20 with PID, 30% became reinfected. In women over 21 years old, 13.2% became reinfected. The frequencies of reinfection did not depend on the severity of the index case: 12.9% of mild PID were reinfected, 13% of moderate PID were reinfected, and 11% of severe PID were reinfected.

Safrin and coworkers followed 51 women for a mean of 37 months after inpatient treatment of PID.[59] Forty-three percent of patients had one or more repeat episodes of PID after the index case, occurring at a median of 2.1 months after admission (range 1–40 months).[59] Women with subsequent episodes of PID tended to be younger at the time of coitarche and had a longer duration of abdominal pain before presentation for admission in the index episode. The mean number of PID episodes before the index case was higher in women with subsequent episodes, reflecting continued risky behavior and the need for education regarding prevention.[59] The risk of subsequent PID was 30% in women with no history of PID, 50% in those with one prior episode of PID, and 72% in those with two or more past histories of PID.[59] Women with STIs in their first episode of PID were more likely to have recurrent PID, but this was not significant in women with a history of PID at the time of admission.[59]

Eschenbach and coworkers also found that a history of previous GC was obtained significantly more frequently among women with either recurrent GC PID or nongonococcal PID than among patients who were experiencing their first PID episode.[45] A history of previous GC was also more common among women with non-GC PID than among control subjects without GC. It is possible that unrecognized tubal damage occurs in GC, even in the absence of clinically overt PID. Unrecognized fallopian tube damage might impair the bacterial clearance mechanism of the fallopian tube, which predisposes to the high rate of recurrent PID.

PEACH STUDY

In the past, it was thought that treating PID with intravenous antibiotics in the inpatient setting might offer some protection to the sequelae of PID. The PEACH study was the largest randomized trial ever conducted in North America to evaluate the effectiveness of ambulatory vs intravenous therapy for PID in terms of preventing sequelae of PID.[29] This study is very generalizable because it recruited women with mild-to-moderate PID, which represents most women with PID. The diagnosis of PID in the PEACH study was made based on clinical criteria, and patients were randomized to inpatient vs outpatient treatment. Long-term outcomes were pregnancy rate, time to pregnancy, recurrence of PID, chronic pelvic pain, and ectopic pregnancy. Short-term clinical and microbiologic improvements were similar between the inpatient and outpatient groups. After a mean follow-up period of 35 months, there were no statistically significant differences between treatment groups in pregnancy rates, time to pregnancy, recurrent PID, chronic pelvic pain, or ectopic pregnancy.[29] A subset analysis of women who had endometritis, at randomization, also showed no difference in long-term outcomes despite inpatient or outpatient therapy.

The PEACH investigators concluded that outpatient therapy provided sufficient tissue levels for adequate PID treatment in both inpatient and outpatient settings.[29] Unfortunately, for patients with adverse sequelae, the PEACH study provides evidence that the damage of PID had probably already occurred at enrollment, either because of preexisting tubal damage or delay in seeking care. In considering healthcare costs, the PEACH study supports the view that outpatient therapy, which is less expensive to the patient and the healthcare system, is equally as effective as more intensive inpatient regimens.

CONCLUSIONS

Cervicitis should be screened for aggressively to prevent PID. Once PID is diagnosed, inpatient and outpatient therapy appear to be equally effective and, unfortunately, equally ineffective at preventing long-term sequelae of PID. The long-term sequelae of PID – infertility, ectopic pregnancy, CPP, and recurrent PID episodes – are costly in terms of medical expense and emotional toll on patients. A high index of suspicion and early intervention are important because long-term sequelae of PID are associated with severe disease, delay in treatment, and recurrent infections.

REFERENCES

1. Centers for Disease Control and Prevention. STD Fact Sheet, July 2004.
2. Westrom L. Incidence, prevalence, and trends of acute pelvic inflammatory disease and its consequences in industrialized countries. Am J Obstet Gynecol 1980;138(7):880–92.
3. Rein DB, Kassler WJ, Irwin KL, et al. Direct medical cost of pelvic inflammatory disease and its sequelae: decreasing, but still substantial. Obstet Gynecol 2000;95:397–402.
4. Washington AE, Katz P. Cost of and payment source for pelvic inflammatory disease: trends and projections, 1983 through 2000. JAMA 1991;266:2565–9.
5. Yeh JS, Hook EW, Goldie SJ. A refined estimate of the average lifetime cost of pelvic inflammatory disease. Sex Transm Dis 2003;30(5):369–78.
6. Eschenbach DA, Wolner-Hanssen P, Hawes SE, et al. Acute pelvic inflammatory disease: associations of clinical and laboratory findings with laparoscopic findings. Obstet Gynecol 1997;89(2):184–92.
7. Westrom L. Pelvic inflammatory disease: bacteriology and sequelae. Contraception 1987;36(1):111–28.
8. Holmes KK, Eschenbach DA, Knapp JS. Salpingitis: overview of etiology and epidemiology. Am J Obstet Gynecol 1980;138:893–900.
9. Westrom L. Effect of acute pelvic inflammatory disease on fertility. Am J Obstet Gynecol 1975;121(5):707–13.
10. Lepine LA, Hillis SD, Marchbanks PA, et al. Severity of pelvic inflammatory disease as a predictor of the probability of live birth. Am J Obstet Gynecol 1998;178(5):977–81.
11. Westrom L, Joesoef R, Reynolds G, et al. Pelvic inflammatory disease and fertility: A cohort study of 1844 women with laparoscopically verified disease and 657 control women with normal laparoscopic results. Sex Transm Dis 1992;19:185–92.
12. Westrom LV. Sexually transmitted diseases and infertility. Sex Transm Dis 1994;21:S32–7.
13. Westrom L. Influence of sexually transmitted diseases on sterility and ectopic pregnancy. Acta Eur Fertil 1985;16(1):21–4.
14. Svensson L, Mardh PA, Westrom L. Infertility after acute salpingitis with special reference to *Chlamydia trachomatis*. Fertil Steril 1983;40(3):322–9.
15. Westrom L, Iosif S, Svensson L, et al. Infertility after acute salpingitis: results of treatment with different antibiotics. Curr Ther Res 1979;26(6S):752–9.
16. Hillis SD, Joesoef R, Marchbanks PA, et al. Delayed care of pelvic inflammatory disease as a risk factor for impaired fertility. Am J Obstet Gynecol 1993;168:1503–9.
17. McCormack WM, Nowroozi K, Alpert S, et al. Characteristics of patients with gonococcal and nongonococcal infection and evaluation of their response to treatment with aqueous

procaine penicillin G and spectinomycin hydrochloride. Sex Transm Dis 1977;4(4):125–31.

18. Svensson L, Westrom L, Ripa KT, et al. Differences in some clinical and laboratory parameters in acute salpingitis related to culture and serologic findings. Am J Obstet Gynecol 1980;138(7 Pt 2):1017–21.
19. Patton DL, Moore DE, Spadoni LR, et al. A comparison of the fallopian tube's response to overt and silent salpingitis. Obstet Gynecol 1989;73(4):622–30.
20. Shepard MK, Jones RB. Recovery of *Chlamydia trachomatis* from endometrial and fallopian tube biopsies in women with infertility of tubal origin. Fertil Steril 1989;52(2):232–8.
21. Kane JL, Woodland RM, Forsey T, et al. Evidence of chlamydial infection in infertile women with and without fallopian tube obstruction. Fertil Steril 1984;42(6):843–7.
22. Jones RB, Mammel JB, Shepard MK, et al. Recovery of *Chlamydia trachomatis* from the endometrium of women at risk for chlamydial infection. Am J Obstet Gynecol 1986;155(1):35–9.
23. Sellors JW, Mahony JB, Chernesky MA, et al. Tubal factor infertility: an association with prior chlamydial infection and asymptomatic salpingitis. Fertil Steril 1988;49(3):451–7.
24. Brunham RC, Maclean IW, Binns B, Peeling RW. *Chlamydia trachomatis*: its role in tubal infertility. J Infect Dis 1985;152(6):1275–82.
25. Moore DE, Spadoni LR, Foy HM, et al. Increased frequency of serum antibodies to *Chlamydia trachomatis* in infertility due to distal tubal disease. Lancet 1982;2:574–7.
26. Henry-Suchet J, Catalan F, Loffredo V, et al. Microbiology of specimens obtained by laparoscopy from controls and from patients with pelvic inflammatory disease or infertility with tubal obstruction: *Chlamydia trachomatis* and *Ureaplasma urealyticum*. Am J Obstet Gynecol 1980;138(7):1022–5.
27. Bernstine R, Kennedy WR, Waldron J. Acute pelvic inflammatory disease: a clinical follow up. Int J Fertil 1987;32(3):229–32.
28. Gerber B, Krause A. A study of second-look laparoscopy after acute salpingitis. Arch Gynecol Obstet 1996;258:193–200.
29. Ness RB, Soper DE, Holley RL, et al. Effectiveness of inpatient and outpatient treatment strategies for women with pelvic inflammatory disease: results from the Pelvic Inflammatory Disease Evalution and Clinical Health (PEACH) Randomized Trial. Am J Obstet Gynecol 2002;186(5):929-37.
30. Haggerty CL, Ness RB, Amortegui A, et al. Endometritis does not predict reproductive morbidity after pelvic inflammatory disease. Am J Obstet Gynecol 2003;188:141–8.
31. Heinonen PK, Leinonen M. Fecundity and morbidity following acute pelvic inflammatory disease treated with doxycycline and metronidazole. Arch Gynecol Obstet 2003;268(4):284–8.
32. Ries E. The mechanism of occlusion of the tube. Am J Obstet Dis Women 1909;60(2):201–12.
33. Schlaff WD, Hassiakos DK, Damewood MD, et al. Neosalpingostomy for distal tubal obstruction: prognostic factors and impact of surgical technique. Fertil Steril 1990;54(6):984–90.
34. Whiteside JL, Katz T, Anthes T, et al. Risks and adverse outcomes of sexually transmitted diseases. J Reprod Med 2001;46(1):34–8.
35. Scholes D, Stergachis A, Heidrich FE, et al. Prevention of pelvic inflammatory disease by screening for cervical chlamydial infection. N Engl J Med 1996;334:1362–6.
36. Eschenbach DA. Acute pelvic inflammatory disease: etiology, risk factors, and pathogenesis. Clin Obstet Gynecol 1976;19:147–69.
37. Rubin GL, Ory HW, Layde PM. Oral contraceptives and pelvic inflammatory disease. Am J Obstet Gynecol 1982;144:630–5.
38. Wolner-Hanssen P, Eschenback DA, Paavonen J, et al. Decreased risk of symptomatic chlamydia pelvic inflammatory disease associated with oral contraceptive use. JAMA 1990;263(1):54–9.
39. Svensson L, Westrom L, Mardh PA. Contraceptives and acute salpingitis. JAMA 1984;251(19):2553–5.
40. Maslow AS, Davis CH, Choong J, et al. Estrogen enhances attachment of *Chlamydia trachomatis* to human endometrial epithelial cells in vitro. Am J Obstet Gynecol 1988;159(4):1006–14.
41. Wolner-Hanssen P. Oral contraceptive use modifies the manifestations of pelvic inflammatory disease. Br J Obstet Gynaecol 1986;93:619–24.
42. Senanayake P, Kramer DG. Contraception and the etiology of pelvic inflammatory disease: new perspectives. Am J Obstet Gynecol 1980;138((7 Pt 2):852–60.
43. Rice PA, Schachter J. Pathogenesis of pelvic inflammatory disease: What are the questions? JAMA 1991;266:2587–93.
44. Ryden G, Fahraeus L, Molin L, Ahman K. Do contraceptives influence the incidence of acute pelvic inflammatory disease in women with gonorrhoea? Contraception 1979;20(2):149–57.
45. Eschenbach DA, Harnisch JP, Holmes KK. Pathogenesis of acute pelvic inflammatory disease: role of contraception and other risk factors. Am J Obstet Gynecol 1977;128(8):838–50.
46. Washington AE, Gove S, Schachter J, et al. Oral contraceptives, *Chlamydia trachomatis* infection, and pelvic inflammatory disease: a word of caution about protection. JAMA 1985;253(15):2246–50.
47. Targum SD, Wright NH. Association of the intrauterine device and pelvic inflammatory disease: a retrospective pilot study. Am J Epidemiol 1974;100(4):262–71.
48. Ness RB, Soper DE, Holley RL, et al. Hormonal and barrier contraception and risk of upper genital tract disease in the PID Evaluation and Clinical Health (PEACH) study. Am J Obstet Gynecol 2001;185(1):121–7.
49. Ness RB, Keder LM, Soper DE, et al. Oral contraception and the recognition of endometritis. Am J Obstet Gynecol 1997;176(3):580–5.
50. Manor E, Schmitz E, Sarov I. TNF-α, IL-1 and PGEα production by human monocyte-derived macrophages infected with *C. trachomatis*. In: Bowie WR, Caldwell HD, Jones RP et al, eds. Chlamydial Infections: Proceedings of the Seventh International Symposium of Human Chlamydia Infections. New York: Cambridge University Press, 1990: 209–12.
51. Pasley JN, Hyoik R, White MJ, Barron AL. Influence of prostaglandin inhibitors on estradiol enhanced chlamydial infection in femal guinea pigs. In: Bowie WR, Caldwell HD, Jones RP, et al, eds. Chlamydial Infections: Proceedings of the Seventh International Symposium of Human Chlamydial Infections. New York: Cambridge University Press, 1990:245–8.
52. Landers DV, Sung ML, Botttles K, et al. Does addition of anti-inflammatory agents to antimicrobial therapy reduce infertility after murine chlamydial salpingitis? Sex Transm Dis 1993;20(3):121–5.
53. Blanco JD, Patterson RM, Ramzy I, et al. Clindamycin and ibuprofen effects on chlamydial salpingitis in mice. Sex Transm Dis 1989;16(4):192–4.
54. Centers for Disease Control and Prevention. Ectopic pregnancy – United States, 1990–1992. MMWR 1995;44:46–8.
55. Marchbanks PA, Annegers JF, Coulam CB, et al. Risk factors for ectopic pregnancy: a population-based study. JAMA 1988;259(12):1823–7.
56. Westrom L, Bengtsson LP, Mardh PA. Incidence, trends, and risks of ectopic pregnancy in a population of women. BMJ 1981;282:15–18.
57. Joesoef MR, Westrom L, Reynolds G, et al. Recurrence of ectopic pregnancy: the role of salpingitis. Am J Obstet Gynecol 1991;165:46–50.
58. Chaparro MV, Ghosh S, Nashed A, et al. Laparoscopy for the confirmation and prognostic evaluation of pelvic inflammatory disease. Int J Gynaecol Obstet 1978;15:307–9.
59. Safrin S, Schachter J, Dahrouge D, et al. Long-term sequelae of acute pelvic inflammatory disease: a retrospective cohort study. Am J Obstet Gynecol 1992;166(4):1300–5.

60. Svensson L, Mardh PA, Ahlgren M, Nordenskjold F. Ectopic pregnancy and antibodies to *Chlamydia trachomatis*. Fertil Steril 1985;44(3):313–17.
61. Walters MD, Eddy CA, Gibbs RS, et al. Antibodies to *Chlamydia trachomatis* and risk for tubal pregnancy. Am J Obstet Gynecol 1988;159(4):942-6.
62. Wang SP, Eschenbach DA, Holmes KK, et al. *Chlamydia trachomatis* infection in Fitz-Hugh–Curtis syndrome. Am J Obstet Gynecol 1980;138(7):1034–8.
63. Chow JM, Yonekura L, Richwald GA, et al. The association between *Chlamydia trachomatis* and ectopic pregnancy. JAMA 1990;263(23):3164–7.
64. Hartford SL, Silva PD, diZerega GS, et al. Serologic evidence of prior chlamydial infection in patients with tubal ectopic pregnancy and contralateral tubal disease. Fertil Steril 1987;47(1):118–21.
65. Hillis S, Black C, Newhall J, et al. New opportunities for chlamydia prevention: applications of science to public health practice. Sex Transm Dis 1995;22(3):197–202.
66. Buchan H, Vessey M, Goldace M, et al. Morbidity following pelvic inflammatory disease. Br J Obstet Gynaecol 1993;100:558-62.
67. Adler MW, Belsey EH, O'Connor BH. Morbidity associated with pelvic inflammatory disease. Br J Vener Dis 1982;58:151–7.
68. Haggerty CL, Peipert JF, Weitzen S, et al. PID Evaluation and Clinical Health (PEACH) Study Investigators. Predictors of chronic pelvic pain in an urban population of women presenting with symptoms and signs of pelvic inflammatory disease. Sex Transm Dis 2005;32:293–9.
69. Haggerty CL, Schulz R, Ness RB; PID Evaluation and Clinical Health Study Investigators. Lower quality of life among women with chronic pelvic pain after pelvic inflammatory disease. Obstet Gynecol 2003;102:934–9.

6. Subclinical Pelvic Inflammatory Disease

Harold C. Wiesenfeld

INTRODUCTION

Acute pelvic inflammatory disease (PID) has long been recognized as an important cause of tubal factor infertility, ectopic pregnancy, and chronic pelvic pain.[1] Despite this well-known relationship, there is a growing body of literature suggesting that the greatest burden of post-infectious tubal infertility results from PID that is unrecognized by the patient and her physician. In this chapter, we will outline the historical evidence linking subclinical PID with adverse reproductive outcomes. Associations between lower genital tract infections and subclinical PID will be explored and the reproductive outcomes of women with subclinical PID will be discussed.

CASE

A 24-year-old primigravid presents to the emergency room of a local hospital with a 2-day history of right lower quadrant pain. Her past medical history was notable for a diagnosis of *Chlamydia trachomatis* infection detected during routine screening at age 19. Her examination revealed moderate right lower quadrant tenderness. A pregnancy test was positive and a pelvic ultrasound reveals a complex right adnexal mass. A laparoscopy is undertaken, revealing an ectopic pregnancy in the right fallopian tube (Figure 6.1). Other findings include pelvic adhesions and perihepatic adhesions indicative of remote PID. During her recovery phase, the patient further denied any known prior history of acute pelvic inflammatory disease.

RECENT TRENDS ON SEVERITY OF PELVIC INFLAMMATORY DISEASE

In the United States between 1979 and 1988, hospitalizations for acute PID decreased by 36%. In the subsequent decade from 1990 to 2000, the number of hospitalizations for women in the United States

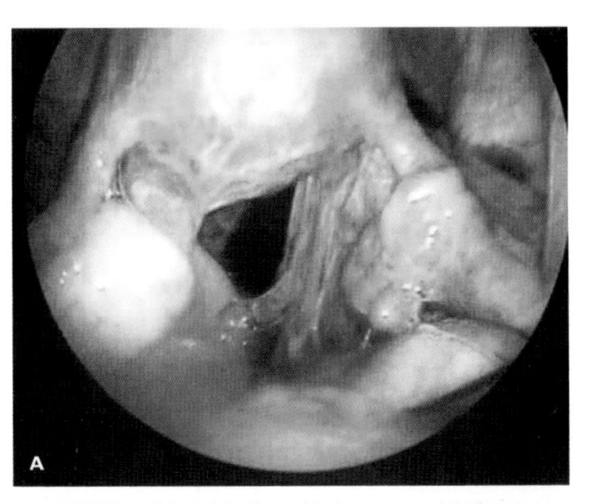

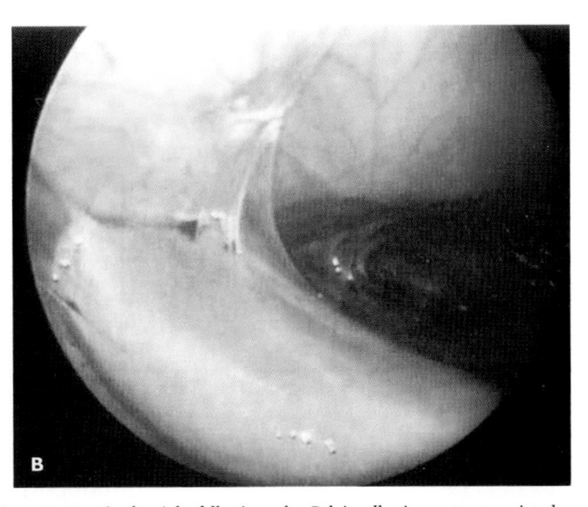

Figure 6.1 View of the pelvis obtained by laparoscopy. (A) There is an ectopic pregnancy in the right fallopian tube. Pelvic adhesions are appreciated in the left adnexa. (B) Perihepatic adhesions consistent with Fitz–Hugh–Curtis syndrome.

between the ages of 15 and 44 dropped further by approximately one-half.[2,3] In the face of this decline, the number of visits to physicians' offices for PID remained stable over the same time period. What are the possible reasons for declining hospitalizations for acute PID in the setting of an overall unchanged number of cases? A number of reasons can be postulated to explain these divergent statistics. First, it is known that many physicians do not follow widely recognized guidelines for the treatment of acute PID.[4,5] Despite such deficiencies, there is no indication that physician knowledge diminished over this time period in a way that would explain the declining trends in hospitalization. Secondly, these data may reflect practice pattern trends to reduce medical costs by managing diseases on an outpatient basis. In a review of hospitalizations for acute PID in Oslo, Norway, Sorbye et al documented a 35% reduction in hospitalized cases of acute PID, comparing two time periods separated by 10 years (1990–1992 and 2000–2002).[6] During that decade, however, there were no changes in policy regarding admission criteria for acute PID, which suggests that provider behavior did not influence the declining numbers of hospitalizations. A third and very plausible explanation is that the severity of cases of PID has changed due to evolving trends in microbiologic etiology. Specifically, the declining rate of *Neisseria gonorrhoeae*, which has not been observed with the prevalence of *C. trachomatis* infection, may have resulted in fewer cases of PID associated with gonorrhea, and a relative increased proportion of cases associated with chlamydia. As cases of PID caused by *N. gonorrhoeae* are typically more clinically severe that those caused by *C. trachomatis*, decreased hospitalizations for acute disease would be expected to be seen if most cases of PID are nongonococcal in etiology. Thus, the presentation of PID is evolving, trending towards less-severe clinical presentations. In this light, much attention is focused on milder forms of pelvic infection, recognizing that atypical, silent, or clinically unrecognized cases of PID are commonplace. As will be described later, these subclinical cases of PID may be associated with reproductive health risks. Mirroring these trends in clinical presentation is the evolution of the minimum criteria

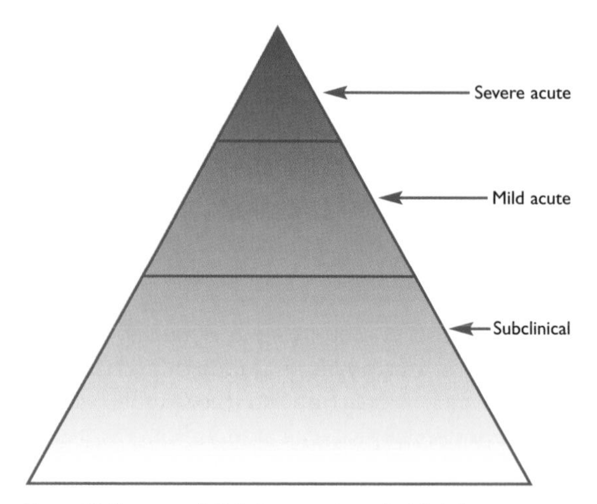

Figure 6.2 Spectrum of clinical presentations of pelvic inflammatory disease.

for the diagnosis of acute PID as devised by the Centers for Disease Control and Prevention (CDC) in their sexually transmitted disease (STD) treatment guidelines. In the 1998 STD treatment guidelines, the CDC's minimum clinical criteria for the diagnosis of acute PID required the presence of all of the following: lower abdominal tenderness, adnexal tenderness, and cervical motion tenderness.[7] These criteria contrast with the far less stringent criteria contained in the 2002 STD treatment guidelines, which require as minimum criteria the presence of either cervical motion tenderness or uterine/adnexal tenderness.[8] The new paradigm of clinical presentations of PID is demonstrated in Figure 6.2, and reflects the shifting spectrum of clinical presentations from acute, symptomatic illness to subclinical disease.

HISTORICAL EVIDENCE LINKING INFERTILITY WITH PRIOR EPISODES OF SUBCLINICAL PELVIC INFLAMMTORY DISEASE

PERSISTENT INFECTION OF THE UPPER GENITAL TRACT

Pelvic pathogens can be recovered from the upper genital tract in women in the absence of symptoms of acute pelvic inflammatory disease. Among the earliest observations is a report by Henry-Suchet and Loffredo in 1980 describing the isolation of *C. trachomatis* from the abdomen in 6 of 23 infertile women without pain or other evidence of acute pelvic infection.[9] A larger study expanded on this preliminary series, further documenting that in women undergoing laparoscopy for infertility, a large proportion had evidence of upper genital tract infection.[10] Among these women who did not have any clinical evidence of acute PID, *C. trachomatis* was recovered from the abdominal cavity from 23.3% of women with tubal damage and laparoscopic evidence of chronic inflammation. The chlamydial isolation rate among women with tubal damage but without inflammation was 15.4%, whereas that among controls who did not have tubal damage was 2%. Further evidence that *C. trachomatis* can persist in the upper genital tract in the absence of symptoms arises from a study of women with acute PID by Sweet and colleagues.[11] Despite clinical response, post-treatment endometrial cultures were positive for *C. trachomatis* in 12 of 13 women treated with a cephalosporin agent that does not have activity against this pathogen. These early findings not only point out the need for antichlamydial therapy for acute PID but also importantly suggest that *C. trachomatis* infection of the upper genital tract can occur in the absence of symptoms of acute PID. Patton et al elegantly studied fallopian tube specimens from women with laparoscopy-confirmed post-infectious tubal infertility, searching for evidence of *C. trachomatis* by culture, in-situ hybridization, immunoperoxidase staining, and transmission electron microscopy.[12] Using these comprehensive techniques, persistent infection with *C. trachomatis* was evident in nearly 80% of women. These results strongly suggest that *C. trachomatis* can cause a persistent and clinically silent infection of the upper genital tract.

SEROLOGIC EVIDENCE OF PRIOR CHLAMYDIAL INFECTION IN WOMEN WITH INFERTILITY

Much of the association between subclinical PID and infertility derives from retrospective studies documenting serologic evidence of prior chlamydial or gonococcal infections. Moore et al tested sera from infertile women for *C. trachomatis* antibody by micro-immunofluorescence.[13] Among 33 infertile women with distal occlusion detected by laparoscopy, 24 (73%) were seropositive for *C. trachomatis* antibodies, compared with 0/35 infertile women without tubal disease. Tjiam et al performed a similar study in the Netherlands of 53 women who were infertile for at least 18 months. All subjects had undergone an infertility evaluation that included documentation of fallopian tube status by hysterosalpingography (HSG) and laparoscopy.[14] Antibodies to *C. trachomatis* were detected in 21.2% (7/33) of women with tubal factor infertility, whereas none of the 20 infertile women without tubal disease tested positive for chlamydial antibodies. In a cohort of 218 infertile women in Colorado who underwent HSG and laparoscopy, Meikle et al reported that *C. trachomatis* antibodies were present in the sera of 78.2% (68/87) of women with tubal disease as determined by laparoscopy, whereas only 36% of infertile women without tubal disease had antichlamydial antibodies.[15] The World Health Organization (WHO) Task Force on the Prevention and Management of Infertility found very similar results in a multicenter case–control study of women in Thailand, Slovenia, and Hungary reporting at least 12 months of infertility. Using an enzyme-linked immunosorbent assay (ELISA), antichlamydial antibodies were present in 71% (32/45) of women, with bilateral tubal occlusion detected by either HSG or laparoscopy, compared with this finding in 32% (31/96) of women with other etiologies for infertility.[16] Some investigators have compared seroprevalences with rates found among fertile women. Sellors et al compared the seroprevalence of antibodies to *C. trachomatis* – measured by enzyme immunoassay – of women with tubal factor infertility with the rates in two control cohorts, one comprising women undergoing tubal sterilization and the other control group undergoing hysterectomy.[17] Three of four women (32/43, 74.4%) with tubal factor infertility had serologic evidence of prior infection with *C. trachomatis*, whereas the seroprevalence among the two control groups was 34%. The authors concluded

Table 6.1. Antibodies to *Chlamydia trachomatis* and tubal factor infertility

	Antibodies to *C. trachomastis*		
	Infertile women		Fertile women
Study (first author)	Tubal factor	Non-tubal factor	
Moore,[13] 1982	73% (24/33)	0% (0/35)	–
Gump,[21] 1983	64% (34/53)	28% (38/134)	
Kane,[56] 1984	35.7% (25/70)	11.5% (6/52)	11% (22/200)
Conway,[57] 1984	75% (36/48)	31% (23/75)	47% (48/103)
Brunham,[32] 1985	72.2% (13/18)	8.6% (6/70)	22.4% (11/49)
Tjiam,[14] 1985	21.2% (7/33)	0% (0/20)	–
Sarov,[58] 1986	87% (26/30)	20% (10/50)	10% (10/100)
Robertson,[20] 1987	73% (35/48)	34% (26/77)	38% (25/63)
Sellors,[17] 1988	74.4% (32/43)	–	33.8% (26/77)
Garland,[59] 1990	65% (22/34)	22% (5/23)	–
Miettinen,[18] 1990	46% (32/69)	7% (2/28)	–
Meikle,[15] 1994	78.2% (68/87)	35.9% (47/131)	–
WHO,[16] 1995	71% (32/45)	32% (31/96)	–
Den Hartog,[60] 2005	54.2% (32/59)	7.9% (20/254)	

that women with evidence of prior chlamydial infection are approximately 6 times more likely to develop tubal factor infertility than women without prior infection. A compilation of studies examining the relationship between the presence of *C. trachomatis* antibodies and tubal factor infertility is presented in Table 6.1.

SEROLOGIC EVIDENCE OF PRIOR GONOCOCCAL INFECTION IN WOMEN WITH INFERTILITY

Fewer data are available linking serologic evidence of past *N. gonorrhoeae* infection and tubal factor infertility (Table 6.2). In the Dutch cohort of infertile women who underwent HSG and laparoscopy investigation to determine fallopian tube status, antibodies to *N. gonorrhoeae* pili antigens were assayed by ELISA.[14] Such antibodies were identified in 60.6% (20/33) women with fallopian tube damage and in 25% (5/20) infertile women with normal fallopian tubes. In the WHO study, antibodies to the alpha pili of *N. gonorrhoeae* were present in 62.2% (28/45) of infertile women with bilateral tubal occlusion compared with 37.5% (36/96) of women with other etiologies of infertility and without tubal occlusion ($p < 0.01$).[16] Miettinen et al identified serologic evidence of past gonococcal infection in 14% of women with infertility and fallopian tube abnormalities, whereas none of the infertile women without tubal damage had prior infection with *N. gonorrhoeae*.[18] Finally, among a cohort of 172 women in Thailand, serum antibodies to the alpha pili of *N. gonorrhoeae* were more

Table 6.2. Antibodies to *Neisseria gonorrhoeae* and tubal factor infertility

	Antibodies to *N. gonorrhoeae*		
	Infertile women		Fertile women
Study (first author)	Tubal factor	Non-tubal factor	
Tjiam,[14] 1985	21% (20/33)	0% (0/20)	–
Robertson,[20] 1987	2% (1/48)	3% (2/77)	16% (10/63)
Miettinen,[18] 1990	14% (11/76)	0% (0/28)	–
WHO,[16] 1995	62.2% (28/45)	37.5% (36/96)	–
Swasdio,[19] 1996	29.1% (16/55)	5.2% (3/58)	3.4% (2/59)

commonly seen among infertile women with tubal damage, as assessed by laparoscopy, than among infertile women with normal fallopian tubes and fertile controls.[19] However, Robertson et al, found no such relationship between serologic evidence of prior *N. gonorrhoeae* infection and infertility.[20]

SEROLOGIC EVIDENCE OF PRIOR SEXUALLY TRANSMITTED DISEASES IN WOMEN WITH ECTOPIC PREGNANCY

Another important late sequela of pelvic inflammatory disease is ectopic pregnancy. The relationship between previous infection with both *C. trachomatis* and ectopic pregnancy has been extensively evaluated by numerous investigations (Table 6.3). In 1983, Gump and colleagues examined 204 infertile women for an association between *C. trachomatis* and infertility.[21] Among the 76 women who subsequently became pregnant, 11 were diagnosed with an ectopic pregnancy. The prevalence of antichlamydial antibodies was greater among those with ectopic pregnancy (9/11, 82%) than among these previously infertile women who had an intrauterine pregnancy (19/65, 29%). Svensson and associates reported a case–control study of 112 women with ectopic pregnancies, of whom 56 were determined to have prior episode(s) of PID based on the presence of tubal adhesions at the time of surgery. Antichlamydial antibodies were found in the sera of 65% (73/112) women with ectopic pregnancies, which was statistically greater than the rate of 21% seen in a control group of pregnant women ($p < 0.001$).[22] Brunham et al divided a cohort of 50 women with ectopic pregnancy into two groups according to the presence or absence of ectopic pregnancy risk factors (tubal ligation or intrauterine contraceptive device), and compared these two groups with a group of 49 women with an intrauterine pregnancy.[23] Serologic evidence of prior *C. trachomatis* infection was present in 18% of women with known risk factors for ectopic pregnancy and 22% of women with intrauterine pregnancy. Thirty-two women with ectopic pregnancy in this cohort had no identifiable risk factor for ectopic pregnancy, and 56% of these women had the *C. trachomatis* antibody. Many in this group of women, lacking known risk factors for ectopic pregnancy, are believed to have previously experienced infection of the fallopian tubes. Most investigators examining the relationship between chlamydia and ectopic pregnancy used pregnant women as their control groups. Others have classified women with ectopic pregnancies into groups with and without prior PID based on the gross appearance of the fallopian tubes at the time of surgical therapy for ectopic pregnancy. Hartford et al demonstrated that antichlamydial antibodies were present in 50% (5/10) of women undergoing laparotomy for ectopic pregnancy who had evidence of damage of the contralateral fallopian tube, compared with 0% (0/14) of women with normal-appearing contralateral tubes.[24] Similarly, Sheffield et al reported nearly a doubling of the prevalence rate of antichlamydial antibodies among women with ectopic pregnancies who had damage of the contralateral fallopian tube, compared with women with ectopic pregnancies and normal tubes.[25] Thus, there is ample retrospective evidence associating prior infection with *C. trachomatis* and ectopic pregnancy.

The association between prior genital infection and ectopic pregnancy is also supported for *N. gonorrhoeae*, although the data are less robust. Robertson et al detected antibodies to gonococcal

Table 6.3. Antibodies to *Chlamydia trachomatis* and ectopic pregnancy

	Antibodies to *C. Trachomatis*	
Study (first author)	Ectopic pregnancy	Intrauterine pregnancy
Gump,[21] 1983	82% (9/11)	29% (19/65)
Svensson,[22] 1985	65% (73/112)	21% (18/86)
Brunham,[23] 1986	56% (18/32)	22% (11/49)
Robertson,[26] 1988	76% (38/50)	38% (19/50)
Walters,[61] 1988	82% (49/60)	58% (35/60)
Chow,[62] 1990	71%	39%
Kihlstrom,[63] 1990	78% (7/9)	13% (7/55)
Ville,[27] 1991	84% (38/45)	46% (34/74)
Chrysostomou,[64] 1992	76% (37/49)	46% (26/56)
Odland,[65] 1993	80% (24/30)	44% (22/50)
Mehanna,[66] 1995	21% (14/66)	12% (6/51)
Sziller,[67] 1998	52% (35/67)	27% (12/45)

pili in 32% (16/50) women with ectopic pregnancy and in only 4% (2/50) of fertile women with intrauterine pregnancies ($p < 0.001$).[26] In a cohort from Gabon, gonococcal pili antibodies were evident twice as often (49% vs 23%) in women with ectopic pregnancy than in pregnant women.[27]

SUBCLINICAL PELVIC INFECTION AND PREGNANCY LOSS

The impact of silent chlamydial infections on the success of embryo implantation has been investigated. Licciardi et al examined *C. trachomatis* immunoglobulin G (IgG) antibodies in the sera of 145 women undergoing in-vitro fertilization (IVF).[28] The presence of chlamydial IgG antibodies was strongly associated with spontaneous abortion. There were no active *C. trachomatis* infections detected in this cohort, yet antichlamydial antibodies were found in 69% (20/29) of women who experienced a spontaneous abortion compared with 24% (9/38) of women with successful pregnancies ($p < 0.001$). Work from the same laboratory demontrated a similar relationship when examining women with recurrent pregnancy loss.[29] High-titer antichlamydial antibodies were found in 13.5%, 12.8%, 12.1%, 41%, and 60% of women with zero, one, two, three, and four spontanous abortions, respectively ($p < 0.01$). The mechanism of pregnancy loss in these women remains to be determined. It is possible that a low-level persistent chlamydial infection, and its associated inflammation of the endometrium, affects implantation. Alternatively, immune activation could interfere with implantation, perhaps via production of antibody to the chlamydial heat shock protein (chlamydial Hsp 60), which has similar features to mammalian heat shock proteins. Such immune activation may cause an autoimmune type of response to the embryo. Lastly, remote infection may have caused irreparable damage to the endometrium, prohibiting successful implantation. Despite lacking a mechanistic explanation, the association between remote chlamydial infection and pregnancy loss suggests that upper genital tract inflammation creates a hostile environment for embryo implantation.

HISTOPATHOLOGY OF SUBCLINICAL PELVIC INFLAMMATORY DISEASE

Some of the most convincing data on the devastating impact of subclinical PID derives from pathologic analysis of the fallopian tubes in women with acute PID and subclinical PID. Patton et al examined the morphologic changes of the fallopian tube mucosa from women undergoing salpingostomy to repair distal tubal occlusion.[30] These women were divided into two groups – those with a history of salpingitis (overt PID) and those without a prior history of salpingitis (subclinical PID). The control group consisted of women with normal tubes undergoing hysterectomy. One-half of the women in each of the PID groups had serologic evidence of prior chlamydial infection, whereas antichlamydial antibodies were not identified in any of the control women. Fallopian tube damage was assessed by light, scanning electron, and transmission electron microscopy. Evidence of fallopian tube damage included flattened mucosal folds, deciliation, and damage to the secretory epithelial cells. The morphologic damage to the fallopian tube was very similar among women with acute PID and subclinical PID. Further, the characterization of the damage was strikingly similar, suggesting very similar pathophysiologic mechanisms. The investigators further assessed tubal damage by measuring ciliary beat frequency. The beat frequency was similar in the tubes from women with acute and subclinical PID. It was 3 times faster in the fallopian tubes of the control women than in the tubes from either the women with acute or silent PID. The results from this important work highlight that fallopian tube damage (as measured morphologically) from acute and subclinical PID is nearly identical and suggest that subclinical pelvic infections are responsible for substantial tubal damage and the potential for subsequent infertility.

LIMITED UTILITY OF HISTORY TAKING FOR INFECTION-MEDIATED INFERTILITY

As *N. gonorrhoeae* and *C. trachomatis* are important causes of acute PID, one can argue that the serologic data linking these two sexually transmitted organisms with infertility and ectopic pregnancy reflect prior episodes of acute PID. However, many women with infertility do not recall a history of acute PID. History taking has limited usefulness in the evaluation of women with tubal factor infertility, as many women with infection-mediated infertility do not recall a history of pelvic infection.[31] Among 204 infertile women studied for the relationship between *C. trachomatis* and infertility, only one-third recalled an illness that was consistent with acute PID.[21] In a cohort of 99 women undergoing infertility evaluation, Brunham et al noted that 60% of women with tubal factor infertility lacked a history of acute PID.[32] Similarly, in another study by Sellors et al, 69% of women with tubal factor infertility denied a history of acute PID, and recall of past PID was unrelated to chlamydial serology.[17] Subclinical disease appears to be common in women with prior gonococcal infection and subsequent infertility and ectopic pregnancy. In a study of Finnish women with infertility, only 45% of women with damaged fallopian tubes and antibodies to *N. gonorrhoeae* had a history of prior PID.[18] In the WHO study investigating the relationship between chlamydia and gonorrhea serology and infertility, two-thirds of women with bilateral tubal occlusion and serologic evidence of past gonococcal or chlamydial infection did not report any symptoms suggestive of acute PID.[16] Recall bias may explain some of these discrepant findings. Importantly, however, a high frequency of antibodies to *C. trachomatis* and *N. gonorrhoeae* in women with infertility or ectopic pregnancy reflects prior acute PID in only a minority of women. Rather, tubal damage that occurs as a result of chlamydial or gonococcal infections indicates that many cases of post-infectious tubal damage arise from subclinical PID rather than acute PID.

IMMUNOPATHOGENESIS OF FALLOPIAN TUBE DAMAGE FROM SUBCLINICAL PELVIC INFLAMMATORY DISEASE

The exact mechanisms of tubal damage resultant from upper genital tract infection remain undefined. Induction of delayed-type hypersensitivity to chlamydial antigens leads to persistent infection in the fallopian tubes with resultant tubal damage. Much attention has been focused on the immunologic response to chlamydial Hsp 60. Toth et al and Awad et al, as well as others, have demonstrated an association between antibodies to chlamydial Hsp 60 and tubal factor infertility.[33,34] *C. trachomatis* Hsp 10, a 10 kDa protein that is genetically linked to chlamydial Hsp 60, has also been shown to be more prevalent among women who were infertile due to hydrosalpinx than among women whose partners had male factor infertility.[35] Evidence of the importance of the host's response to chlamydial Hsp to the pathogenesis of PID extends from a strong association between antibodies to chlamydial Hsp 60 and Fitz-Hugh–Curtis syndrome. Among women with salpingitis, antibodies to chlamydial Hsp 60 were found more commonly among women with, than without, concomitant perihepatitis, suggesting that the chlamydial Hsp 60 antigen induces a severe inflammatory response.[36] On a population-based sample from northern Finland, Karinen demonstrated an association between antibodies to chlamydial Hsp 60 and Hsp 10 antigens and female subfertility, defined as time to first pregnancy exceeding 12 months.[37] Clearly, much more information is needed to delineate the pathogenesis of PID, and key to this understanding is the identification of the early immunologic responses to pelvic infection.

SUBCLINICAL PELVIC INFLAMMATORY DISEASE IN WOMEN WITH LOWER GENITAL TRACT INFECTION

As previously noted, there are substantial historical data demonstrating the association between subclinical PID and fallopian tube damage. Data showing a concurrent relationship between lower genital tract infection and subclinical PID are necessary as a first step to support the retrospective studies published to date. Several investigators have examined the relationship between lower genital tract infections and endometritis. In this section, we will explore the findings of concomitant upper genital tract inflammation in women with lower genital tract infection.

N. gonorrhoeae and *C. trachomatis* are considered key organisms in the pathogenesis of many cases of pelvic inflammatory disease. In a small study of 35 women with suspected cervicitis, Paavonen et al demonstrated that 14 (40%) had histologic endometritis, and that endometritis was correlated with the presence of chlamydial or gonococcal cervicitis.[38] Korn et al determined the rate of plasma cell endometritis in a cohort of 111 women with lower genital tract infection.[39] Using criteria of the presence of any plasma cells in the endometrial specimen, 56% (15/27) of women with gonorrhea and 57% (17/30) of women with chlamydia had plasma cell endometritis.

Wiesenfeld et al performed a cross-sectional study evaluating the relationship between lower genital tract infection and subclinical PID (Table 6.4).[40] Among 556 women between the ages of 15 and 30 enrolled from STD and ambulatory care clinics, 57 were diagnosed with cervical *N. gonorrhoeae* infection, 103 were infected with *C. trachomatis*, and 377 were diagnosed with bacterial vaginosis. None of the participants had clinical evidence of acute PID. All women underwent endometrial biopsy, and the diagnostic criteria for subclinical PID required the presence of neutrophils and plasma cells in the endometrial sample, as described by Kiviat et al.[41] Subclinical PID was detected in 27% of women with *C. trachomatis* infection and 26% of women diagnosed with gonorrhea. After controlling for potential confounding factors, the odds ratio for subclinical PID among women with chlamydial cervicitis was 3.4 (95% confidence interval (CI) 1.8, 6.3), whereas that for gonococcal cervicitis was 2.4 (95% CI 1.1, 5.1). In the absence of clinical evidence of acute PID, *C. trachomatis* and *N. gonorrhoeae* infection of the cervix is associated with concomitant upper genital tract inflammation.

Given the association between bacterial vaginosis and PID, several investigators have examined whether women with bacterial vaginosis are at risk for subclinical PID. Bacterial vaginosis-associated microorganisms have been isolated from the upper genital tract of women with pelvic inflammatory disease.[42] Korn et al investigated the relationship between bacterial vaginosis and plasma cell endometritis in a cohort of women without signs or symptoms of acute PID.[43] Twenty-two women with bacterial vaginosis and without clinical evidence of PID or infection with either *N. gonorrhoeae* or *C. trachomatis* were compared with a control group of 19 women without gonorrhea, chlamydia, or bacterial vaginosis. Plasma cell endometritis, defined as the presence of any plasma cells in the endometrial sample, was diagnosed in 10/22 (45%) of the women with bacterial vaginosis and in only 1/19 (5%) of controls ($p < 0.05$). Bacterial vaginosis-associated organisms were recovered from the endometria more frequently

Table 6.4. Association between lower genital tract infections and subclinical pelvic inflammatory disease

	Subclinical PID[a]		Plasma cell endometritis[b]	
	OR	95% CI	OR	95% CI
Vaginal smear:				
Bacterial vaginosis	2.7	1.02, 7.2	1.6	0.8, 3.2
Intermediate flora	1.5	0.4, 4.7	1.6	0.7, 3.7
Normal flora	Ref		Ref	
Gonorrhea (cervix)	2.4	1.1, 5.1	1.7	0.8, 3.5
Chlamydia (cervix)	3.4	1.8, 6.3	1.7	0.96, 3.1
Trichomoniasis	1.8	0.9, 3.8	0.9	0.4, 3.8

From Wiesenfeld et al.[40]

PID = pelvic inflammatory disease; OR = odds ratio; CI = confidence interval; Ref = reference group

[a] Subclinical PID defined on endometrial sampling as the presence of ≥5 neutrophils per 400× field of superficial epithelium AND ≥1 plasma cell per 100× field of endometrial stroma.

[b] Plasma cell endometritis defined on endometrial sampling in the presence of ≥1 plasma cell per 100× field of endometrial stroma.

from those women with bacterial vaginosis than from those without bacterial vaginosis. Moreover, these organisms were isolated nearly twice as often from women with plasma cell endometritis as from those without endometritis, suggesting that the microbiologic findings from the endometrium did not reflect contamination from the lower genital tract. In a study using a larger cohort of women, published later by the same group of investigators, comprising women attending an inner-city hospital or an STD clinic, 24 of 57 women with bacterial vaginosis (and negative tests for *N. gonorrhoeae* and *C. trachomatis*) had plasma cell endometritis.[39] Only 3 of 24 women without any lower genital tract infection had plasma cell endometritis. In a cohort of women without clinical evidence of acute PID, Wiesenfeld et al identified plasma cell endometritis in 39% (148/377) of women with bacterial vaginosis, which was significantly greater than the 29% rate of endometritis in women without bacterial vaginosis ($p < 0.05$).[40] When controlling for confounding variables, plasma cell endometritis was not related to bacterial vaginosis. However, using stricter histopathologic criteria (the presence of both neutrophils and plasma cells), endometritis was statistically associated with bacterial vaginosis. As with the sexually transmitted pathogens *C. trachomatis* and *N. gonorrhoeae*, bacterial vaginosis is not only implicated in the pathogenesis of acute PID but also suspect in the development of subclinical PID.

ENDOMETRIAL PATHOLOGY IN SUBCLINICAL PELVIC INFLAMMATORY DISEASE

Whereas direct visualization of the pelvic structures is widely considered the gold standard diagnostic test for confirming the presence of PID, endometrial histopathology is becoming a popular tool to detect upper genital tract inflammation. Endometrial biopsy is less invasive and less costly than laparoscopy, and has far fewer risks. Its main limitation is that pathologic interpretation takes at least 1–2 days, precluding its use to timely influence therapeutic management. However, its utility in confirming or refuting the presence of upper genital tract inflammation is a considerable advantage. Investigators have used several different histologic criteria to define endometritis (i.e. upper genital tract inflammation). Some investigators rely solely on the presence of a single plasma cell in the entire endometrial specimen.[43–45] Outcomes to correlate with histology in women with subclinical PID are lacking. Therefore, attention should be directed to studies of endometrial histology in women with laparoscopy-confirmed acute PID. Paavonen et al compared endometrial pathology with laparoscopy-confirmed PID among 27 women with suspected acute PID. Two-thirds of the women had acute salpingitis evident at laparoscopy.[38] The sensitivity of the finding of plasma cells for the diagnosis of acute PID was 89%, with a specificity of 67%.

The most comprehensive evaluation of endometrial histopathology in women with pelvic inflammatory disease has been performed by Kiviat et al.[41] Sixty-nine women with clinically suspected acute PID underwent endometrial biopsy, laparoscopy, and endosalpingeal cytology along with cultures from the cervix, endometrium, fallopian tube, and cul-de-sac. Several histologic features of the endometrium were analyzed according to the presence of upper genital tract infection and salpingitis. The best histologic criteria that predicted upper genital tract infection and salpingitis were the combined presence of at least 5 neutrophils per 400× field in the endometrial surface epithelium and one or more plasma cells per 120× field of endometrial stroma. These stringent criteria had a sensitivity of 92% and a specificity of 87% for predicting pelvic inflammatory disease. A number of studies utilizing endometrial histology in PID studies have used these criteria to diagnose endometritis.[40,46–48]

Although the best validated criteria for the diagnosis of histologic endometritis have been those outlined by Kiviat et al, as noted above, a number of different histopathologic criteria have been used in the literature to document upper genital tract inflammation. The presence of plasma cells in the endometrium, referred to as plasma cell endometritis, has been associated with lower genital tract infection in cohorts of women at risk for

STDs.[39,43] Paukku et al studied the association between *C. trachomatis* infection and plasma cell endometritis by reexamining endometrial biopsy specimens from women originally diagnosed with and without plasma cell endometritis.[49] The endometrial tissue was processed with methyl green–pyronin, a stain that highlights plasma cells. Detection of *C. trachomatis* within the biopsy specimen was performed using DNA extraction and polymerase chain reaction (PCR) of paraffinized endometrial tissue to amplify *C. trachomatis* DNA and by immunohistochemistry. Overall, 5/21 (24%) of samples with plasma cell endometritis, determined by the presence of at least one plasma cell per 120× field, were positive for *C. trachomatis*, compared with 1/28 (4%) of specimens that did not have plasma cell endometritis. This study was limited by its small size and by potential selection bias. Furthermore, over 50% of the women whose biopsies revealed plasma cell endometritis had a fever > 38°C and a similar percentage had lower abdominal pain, suggesting that many of these women did not have subclinical PID but rather may have been presenting with acute PID. Contradicting these results, Stern et al concluded that there was no concordance between the presence of plasma cells in the endometrium and chlamydial infection in a study using nested PCR to detect the presence of *C. trachomatis*.[45]

The question that remains to be asked is whether endometrial plasma cells are a normal finding in women without clinical evidence of pelvic inflammatory disease, or whether their presence signifies a subclinical inflammatory process. Plasma cells appear with an eccentric nucleus with a paranuclear pale-staining area and a clumped chromatin pattern (Figure 6.3). Traditionally, plasma cells have not been considered as normal constituents of the endometrium.[50] The presence of plasma cells in the endometrial sample may be unappreciated, perhaps because their appearance is similar to lymphocytes and stromal cells. As such, some advocate the use of special stains, particularly methyl green–pyronin, to highlight the presence of plasma cells. The presence of plasma cells in the endometrium is readily evident using methyl green–pyronin stain. There is recent evidence suggesting that plasma cells are commonly found in the endometrium, and their presence, in the absence of other inflammatory cells (e.g. neutrophils), may not signify an ongoing inflammatory process. In a cohort of women 3 months postpartum, 31% of 316 specimens demonstrated plasma cell endometritis.[51] This high rate of plasma cell

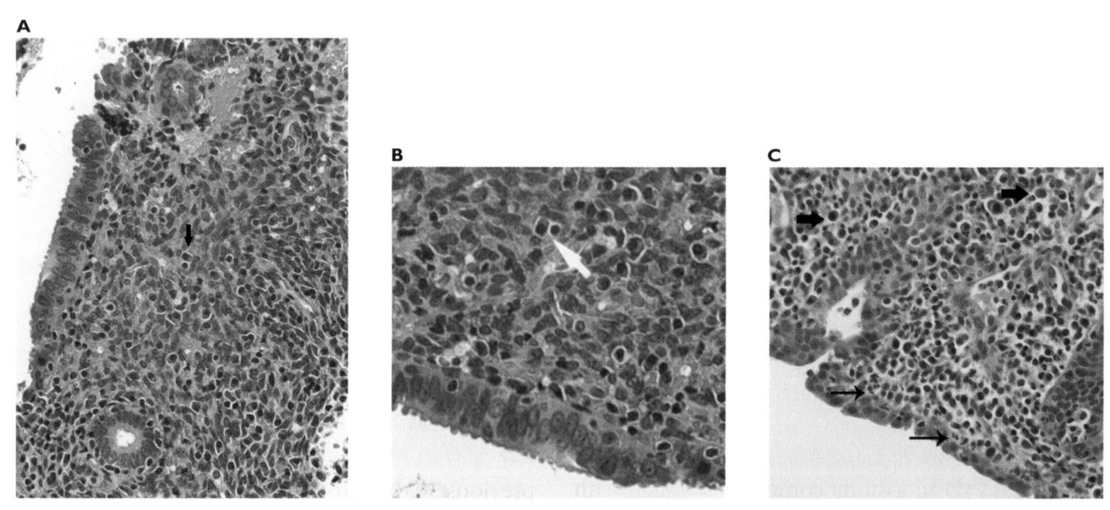

Figure 6.3 Endometrial histopathology in a woman with gonococcal cervicitis. A. lower power field- numerous neutrophils can be seen. B. high power field demonstrating plasma cells within the endometrial stroma (white arrow). C. Neutrophils in the submucosa (narrow arrow) and plasma cells in the endometrial stroma (wide arrows) are evident.

endometritis in a cohort of women 3 months postpartum raises the suspicion that this endometrial histopathologic diagnosis may not represent a pathogenic process. In Wiesenfeld's study of 556 women without clinical evidence of acute PID, infection with *N. gonorrhoeae, C. trachomatis*, and bacterial vaginosis was associated with endometritis when the criteria of the combined presence of neutrophils and plasma cells was used.[40] However, these lower genital tract infections were not associated with plasma cell endometritis. To determine if endometrial plasma cells are found in healthy women, we performed a cross-sectional study of women with proven fertility undergoing tubal ligation and, as such, deemed to be at low risk for PID.[52] At the time of surgery, an endometrial biopsy was performed and the tissue was stained with hematoxylin–eosin and methyl green–pyronin, the latter to highlight the presence of plasma cells. None of the women had laparoscopic evidence of acute PID. Endometrial plasma cells were identified in one-third of the asymptomatic fertile women in our cohort, and were not associated with lower genital tract infection, including bacterial vaginosis. Thus, plasma cells can be commonly found in endometrial samples from healthy women, and their presence may not represent ongoing upper genital tract inflammation. Histopathologic changes in the endometrium of women with subclinical PID need to be correlated with long-term outcomes (i.e. infertility) to determine the optimum histologic criteria of subclinical PID.

CLINICAL FINDINGS IN WOMEN WITH SUBCLINICAL PELVIC INFLAMMATORY DISEASE

Given the epidemic proportions of women with bacterial vaginosis, gonorrhea, or chlamydia, there are probably vastly more women with subclinical PID than with acute PID. Yet, the identification of women with subclinical PID has remained elusive. Cates et al attempted to identify clinical predictors of subclinical PID in a study comparing women with tubal infertility due to PID (overt PID), women with tubal infertility without a history of PID (atypical or subclinical PID), and women without infertility or PID.[53] Sociodemographic characteristics of women with subclinical PID were more similar to those of fertile women than of women with post-PID infertility. Behavioral characteristics such as number of sexual partners, illicit drug use, and douching were identified in women with subclinical PID at rates intermediate between the rates in fertile women and women with infertility due to overt PID. We similarly compared women with acute PID, subclinical PID, and controls (women without upper genital tract inflammation).[54] Many demographic characteristics, such as age, race, and education, of women with subclinical PID were found at intermediate rates compared with women with acute PID and women without PID. Despite these findings, there are no strong sociodemographic predictors that can be used to identify women with subclinical PID.

PID can present clinically with a range of symptomatology, and clinical findings have limited predictive value in the diagnosis of PID.[55] It has been suggested that women with subclinical PID may have subtle symptoms and signs of PID that may alert the provider of an ongoing inflammatory process of the endometrium and/or fallopian tubes. We explored the symptomatology and physical findings of women with subclinical PID in comparison with symptoms of women with acute PID.[54] Subclinical PID was identified in a cohort of women without the diagnostic symptoms of acute PID but who had lower genital tract infection (gonorrhea, chlamydia, or bacterial vaginosis) and histologic evidence of upper genital tract inflammation. None of these women met the clinical definition of acute PID outlined in the CDC's 1998 STD treatment guidelines.[7] These women were compared with women with symptoms of acute PID, confirmed by the presence of endometrial inflammation on histology. A group of women without endometrial inflammation was also used as a comparative group (Table 6.5). The symptomatology of women with subclinical PID closely resembled that of women without endometritis, aside from a slightly higher rate of self-reporting of abdominal pain within the previous 30 days from enrollment. As expected, the symptoms reported by women with acute PID were far more common than in women with subclinical PID.

Table 6.5. Symptoms among women with acute pelvic inflammatory disease (PID) and women with subclinical PID

Symptom	Acute PID $n = 168$	Subclinical PID $n = 75$	Controls (no endometritis) $n = 360$	Acute vs subclinical PID OR (95% CI)	Subclinical PID vs controls OR (95% CI)	p (trend)
Urinary frequency	81 (48%)	8 (11%)	48 (13%)	9.0 (3.9, 21.5)	0.8 (0.2, 1.8)	<0.001
Abnormal discharge	103 (61%)	25 (33%)	114 (32%)	3.8 (2.0, 7.0)	1.1 (0.6, 1.9)	<0.001
Intermenstrual bleeding	69 (41%)	11 (15%)	43 (12%)	4.1 (1.9, 88)	1.2 (0.6, 2.7)	<0.001
Bleeding with sex	22 (13%)	5 (7%)	20 (6%)	2.1 (0.7, 7.4)	1.2 (0.4, 3.6)	<0.003
Abdominal pain <30 days	93 (55%)	10 (13%)	24 (7%)	8.1 (3.7, 18)	2.2 (0.9, 5.0)	<0.001
Low back pain	62 (37%)	7 (9%)	42 (12%)	5.7 (2.4, 15.5)	0.8 (0.3, 1.9)	0.4

From Wiesenfeld et al.[54]
OR = odds ratio; CI = confidence interval.

We also examined physical findings and microbiologic results in women with subclinical PID, women with acute PID, and women without endometritis (Table 6.6). Adnexal tenderness was more common in women with subclinical PID than in women without subclinical PID (11% vs 3%, OR = 4.7; 95% CI 1.6, 13.8). Pelvic tenderness was uniformly present in women with acute PID. Although 4–5 times more common in women with subclinical PID than in women without subclinical PID, pelvic organ tenderness was nonetheless uncommon in women with subclinical PID. The infrequent finding of cervical, uterine, or adnexal tenderness demonstrates that the great majority of women neither experience symptoms nor demonstrate findings on physical examination suggestive of PID. Given the absence of symptoms and signs of PID, the diagnosis of subclinical PID relies on endometrial histopathology. Unfortunately, endometrial biopsy is not available in a timely manner to influence diagnosis. The hidden nature of subclinical PID makes the identification of this disease very difficult, even by experienced clinicians.

Microbiologic findings in women with subclinical PID, compared with those in women with acute PID, may provide insight on the pathogenesis of subclinical PID. Rates of endometrial recovery of *C. trachomatis* and *N. gonorrhoeae* are intermediate between the rates identified in women with acute PID and women without PID.[54] In the comparative study of women with acute PID, subclinical PID, and without PID, the recovery rates of *C. trachomatis* from the endometrium were 20%, 10%, and 2%, respectively (p for trend < 0.001). Rates for isolation of *N. gonorrhoeae* from the endometrium in these 3 groups of women were 9%, 3%, and 0.3% (p for trend < 0.001). These microbiologic data regarding intermediate rates of recovery of *N. gonorrhoeae*

Table 6.6. Physical findings in women with acute pelvic inflammatory disease and subclinical PID

Finding	Acute PID $n = 168$	Subclinical PID $n = 75$	Controls (no endometritis) $n = 360$	p (trend)	Subclinical PID vs controls OR (95% CI)
Cervical motion tenderness	155 (93%)	8 (11%)	10 (3%)	<0.001	4.2 (1.4, 12)
Uterine tenderness	160 (95%)	11 (15%)	12 (3%)	<0.001	5.0 (2.0, 12.7)
Adnexal tenderness	131 (78%)	8 (11%)	9 (3%)	<0.001	4.7 (1.6, 13.8)

From Wiesenfeld et al.[54]
OR = odds ratio; CI = confidence interval.

and *C. trachomatis* support the hypothesis that the pathogenesis of acute and subclinical PID is similar.

The difficulty in detecting ongoing upper genital tract inflammation in women with lower genital tract infection is appreciable. Even with a heightened sense of suspicion for upper tract disease, most women with subclinical PID would not be identified merely by reported symptomatology or clinical findings. The diagnosis of subclinical PID rests on the identification of inflammation in the upper genital tract. This is most easily accomplished using endometrial sampling techniques. Endometrial pathology requires skilled pathologists. Further, the results are not available in a timely manner to influence clinical management at the time of presentation. As such, further work is needed to elucidate predictors of upper genital tract inflammation in an effort to achieve timely diagnosis of subclinical PID. Innovative techniques are needed to identify those women who have subclinical PID, which may provide prognostic information to the patient and may influence antibiotic management.

ENDOMETRITIS IN HIV-INFECTED WOMEN

It may be expected that women with immune dysfunction may be at risk for upper genital tract inflammation. Eckert et al characterized histologic endometritis in a cohort of human immunodeficiency virus (HIV)-infected women who did not have clinical evidence of acute PID.[47] None of the 42 women enrolled in the study were infected with *C. trachomatis* or *N. gonorrhoeae*, and 29% had bacterial vaginosis. Histologic endometritis was indentified in 16/42 (38%) of the cohort, indicating a high rate of subclinical PID in this cohort of HIV-infected women. These results suggest that subclinical PID in HIV-infected women may be related to pathogens other than (or in addition to) *N. gonorrhoeae* and *C. trachomatis*, or that these women may have altered immune function predisposing to upper genital tract inflammation. Further work is needed to determine the impact of HIV on subclinical PID and the sequelae of subclinical PID in HIV-infected women.

DO ANTIBIOTICS CLEAR ENDOMETRIAL INFLAMMATION?

Further evidence of the abnormal nature of histologic endometritis in women without PID stems from a treatment study of women with subclinical PID by Eckert et al.[48] This prospective trial enrolled women without clinical evidence of PID who presented for evaluation at an STD clinic or who had abnormal uterine bleeding. Endometrial biopsies were performed prior to oral antibiotic treatment, which consisted of single doses of cefixime and azithromycin, and a 1-week course of metronidazole. Of the 48 women who had endometrial biopsies before and after treatment, 18 had histologic endometritis before treatment, whereas only 2 had endometritis following therapy ($p < 0.001$). These results demonstrate that antibiotic therapy can eliminate inflammatory changes of the upper genital tract in women without clinical evidence of acute PID. Moreover, these data indicate that such histologic changes are not normal findings in otherwise healthy women, and imply that these histopathalogic findings represent ongoing upper genital tract inflammation.

REPRODUCTIVE SEQUELAE OF SUBCLINICAL PELVIC INFLAMMATORY DISEASE

The data available to date on subclinical PID reveal that this disorder is commonly found in women with seemingly uncomplicated lower genital tract infection. Moreover, the presenting symptoms are nearly uniformly vague and mostly absent. Likewise, physical findings of pelvic infection are absent, making the identification of this condition difficult. There are substantial retrospective data that strongly imply that subclinical PID is associated with subsequent fallopian tube damage, as many women with tubal factor infertility or ectopic pregnancy have evidence of remote infection. Current prospective studies are underway examining whether women with subclinical PID are at risk for tubal factor infertility. Preliminary data indicate that women with subclinical PID are at increased risk for subsequent involuntary infertility (HC Wiesenfeld, unpublished data) Should this hypothesis be proven in a prospective manner, subsequent research would be focused on determining the most favorable therapeutic regimen to optimize fertility in women with subclinical PID. Subclinical PID is present in a substantial proportion of women with otherwise uncomplicated gonococcal or chlamydial cervicitis and bacterial vaginosis. Given the STD epidemic around the world, far more women may be at risk for infertility from subclinical PID than from acute PID.

REFERENCES

1. Westrom L, Joesoef R, Reynolds G, et al. Pelvic inflammatory disease and fertility. A cohort study of 1844 women with laparoscopically verified disease and 657 control women with normal laparoscopic results. Sex Transm Dis 1992;19:185–92.
2. Rolfs RT, Galaid EI, Zaidi AA. Pelvic inflammatory disease: trends in hospitalizations and office visits, 1979 through 1988. Am J Obstet Gynecol 1992;166(3):983–90.
3. Centers for Disease Control and Prevention. Sexually Transmitted Disease Surveillance, 2003. Atlanta, GA, 2004.
4. Hessol NA, Priddy FH, Bolna G, et al. Management of pelvic inflammatory disease by primary care physicians: a comparison with Centers for Disease Control and Prevention guidelines. Sex Transm Dis 1996;23:157–63.
5. Grimes DA, Blount JH, Patrick J, Washington AE. Antibiotic treatment of pelvic inflammatory disease. Trends among private physicians in the United States, 1966 through 1983. JAMA 1986;256(23):3223–6.
6. Sorbye IK, Jerve F, Staff AC. Reduction in hospitalized women with pelvic inflammatory disease in Oslo over the past decade. Acta Obstet Gynecol Scand 2005;84(3):290–6.
7. Centers for Disease Control and Prevention. 1998 Guidelines for treatment of sexually transmitted diseases. MMWR 1998;47(RR-1):1–116.
8. Centers for Disease Control and Prevention. Sexually transmitted diseases treatment guidelines 2002. MMWR 2002;51(No. RR-6):1–78.
9. Henry-Suchet J, Loffredo V. Chlamydia and mycoplasma genital infection in salpingitis and tubal sterility. Lancet 1980;i(8167):539.
10. Henry-Suchet J, Catalan F, Loffredo V, et al. *Chlamydia trachomatis* associated with chronic inflammation in abdominal specimens from women selected for tuboplasty. Fertil Steril 1981;36:599–605.
11. Sweet RL, Schachter J, Robbie MO. Failure of beta-lactam antibiotics to eradicate *Chlamydia trachomatis* in the endometrium despite apparent clinical cure of acute salpingitis. JAMA 1983;250(19):2641–5.
12. Patton DL, Askienazy-Elbhar M, Henry-Suchet J, et al. Detection of *Chlamydia trachomatis* in fallopian tube tissue in women with postinfectious tubal infertility. Am J Obstet Gynecol 1994;171(1):95–101.
13. Moore DE, Spadoni LR, Foy HM, et al. Increased frequency of serum antibodies to *Chlamydia trachomatis* in infertility due to distal tubal occlusion. Lancet 1982;2(8298):574–7.
14. Tjiam KH, Zeilmaker GH, Alberda AT, et al. Prevalence of antibodies to *Chlamydia trachomatis, Neisseria gonorrhoeae,* and *Mycoplasma hominis* in infertile women. Genitourin Med 1985;61:175–8.
15. Meikle SF, Calonge BN, Zhang X, et al. *Chlamydia trachomatis* antibody titers and hysterosalpingography in predicting tubal disease in infertility patients. Fertil Steril 1994;62(2):305–12.
16. World Health Organization Task Force on the Prevention and Management of Infertility. Tubal infertility: serologic relationship to post chlamydial and gonococcal infection. Sex Transm Dis 1995;22:71–7.
17. Sellors JW, Mahony JB, Chernesky MA, Rath DJ. Tubal factor infertility: an association with prior chlamydial and asymptomatic salpingitis. Fertil Steril 1988;49:451–7.
18. Miettinen A, Heinonen PK, Teisala K, et al. Serologic evidence for the role of *Chlamydia trachomatis, Neisseria gonorrhoeae,* and *Mycoplasma hominis* in the etiology of tubal factor infertility and ectopic pregnancy. Sex Transm Dis 1990;17:10–14.
19. Swasdio K, Rugpao S, Tansathit T, et al. The association of *Chlamydia trachomatis*/gonococcal infection and tubal factor infertility. J Obstet Gynaecol Res 1996;22:331–40.
20. Robertson JN, Ward ME, Conway D, Caul EO. Chlamydial and gonococcal antibodies in sera of infertile women with tubal obstruction. J Clin Pathol 1987;40:377–83.
21. Gump DW, Gibson M, Ashikaga T. Evidence of prior pelvic inflammatory disease and its relationship to *Chlamydia trachomatis* antibody and intrauterine contraceptive device use in infertile women. Am J Obstet Gynecol 1983;146:153–9.
22. Svensson L, Mardh PA, Ahlgren M, Nordenskjold M. Ectopic pregnancy and antibodies to *Chlamydia trachomatis.* Fertil Steril 1985;44:313–17.
23. Brunham RC, Binns B, McDowell J, Paraskevas M. *Chlamydia trachomatis* infection in women with ectopic pregnancy. Obstet Gynecol 1986;67:722–6.
24. Hartford SL, Silva PD, diZerega GS, Yonekura ML. Serologic evidence of prior chlamydial infection in patients with tubal ectopic pregnancy and contralateral tubal disease. Fertil Steril 1987;47:118–21.
25. Sheffield PA, Moore DE, Voigt LF, et al. The association between *Chlamydia trachomatis* serology amd pelvic damage in women with tubal ectopic gestations. Fertil Steril 1993;60:970–5.
26. Robertson JN, Hogston P, Ward ME. Gonococcal and chlamydial antibodies in ectopic and intrauterine pregnancy. Br J Obstet Gynaecol 1988;95:711–16.
27. Ville Y, Leruez M, Glowaczower E, et al. The role of *Chlamydia trachomatis* and *Neisseria gonorrhoeae* in the aetiology of ectopic pregnancy in Gabon. Br J Obstet Gynaecol 1991;98:1260–6.
28. Licciardi F, Grifo JA, Rosenwaks Z, Witkin SS. Relation between antibodies to *Chlamydia trachomatis* and spontaneous abortion following in vitro fertilization. J Assist Reprod Genet 1992;9:207–10.
29. Witkin SS, Ledger WJ. Antibodies to *Chlamydia trachomatis* in sera of women with recurrent spontaneous abortions. Am J Obstet Gynecol 1992;167(1):135–9.
30. Patton DL, Moore DE, Spadoni LR, et al. A comparison of the fallopian tube's response to overt and silent salpingitis. Obstet Gynecol 1989;73(4):622–30.
31. Hubacher D, Grimes D, Lara-Ricalde R, et al. The limited clinical usefulness of taking a history in the evaluation of women with tubal factor infertility. Fertil Steril 2004;81:6–10.
32. Brunham RC, Maclean IW, Binns B, Peeling RW. *Chlamydia trachomatis*: its role in tubal infertility. J Infect Dis 1985;152:1275–82.
33. Toth M, Jeremias J, Ledger WJ, Witkin SS. In vitro tumor necrosis factor production in women with salpingitis. Surg Gynecol Obstet 1992;124:359–62.

34. Awad MR, El-Gamel A, Hasleton P, et al. Genotypic variation in the transforming growth factor-beta 1 gene: association with transforming factor-beta 1 production, fibrotic lung disease, and graft fibrosis after lung transplantation. Transplantation 1998;66:1014–20.
35. Spandorfer SD, Neuer A, LaVerda D, et al. Previously undetected *Chlamydia trachomatis* infection, immunity to heat shock proteins and tubal occlusion in women undergoing in-vitro fertilization. Hum Reprod 1999;14(1):60–4.
36. Money DM, Hawes SE, Eschenbach DA, et al. Antibodies to the chlamydial 60 kd heat-shock protein are associated with laparoscopically confirmed perihepatitis. Am J Obstet Gynecol 1997;176(4):870–7.
37. Karinen L, Pouta A, Hartikainen AL, et al. Antibodies to *Chlamydia trachomatis* heat shock proteins Hsp60 and Hsp10 and subfertility in general population at age 31. Am J Reprod Immunol 2004;52(5):291–7.
38. Paavonen J, Kiviat N, Brunham RC, et al. Prevalence and manifestations of endometritis among women with cervicitis. Am J Obstet Gynecol 1985;152(3):280–6.
39. Korn AP, Hessol NA, Padian NS, et al. Risk factors for plasma cell endometritis among women with cervical *Neisseria gonorrhoeae*, cervical *Chlamydia trachomatis*, or bacterial vaginosis. Am J Obstet Gynecol 1998;178(5):987–90.
40. Wiesenfeld HC, Hillier SL, Krohn MA, et al. Lower genital tract infection and endometritis: insight into subclinical pelvic inflammatory disease. Obstet Gynecol 2002;100(3):456–63.
41. Kiviat NB, Wolner-Hanssen P, Eschenbach DA, et al. Endometrial histopathology in patients with culture-proved upper genital tract infection and laparoscopically diagnosed acute salpingitis. Am J Surg Pathol 1990;14:167–75.
42. Sweet RL, Schachter J, Landers DV, et al. Treatment of hospitalized patients with acute pelvic inflammatory disease: comparison of cefotetan plus doxycycline and cefoxitin plus doxycycline. Am J Obstet Gynecol 1988;158(3 Pt 2):736–41.
43. Korn AP, Bolan G, Padian N, et al. Plasma cell endometritis in women with symptomatic bacterial vaginosis. Obstet Gynecol 1995;85:387–90.
44. Korn AP, Landers DV, Green JR, Sweet RL. Pelvic inflammatory disease in human immunodeficiency virus-infected women. Obstet Gynecol 1993;82(5):765–8.
45. Stern RA, Svoboda-Newman SM, Frank TS. Analysis of chronic endometritis for *Chlamydia trachomatis* by polymerase chain reaction. Hum Pathol 1996;27(10):1085–8.
46. Eckert LO, Hawes SE, Wolner-Hanssen PK, et al. Endometritis: the clinical–pathologic syndrome. Am J Obstet Gynecol 2002;186(4):690–5.
47. Eckert LO, Watts DH, Thwin SS, et al. Histologic endometritis in asymptomatic human immunodeficiency virus-infected women: characterization and effect of antimicrobial therapy. Obstet Gynecol 2003;102:962–9.
48. Eckert LO, Thwin SS, Hillier SL, Kiviat NB, Eschenbach DA. The antimicrobial treatment of subacute endometritis: a proof of concept study. Am J Obstet Gynecol 2004;190(2):305–13.
49. Paukku M, Puolakkainen M, Paavonen T, Paavonen J. Plasma cell endometritis is associated with *Chlamydia trachomatis* infection. Am J Clin Pathol 1999;112:211–15.
50. Sherman ME, Mazur MT, Kurman RJ. Benign diseases of the endometrium. In: Kurman RJ, ed. Blaustein's Pathology of the Female Genital Tract, 5th edn. New York: Springer-Verlag, 2002:421–67.
51. Andrews WW, Hauth JC, Cliver S, et al. Endometrial microbial colonization and plasma cell endometritis are common three months postpartum. In: 20th Annual Meeting of the Society for Maternal–Fetal Medicine, Miami Beach, FL; 2000.
52. Achilles SL, Amortegui AJ, Wiesenfeld HC. Endometrial plasma cells: do they indicate subclinical pelvic inflammatory disease? Sex Transm Dis 2005;32(3):185–8.
53. Cates W Jr, Joesoef MR, Goldman MB. Atypical pelvic inflammatory disease: can we identify clinical predictors? Am J Obstet Gynecol 1993;169(2 Pt 1):341–6.
54. Wiesenfeld HC, Sweet RL, Ness RB, et al. Comparison of acute and subclinical pelvic inflammatory disease. Sex Transm Dis 2005;32(7):400–5.
55. Kahn JG, Walker CK, Washington AE, et al. Diagnosing pelvic inflammatory disease. A comprehensive analysis and considerations for developing a new model. JAMA 1991;266(18):2594–604.
56. Kane JL, Woodland RM, Forsey T, et al. Evidence of chlamydial infection in infertile women with and without fallopian tube obstruction. Fertil Steril 1984;42(6):843–8.
57. Conway D, Glazener CM, Caul EO, et al. Chlamydial serology in fertile and infertile women. Lancet 1984;8370:191–3.
58. Sarov I, Kleinman D, Holcberg G, et al. Specific IgG and IgA antibodies to Chlamydia trachomatis in infertile women. Int J Fertil 1986;31(3):193–7.
59. Garland SM, Lees MI, Skurrie IJ. Chlamydia trachomatis – role in tubal infertility. Aust NZ J Obstet Gynaecol 1990;30:83–6.
60. den Hartog JE, Land JA, Stassen FR, et al. Serological markers of persistent *C. trachomatis* infections in women with tubal factor subfertility. Hum Reprod 2005;20:986–90.
61. Walters MD, Eddy CA, Gibbs RS, et al. Antibodies to *Chlamydia trachomatis* and risk for tubal pregnancy. Am J Obstet Gynecol 1988;159:942–6.
62. Chow JM, Yonekura ML, Richwald GA, et al. The association between *Chlamydia trachomatis* and ectopic pregnancy. A matched-pair, case–control study. JAMA 1990;263(23):3164–7.
63. Kihlstrom E, Lindgren R, Ryden G. Antibodies to *Chlamydia trachomatis* in women with infertility, pelvic inflammatory disease and ectopic pregnancy. Eur J Obstet Gynecol Reprod Biol 1990;35:199–204.
64. Chrysostomou M, Karafyllidi P, Papadimitriou V, et al. Serum antibodies to *Chlamydia trachomatis* in women with ectopic pregnancy, normal pregnancy or salpingitis. Eur J Obstet Gynecol Reprod Biol 1992;44:101–5.
65. Odland JO, Anestad G, Rasmussen S, et al. Ectopic pregnancy and chlamydial serology. Int J Gynecol Obstet 1993;43:271–5.
66. Mehanna MTR, Rizk MA, Eweiss NYM, et al. Chlamydial serology among patients with tubal factor infertility and ectopic pregnancy in Alexandria Egypt. Sex Transm Dis 1995;22:317–21.
67. Sziller I, Witkin SS, Ziegert M, et al. Serological responses of patients with ectopic pregnancy to epitopes of the *Chlamydia trachomatis* 60 kDa heat shock protein. Hum Reprod 1998;13:1088–93.

7. Tubo-Ovarian Abscess

Richard L. Sweet

INTRODUCTION

Pelvic inflammatory disease (PID) is primarily an ascending infection with intracanalicular spread of microorganisms from the cervix and/or vagina to involve the endometrial cavity, fallopian tubes, and peritoneal cavity.[1] The ovary's proximity to the distal fallopian tube makes it accessible for spread of infection from the fallopian tube, especially at the time of ovulation, when a portal of entry into the deep ovarian tissue is available.[2] The resultant inflammatory response may wall off the infectious process involving the ovary and distal tube and initiate the tissue destruction involving the fallopian tube and ovary, which leads to formation of a tubo-ovarian abscess. Initially, abscess formation is a beneficial process as it localizes the infectious process. However, unrecognized and untreated abscesses may lead to substantial morbidity and in some instances mortality, especially with rupture of the abscess.

Tubo-ovarian abscess (TOA) is a well-recognized early complication or sequela of acute PID.[3] Although the prevalence of TOA among hospitalized patients with acute PID is generally reported to be 10–15%, rates as high as 34% have been reported.[4–11]These prevalence rates were derived to a large extent prior to the recognition that acute PID is a polymicrobial disease in which anaerobic bacteria play a major role. However, even with the introduction of many new and potent broad-spectrum antimicrobial agents and the recommendation for polymicrobic coverage with antimicrobial agents that are effective against *Neisseria gonorrhoeae*, *Chlamydia trachomatis*, and the bacterial vaginosis-associated microorganisms, including Gram-negative anaerobic bacteria, TOA remains a not infrequent diagnostic and therapeutic challenge for physicians providing health care to women.

Although TOA is generally believed to be an end stage in the progression of acute PID,[9,10] several studies have demonstrated that only one-third to one-half of patients presenting with TOAs acknowledge a prior history of PID.[6,10,12,13] There are two possible explanations for this finding: either acute PID may progress rapidly to abscess formation during the initial infection, probably dependent upon which microorganisms are involved, or subclinical PID is more frequent than suspected (see Chapter 6).

No specific risk factors for the development of TOA have been identified.[2] Studies in the 1970s, when the primary etiologic agent of PID was believed to be *N. gonorrhoeae*, which used doxycycline as single-agent therapy for PID, demonstrated the development of TOA during initial antibiotic treatment.[14] This occurrence suggested that failure to provide antimicrobial coverage for anaerobic bacteria (especially Gram-negative rods such as *Bacteroides* and *Prevotella* species) was a factor in the abscess formation. Whereas early retrospective studies reported a high rate (20–54%) of intrauterine device (IUD) use among patients with TOA,[15–17] more recent studies failed to confirm such an association.[6,12,18] The presence of actinomycetes, most commonly *Actinomyces israelii*, has been proposed as a predisposing factor for the development of TOAs.[23] Burkman et al reported that 7/8 (87.5%) PID patients with actinomycetes present had a TOA, whereas only 11/38 (28.9%) PID patients without this organism were diagnosed with a TOA.[23] However, several additional studies failed to recover actinomycetes in TOA patients.[16,19,20]

MICROBIOLOGY OF TUBO-OVARIAN ABSCESSES

Similar to acute PID, the microbiology of TOAs is predominantly a mixed flora of anaerobes and facultative or aerobic organisms.[6,20,21] Unlike acute PID, the sexually transmitted organisms *N. gonorrhoeae* and *C. trachomatis* are uncommonly found in TOAs.[2,21,22] Anaerobic organisms are particularly prevalent in these abscesses, having been recovered from 63% to 100% of adnexal abscesses when appropriate anaerobic microbiologic technology was used.[6,20,22–27] Initially the major role played by anaerobes in TOAs was demonstrated by Altemeier in the early 1940s, when he reported the isolation of anaerobic organisms from 92% of TOA specimens that had been previously reported by the clinical laboratory as "no growth".[25] Subsequently, Landers and Sweet reported that the most common organisms isolated from TOA aspirates were *Escherichia coli* (37%), *Bacteroides fragilis* (22%), other *Bacteroides* (now *Prevotella*) species (26%), aerobic streptococci, *Peptococcus* (11%), and *Peptostreptococcus* (18%).[6] Thus, this study also demonstrated that anaerobic bacteria were the predominant organisms isolated directly from TOAs.[6] These are many of the similar organisms involved in the biphasic aerobic–anaerobic animal model of intra-abdominal sepsis and abscess formation developed by Weinstein and colleagues.[28] In this model, the organisms recovered from the abscesses were predominantly anaerobes, especially *B. fragilis* and other *Bacteroides* species. Thus, anaerobic organisms, in particular *B. fragilis*, seem to be strongly associated with abscess formation. The all too frequently noted concept of the "sterile abscess" is a misnomer. These reported sterile abscesses probably reflect either inappropriate specimen procurement or lack of appropriate anaerobic microbiology techniques. The report by Landers and Sweet[6] probably underestimates the prevalence of anaerobic bacteria, especially *B. fragilis* and *Prevotella* species, because many of the abscesses were managed prior to establishment of the research anaerobic microbiology laboratory at their institution. In addition to utilization of modern anaerobic technology, optimization of microbiologic results in TOAs requires obtaining an appropriate specimen. Ideally, when dealing with abscess formation, the best specimen for microbiologic assessment is the abscess wall, not the purulent contents of the abscess.

One of the virulence factors associated with *B. fragilis* seems to be related to its capsular polysaccharide. A number of *Bacteroides* species failed to produce significant numbers of abscesses in experimental rats; however, when encapsulated *B. fragilis* was used alone, 95% of the rats developed abscesses.[29] In contradistinction, it has been demonstrated that unencapsulated members of the *B. fragilis* group were not able to induce abscesses by themselves in the rat model. It has further been shown that encapsulated strains of *B. fragilis* are more resistant to opsonophagocytosis than other *Bacteroides* species.[30] Thus, not only are *B. fragilis* strains by themselves capable of causing abscesses, but even the capsular polysaccharide of *B. fragilis* potentiates abscess formation. More recently, Tzianabos and coworkers demonstrated that not only does the capsular polysaccharide complex of *B. fragilis* promote formation of the intra-abdominal abscesses, but when administered systemically it can prevent abscess induction in the rat model of intra-abdominal sepsis.[31] These authors noted that the host response of abscess formation is mediated by a distinct structural motif associated with polysaccharide antigens and is controlled by the cellular immune system.[31] In addition, the virulence of anaerobes may be due to the variety of enzymes they produce.[32] Examples of such enzymes include collagenases and hyaluronidases, which may prevent walling-off of infection, and heparinase, which may promote clotting in small vessels and may further decrease blood supply to infected tissue and consequently decrease oxygenation of the infected area. Superoxide dismutase, which is produced by some anaerobes, may assist these anaerobes in surviving under aerobic conditions. Recent investigations have emphasized the emergence of and recognition of *Prevotella bivia* (formerly *Bacteroides bivius*) and *P. disiens* (formerly *B. disiens*) as major pathogens in infections of the upper female genital tract.[6] *P. bivia* and, to a lesser degree, *P. disiens* are major components of the normal vaginal–cervical flora and, thus, are not unexpectedly frequently present as pathogens on obstetric and gynecologic services.

In the past, *N. gonorrhoeae* (GC) was considered to be "the" major pathogen in the etiology of PID. Current opinion holds that the etiology of acute PID is polymicrobic, with *N. gonorrhoeae*, *C. trachomatis*, and mixed anaerobic and aerobic bacteria involved. Whereas recovery of anaerobic and aerobic bacteria is common in TOAs, the recovery of *N. gonorrhoeae*, *C. trachomatis*, or other sexually transmitted disease (STD) organisms from TOAs is very uncommon. Landers and Sweet recovered *N. gonorrhoeae* from only 3.8% of 53 TOA aspirates, whereas the overall recovery rate of this organism from the endocervix was 31%.[6] *C. trachomatis* is now recognized as a major etiologic agent in acute salpingitis. However, a role for this organism in TOAs has not been established. In our experience, *C. trachomatis* has not been isolated from a tubo-ovarian abscess. McNeeley and coworkers reported that women with TOAs less frequently harbored *N. gonorrhoeae* and/or *C. trachomatis* in their cervix than women with uncomplicated PID (38% vs 25%).[33] However, these authors did not provide microbiologic data on specimens from the TOAs. In addition, neither *N. gonorrhoeae* nor *C. trachomatis* alone produces abscesses in animal models.[34]

Chow et al[35] and Monif et al[36] have hypothesized that initial infection with *N. gonorrhoeae* leads to anaerobic invasion and superinfection of the fallopian tube. It has further has been suggested that facultative and anaerobic bacteria suppress the growth of *N. gonorrhoeae*, preventing recovery of the gonococcus from such infection.[37] Whether such a process occurs during abscess formation has not been established, nor has a similar role been demonstrated for *C. trachomatis*.

As noted above, actinomycetes, most commonly *Actinomyces israelii*, a Gram-positive anaerobe, have occasionally been recovered from patients with PID, especially in association with TOAs. In addition a relationship between actinomycetes and IUD use has been proposed by several investigators.[38–40] Other authors have refuted this suggestion.[41] Burkman et al noted that PID associated with the presence of actinomycetes was more likely to be of increased clinical severity in particular if associated with TOAs.[7] This organism has not been recovered in several TOA series.[6,19,20] However, it is very difficult to culture, often requiring maintenance of anaerobic conditions for as long as 2 weeks. Most actinomycetes are actually identified by histology in pathology specimens or by cytology on Papanicolaou (Pap) smears. Figure 7.1 demonstrates sulfur granules seen with actinomycetes. Thus, the exact role of actinomycetes in abscess formation remains unclear, as does the mechanism of their apparent relationship to the

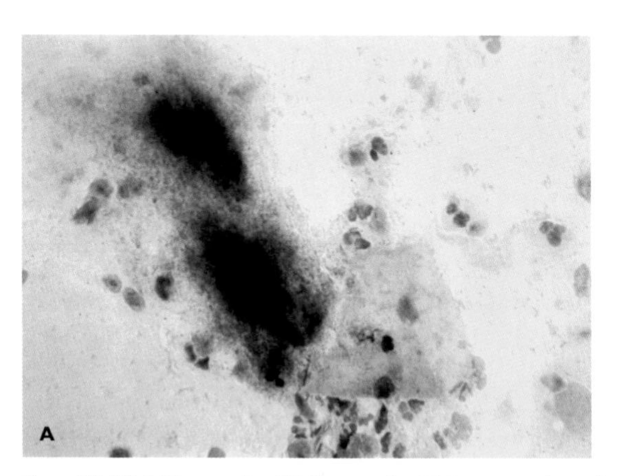

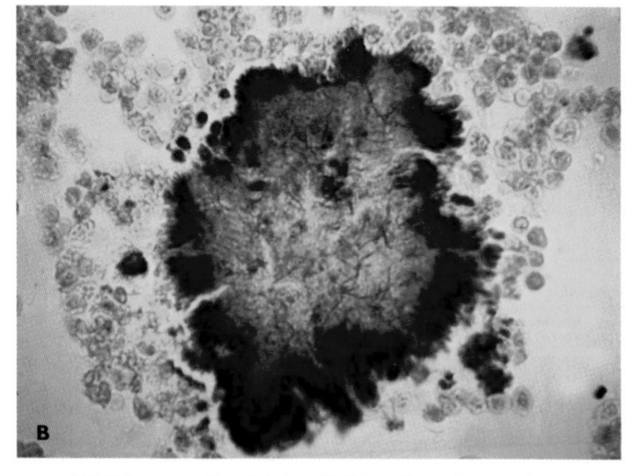

Figure 7.1 (A) Sulfur granules of *Actinomyces israelii* demonstrated on a Pap smear. (B) Sulfur granules of *A. israelii* 400× using a Gram stain. Reproduced with permission from Sweet RL, Gibbs RS. Atlas of Infectious Diseases of the Female Genital Tract. Philadelphia: Lippincott, Williams and Wilkins 2005.[127]

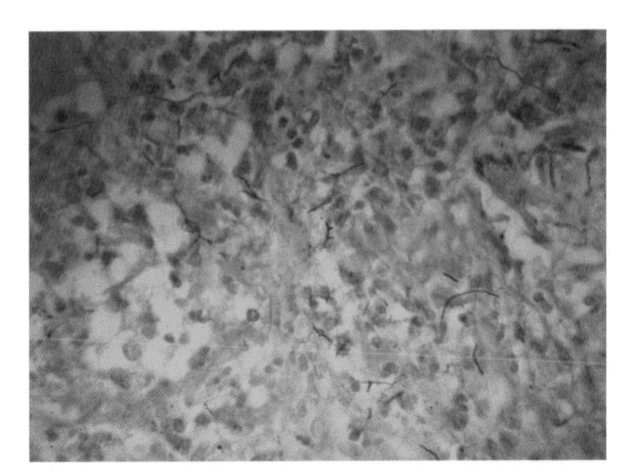

Figure 7.2 *Actinomyces israelii* in the wall of a tubo-ovarian abscess. Reproduced with permission from Sweet RL, Gibbs RS. Atlas of Infectious Diseases of the Female Genital Tract. Philadelphia: Lippincott, Williams and Wilkins 2005.[127]

IUD. Whether *A. israelii* is a sole pathogen or a marker for mixed anaerobic–facultative infection also is unclear. In Figure 7.2, *A. israelii* can be seen in the wall of a tubo-ovarian abscess.

PATHOGENESIS OF TUBO-OVARIAN ABSCESSES

Elucidation of the mechanism for TOA formation has been difficult to establish because of the variety of presentations and degrees of tubal damage present when the infection is noted. Studies carried out with *N. gonorrhoeae* have demonstrated that once the gonococcus ascends to the fallopian tube, it attaches to mucosal epithelial cells, penetrates the epithelial cells via phagocytosis, and causes destruction of the epithelial cells. The resultant tissue destruction in the endosalpinx leads to the production of a purulent exudate. In addition, the gonococci may extend from the mucosa through the subepithelial tissue to involve the muscularis and the serosa of the fallopian tube in the inflammatory process.[42] With *C. trachomatis*, the pathogenesis of tissue damage involves the cell-mediated response to the organism and a hypersensitivity-like reaction.[43] The pathogenic process for anaerobic and facultative bacteria is similar to that seen with *N. gonorrhoeae* in that the end result is tissue damage and production of a purulent exudate. Hare and Barnes demonstrated that *B. fragilis* is more virulent than the gonococcus in a fallopian tube explant system. Within 4 days of inoculation into the explant system, *B. fragilis* destroyed the tubal epithelium.[44] In the early stages of the inflammatory process, the tubal lumen is open, and the purulent exudate exudes from the fimbriated end, resulting in peritonitis. During this initial inflammatory phase or during a recurrent infection, the ovary (as well as other pelvic structures) may become involved in an attempt to localize the inflammatory process. Presumably, an ovulation site in the ovary serves as the portal of entry for organisms into the ovary, with subsequent tissue invasion. Eventually, as a result of the inflammatory process, tissue planes become lost, and the separation of tube and ovary is obscured as the abscess forms. The abscess may remain localized, with involvement of tube and ovary alone. It may involve other contiguous pelvic structures, such as bowel, bladder, or the opposite adnexa, which may be undergoing similar inflammatory changes. At any point in the progression, rupture may occur.

Interestingly, the mechanism whereby a mixture of facultative and anaerobic bacteria results in the formation of TOAs appears to be similar to that demonstrated in an animal model of intra-abdominal sepsis originally described by Weinstein and colleagues,[28] where facultative bacteria dominate the early phase of infection (acute peritonitis) and bacterial metabolic products result in an environment of low oxygen tension that favors the growth of anaerobic bacteria, leading to abscess formation.[34,45]

In addition, a variety of potential factors have been identified in the pathogenesis of abscess formation,[46] including exotoxins that produce tissue necrosis, enzymes such as collagenase and heparinase, polysaccharide from bacterial cell wall, and inflammatory response to antigenic stimuli.

C. trachomatis does not (unlike *N. gonorrhoeae* and anaerobic bacteria) produce its damage through an acute inflammatory and exudative process. Rather, it acts via the cell-mediated immune response to chlamydial heat shock protein to produce damage to the fallopian tube.[43] Although this hypersensitivity-type response leads

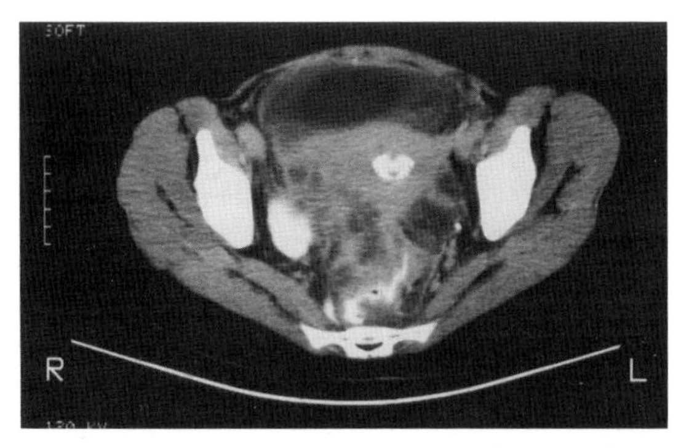

Figure 7.3 Dalkon shield intrauterine contraceptive device in a tubo-ovarian abscess seen with a CT scan.

to tubal scarring, tubal factor infertility, and ectopic pregnancy, it has not been demonstrated to result in abscess formation.[1] Thus it is not surprising that *C. trachomatis* has not been recovered from tubo-ovarian abscesses.

INTRAUTERINE DEVICE USE AND TUBO-OVARIAN ABSCESSES

IUD usage in patients presenting with TOAs has been frequently reported and ranges from 20% to 54%.[12,13,16,18,20,47] In the mid-1970s, studies noted a strong association between IUD use and the presence of unilateral TOAs (Figure 7.3). Taylor et al reported on 16 patients who developed unilateral TOAs while wearing or soon after the removal of an IUD.[17] Dawood and Birnbaum, in the same year, reported four additional cases and emphasized that the IUD association with unilateral TOAs was a distinct clinical entity.[15] Subsequent investigation by Golde et al suggested that unilateral TOAs were a distinct entity, with or without an IUD.[20] They did, however, report that 62.5% of IUD users with TOAs had unilateral disease, compared with 32.1% in nonusers. Subsequent investigators compared the incidence of unilateral abscesses among IUD users and nonusers.[6,12,13,18,47] These results and those of Golde et al are summarized in Table 7.1. In these studies, the incidence of unilateral TOAs ranged from 20 to 71%. The incidence of unilateral TOAs in IUD users was 25–89%. Thus, there was little difference in the incidence of unilateral TOAs with or without IUD use in the majority of these studies.

The pathogenesis of IUD-related salpingitis and adnexal abscess formation has yet to be clearly elucidated. Several hypotheses have been suggested. However, none of these alone can account for the diversity of clinical manifestations associated with IUD-related infections. In 1973, Burnhill suggested that a syndrome of progressive endometritis was associated with IUDs, in which menorrhagia, metrorrhagia, and leukorrhea were noted and were followed by progressive endometritis, parametritis, peritonitis, and pelvic abscess formation.[48] This scenario is similar to that proposed as the mechanism for development of subclinical PID as reviewed in Chapter 6. Bacterial colonization of the endometrium is not merely a result of contamination at the time of insertion.[49] The IUD tail, projecting through the cervical canal, allows easy access of vaginal bacteria to the upper genital tract.

Table 7.1 Incidence of unilateral tubo-ovarian abscesses (TOAs) in intrauterine device (IUD) users and nonusers

Study	No. of TOAs	No. of unilateral TOAs (%)	No. of TOAs in IUD users (% unilateral)	No. of TOAs in nonusers (% unilateral)
Landers and Sweet[6]	232	164 (71)	76 (71)	156 (70.5)
Ginsberg et al[12]	160	90 (56)	75 (61)	85 (52)
Edelman and Berger[13]	318	65 (20)	67 (25)	251 (19)
Golde et al[20]	85	35 (43.5)	32 (62.5)	53 (32)
Scott[47]	66	28 (42)	19 (42)	47 (43)
Manaral[8]	41	29 (71)	9 (89)	32 (66)
Total	902	411 (46)	278 (55)	624 (42)

Reprinted with permission from Sweet RL, Gibbs RS. Infectious Diseases of the Female Genital Tract, 4th edn. Philadelphia: Lippincott, Williams and Wilkins, 2002: 193.

In 1981, Sparks et al published a report on a series of 22 IUD users undergoing hysterectomy who were evaluated by a multiple biopsy technique.[50] Bacteria was found in the uterus in 15 of 17 women with tailed IUDs, whereas all five uteri with a tailless IUD were sterile.

Persistence of bacterial flora in the uterine cavity, combined with a breakdown of the host defense mechanisms associated with the presence of a foreign body and mechanical breakdown of the mucosal surface, may be enough to cause a chronic endometritis with progressive spread either by intracanalicular spread from the endometrium to the fallopian tube(s) and/or ovary or, less likely, via lymphatics in the parametrium and broad ligament to involve the adnexa.

Recently, current theories for the pathogenesis of TOAs have been challenged.[51] Canas et al reported a case of TOA 12 years after total abdominal hysterectomy.[51] Neither the predominant theory of ascending infection as the mechanism of TOA formation, nor alternative pathways such as subacute infection for 12 years, vaginal fistula as a pathway for ascending infection, hematogenous spread, or intra-abdominal source of spread, explain the occurrence of this TOA 12 years after total abdominal hysterectomy. Thus, additional methods of pathogenesis probably exist.

Several unusual presentations with TOAs have been additionally reported. Roth and Rivlin presented a case of bilateral TOAs that developed 50 days postoperatively following a thermal endometrial ablation.[52] Possible explanations for this occurrence proposed by the authors include dissemination of vaginal flora, tubal inoculation of vaginal organisms and transient tubal occlusion leading to a nidus for abscess formation, or pre-existing subclinical salpingitis that was exacerbated by the ablation.[52] Recently, Das and colleagues described development of a pelvic abscess following use of microwave endometrial ablation, a second-generation ablation technique.[53] These authors ascribed the pathogenesis of this acute abscess to infection of a pre-existing endometrioma secondary to an ascending route of infection during the operative procedure. Although unlikely in this patient, infection of pre-existing PID or infection of a traumatic hematoma induced by the procedure are alternative pathogenic mechanisms. Almost 30 years ago Heaton and Ledger reported 12 postmenopausal women with a TOA.[54] They suggested several possible etiologies for these TOAs, including postmenopausal bleeding with ascending infection, recurrence of PID, seeding from an inflammatory process of the gastrointestinal tract (e.g. ruptured appendicitis or diverticulitis), instrumentation (e.g. dilation and curettage (D & C) or endometrial biopsy), seeding from an infected tumor, degenerating leiomyomas that become infected, and hematogenous seeding after bacteremia from another site of infection.

CLINICAL PRESENTATION AND DIAGNOSIS

CLINICAL FINDINGS

The presenting signs and symptoms in patients with TOAs are similar to those associated with uncomplicated PID.[1,4,6] Thus, the diagnosis of TOA relies on clinical findings and imaging studies demonstrating the presence of an inflammatory adnexal mass.[1,4,6] TOAs present most commonly during the third and fourth decades of life.[4,10,19,55,56] The parity of these patients is variable, with approximately 25–50% being nulliparous.[4,6,10,12,13]

Abdominal or pelvic pain is the most frequent presenting complaint among TOA patients and was the major complaint noted in more than 90% of TOA patients reported in the literature.[5,6,10,19,55] In a study of 232 patients with TOAs, Landers and Sweet reported that a complaint of fever and chills was present in 50%, vaginal discharge in 28%, nausea in 26% and abnormal vaginal bleeding in 21%.[6] Whereas most patients with TOAs have fever and leukocytosis, a substantial number do not.[6] Temperatures of at least 37.8°C (100.4°F) and usually higher have been reported in 60–80% of patients, and leukocytosis, although often undefined, was reported in 66–80% of patients.[4–6,12,19,55] An important clinical finding is that many patients harboring TOAs may present with normal temperatures and white blood cell (WBC) counts. In the series reported by Landers and Sweet, 35% of patients with surgically confirmed TOAs were afebrile, and 23% had WBC counts in the normal range.[6] Thus, clinicians should be aware that absence of fever and/or leukocytosis does not, by itself, exclude a diagnosis of TOA.

Several additional laboratory tests have been proposed as adjuncts for improving the diagnostic accuracy in patients with suspected TOA. Erythrocyte sedimentation rate (ESR) is associated with the inflammatory process and has been used as a tool to assess the severity of infection and to demonstrate resolution of infection. However, the ESR elevation frequently lags behind the inflammatory damage and the ESR may continue to rise while the infection is resolving.[2] Serum C-reactive protein (CRP), an acute-phase reactant, has recently been investigated as a diagnostic indicator for TOA. Lehtinen et al reported that CRP was more sensitive than elevation in either ESR or degree of leukocytosis.[57] Subsequently, Mercer et al demonstrated that serial daily CRP determinations can be utilized in predicting resolution of TOAs.[58] However, these studies were small, and additional studies are needed to assess the value of ESR and/or CRP in the diagnosis of TOA or as predictors of short- and long-term outcome in the management of TOAs.

In general, the presenting clinical findings for patients with uncomplicated PID (i.e. no inflammatory mass) and those with tubo-ovarian abscesses are similar. Differentiation requires identification that an inflammatory adnexal mass is present (Figure 7.4). This illustrates the importance of recognizing the presence of an adnexal or pelvic mass in patients presenting with the signs and symptoms of acute PID. Physical examination alone may often be insufficient because pain and tenderness may preclude an adequate pelvic examination. Several relatively noninvasive imaging techniques are currently available to aid in the diagnosis of pelvic abscesses and should be utilized whenever an abscess is suspected. Differentiation of a TOA from inflammatory masses with adherent bowel or omentum is appreciably improved with such techniques. Laparoscopy may also be helpful as a diagnostic clinical tool, especially when the diagnosis is in question.

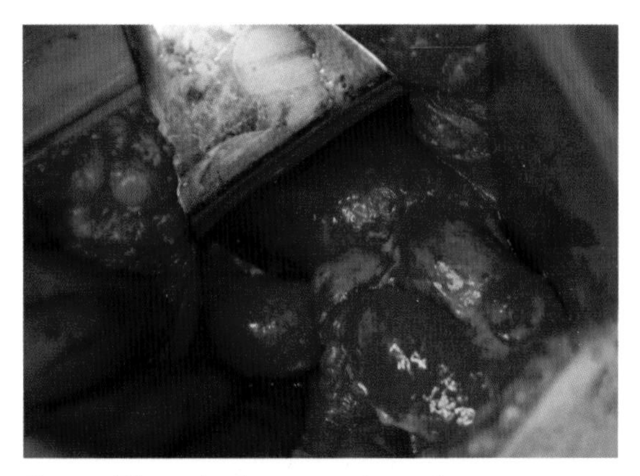

Figure 7.4 Tubo-ovarian abscessess at exploratory laparotomy. Reproduced with permission from Sweet RL, Gibbs RS. Atlas of Infectious Diseases of the Female Genital Tract. Philadelphia: Lippincott, Williams and Wilkins 2005.[127]

IMAGING TECHNIQUES

Several noninvasive imaging techniques are available that can facilitate the diagnosis and management of patients suspected of having abdominal or pelvic abscesses, including TOAs.[59–69] Among these are radionuclide scanning, scintigraphy, ultrasound (sonography), computed tomography (CT), and magnetic resonance imaging (MRI). The commonly employed radionuclide scans using gallium-67 (^{67}Ga)- and indium-111 (^{111}In)-labeled WBCs have been shown to be highly accurate in the localization of intra-abdominal abscesses.[62–65] Although easy to perform, radionuclide scans are expensive, require 24–48 hours' delay before interpretation (^{67}Ga), and produce false-positive scans due to the high affinity of these radionuclides for inflammatory tissue, such as infected or neoplastic tissue, rather than just discrete abscesses. The sensitivity of gallium scanning for detecting intra-abdominal sepsis is poor, and thus this procedure is not generally used for this purpose. The most accurate radionuclide technique for diagnosing abscesses appears to be ^{111}In-labeled WBC scans, which have a reported accuracy of 87%.[64] More recently, additional WBC labeling agents have been assessed. Technetium-99m hexamethylpropyleneamine oxime (^{99m}Tc-HMPAO) appears to be the most promising.[70] The major advantage of this technique is that a waiting period of only 4 hours is required before scanning can be performed after administering the agent, compared with 24 hours for ^{111}In-oxine tagged WBC with equivalent sensitivity.[71] None of the radionuclide scanning techniques have been well studied for diagnostic accuracy in patients with TOAs and, consequently, are infrequently used for diagnosing TOAs.

An additional technique is scintigraphy with radiolabeled polyclonal immunoglobulin G (IgG). For detecting acute infectious processes, the sensitivity and specificity of scanning with ^{111}In-labeled polyclonal IgG are 90% and 95–100%, respectively.[72,73] However, for detecting subacute or chronic infections the sensitivity drops to 74%, whereas the specificity remains high.[74]

Whereas it appears that radionuclide scanning is most useful in patients with localized signs of infection, when radionuclide scanning identifies a focus of intra-abdominal infection, further evaluation by CT or ultrasound is often required for more definitive localization of the infectious process or for guidance of percutaneous catheter drainage.[75] Thus, for suspected pelvic (and intra-abdominal) abscesses, the most appropriate imaging investigations remain ultrasound or CT.[75,76] These high-resolution imaging techniques have substantially impacted the ability to diagnose TOAs.

Ultrasonography has become the most frequently used confirmatory test when the diagnosis of a TOA is suspected; this relatively inexpensive scan can be utilized both for confirming the clinical suspicion of TOA and for measuring response to therapy. A number of retrospective studies have assessed the accuracy of ultrasound in the diagnosis of pelvic abscesses.[60,66–69] The largest of these, by Taylor et al, which included 220 patients with surgically proven abdominal or pelvic abscesses, demonstrated that 36 of 40 abdominal and 32 of 33 pelvic abscesses were correctly identified, while 112 of 113 suspected abdominal and 33 of 34 suspected pelvic abscesses were correctly ruled out.[66] In a report by Landers and Sweet, a series of 98 patients were evaluated with ultrasound, of whom 31 had surgically confirmed TOAs.[6] Twenty-nine of the 31 surgically confirmed TOAs had been reported as complex adnexal masses or cystic-type masses with multiple internal echoes and were felt to be consistent with an abscess. The remaining two were simple cystic masses. A mass was correctly identified in all surgically confirmed TOAs and in 90% of the 67 patients with clinically diagnosed TOAs.[6] Ultrasound of a TOA reveals a discrete mass, with internal echoes indicating its complex nature. A sonogram of a surgically documented TOA is shown in Figure 7.5. Ultrasound is also useful in assessing response to therapy by detecting changes in the size and architecture of these masses. As technology has improved the quality of ultrasound, and ultrasonographers have gained experience with techniques that combine the use of real-time and static imaging, the accuracy of this technique in the diagnosis and management of TOAs has been increased. In a study by Jasinski et al, comparing the sensitivity of ultrasound and CT in the diagnosis of intra-abdominal abscesses, the sensitivity of ultrasound for pelvic abscesses was 75% (42/56) and that of CT was 93% (14/15).[77] These authors ascribed this difference to difficulty in imaging postoperative abscesses in oncology patients by ultrasound. In summary, transabdominal ultrasound has a sensitivity $\geq$ 90% for detecting pelvic abscesses[76] and is the least costly approach for imaging the pelvis.[2] The advent of endovaginal ultrasonography has further enhanced the sensitivity and specificity of ultrasound confirmation of pelvic abscesses.[59] Thus, it is not surprising that ultrasound is the most frequently employed imaging technique for identifying TOAs.

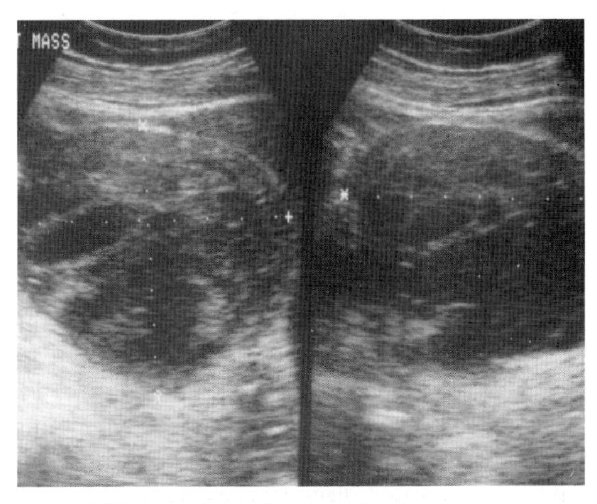

Figure 7.5 Ultrasound image of a tubo-ovarian abscess.

CT scans have been used extensively, in both the diagnosis and the treatment of abdominal abscesses. For intra-abdominal abscesses, CT appears to be superior to ultrasound but is more costly.[78] CT has been shown to have a sensitivity of 78–100%, compared with a sensitivity of 75–82% for ultrasound.[78,79] However, there is little information available on the accuracy of these scans, specifically for the diagnosis of TOAs or other pelvic abscesses. Moir and Robins compared the accuracy of ultrasound, gallium, and CT scanning in the diagnosis of abdominal abscesses.[69] They demonstrated that the sensitivities of ultrasound, gallium, and CT were 82, 96, and 100%, respectively. Specificities was reported as 91, 65, and 100%, respectively. As noted above, Jasinski et al demonstrated that for the diagnosis of intra-abdominal, including pelvic, abscesses, CT scan was more sensitive (93%) than was ultrasound (75%).[77] Whether this difference would hold true for TOAs is not clear. Moreover, this difference was primarily due to difficulties with ultrasound in postoperative oncology patients. Thus, CT scans appear to be very accurate, at least in the abdomen, in detecting the presence of an abscess. It remains uncertain whether the sensitivity and specificity in the pelvis are similar and whether the increased accuracy of CT justifies the additional expense. Currently, we obtain an ultrasound as the initial diagnostic aid and reserve CT scans for those patients in whom ultrasound using endovaginal probes fails to provide adequate information. A large pelvic abscess is seen on a CT scan in Figure 7.6.

MRI may play a role in diagnosing intra-abdominal and pelvic abscesses. Clearly, MRI has proven to be a valuable technique for diagnostic imaging. It has the advantage of discriminating between differing contiguous tissue densities without the need for ionizing radiation. To date, there is a very limited experience with MRI in the evaluation of pelvic masses. In addition, MRI is quite expensive. Only MRI clinical experience can determine if the theoretic advantages in accuracy with MRI are applicable to clinical use in differentiating pelvic masses and whether the increased cost is balanced by increased diagnostic accuracy. Figure 7.7 is an MRI study demonstrating a TOA.

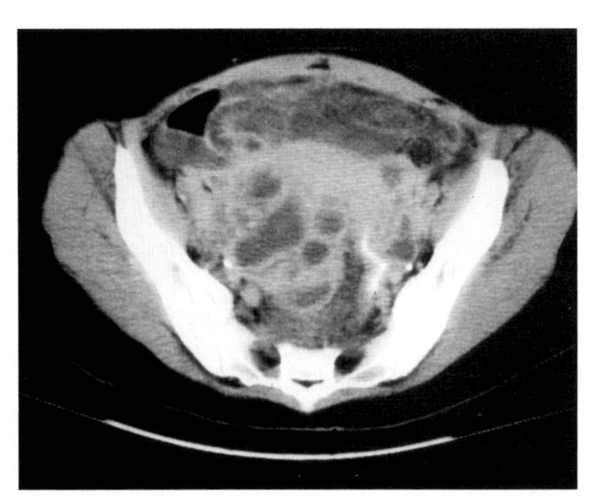

Figure 7.6 CT scan of a tubo-ovarian abscess.

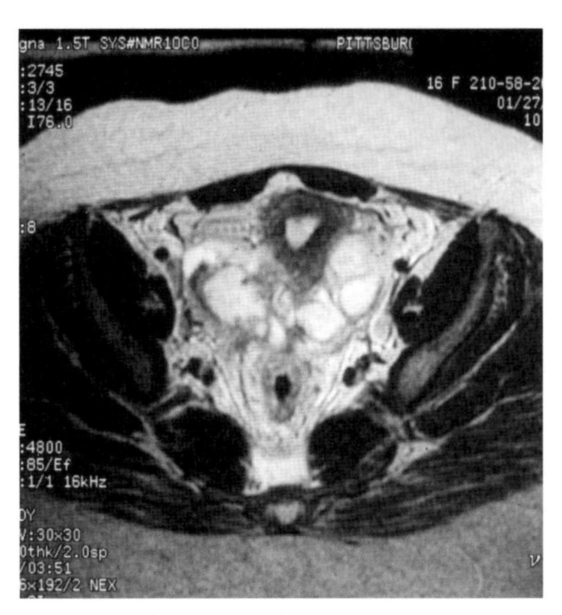

Figure 7.7 MRI of a tubo-ovarian abscess.

TREATMENT APPROACH

MEDICAL THERAPY OF TUBO-OVARIAN ABSCESS

Contemporary management of TOAs has evolved from the traditional dictum that that abscesses cannot be adequately eradicated by antibiotics alone and require surgical drainage or extirpation. Saini and coworkers at the Tufts New England Medical Center noted an improved survival of patients with intra-abdominal abscesses and attributed the improvement to the combination of earlier diagnosis and improved localization of abscesses (with the use of newer imaging techniques such as real-time sonography and CT), earlier drainage, and the use of broad-spectrum antimicrobial regimens effective against anaerobes, especially *B. fragilis*.[80] Current management addresses the issue of whether or not a TOA can be treated conservatively (without surgical intervention), without significant risk to patients, in the hope of preserving fertility and/or ovarian function. It is well accepted that rupture of a TOA is an acute emergency that requires immediate surgical intervention. However, the management of the unruptured TOA has changed dramatically over the past 30 years. Options range from prompt surgical intervention, with complete removal of the uterus and adnexa,[5,81] to treatment with intravenous antibiotics where surgery is reserved for patients who fail to respond or in whom rupture of the TOA is suspected.[6,10,12] An approach frequently used when antibiotics first became available (1950s and 1960s) was long-term antibiotic therapy up to 21 days for the acute stage, followed by 3–6 months of "cooling off", and performance of a total abdominal hysterectomy and bilateral salpingo-oophorectomy during the "chronic, burned-out" stage. As an alternative in patients with unilateral TOAs requiring surgical intervention, it has been suggested that unilateral adnexectomy may be appropriate in hopes of preserving future fertility and hormonal production.[21] In addition, Landers and Sweet questioned whether unilateral adnexectomy is indicated for patients with persistent unilateral TOA in hopes of preventing future flare-ups and improving future fertility on the contralateral uninvolved side.[6]

At the opposite end of the spectrum, a much more aggressive early surgical intervention was proposed. Kaplan et al treated 71 patients with total abdominal hysterectomy and bilateral salpingo-oophorectomy within 24–72 hours of instituting antibiotics.[81] However, this aggressive approach was associated with bowel injury (serosal tears) in 8.4% of patients.[81] Such an approach, although often curative, eliminates future reproductive and/or hormonal function. Thus, it seems prudent to question whether such an aggressive approach is necessary in all patients with TOAs.

Multiple studies have since demonstrated favorable results, utilizing a more conservative approach aimed at preservation of future reproductive potential.[6,10,12,21,33,82] Studies utilizing conservative medical therapy as the initial approach to the management of unruptured TOA are summarized in Table 7.2. Franklin et al reported their findings for

Table 7.2 Studies utilizing conservative medical therapy as the initial approach to management of tubo-ovarian abscess

Study	No. of TOAs treated	No. with response (%)	No. with subsequent pregnancy of patients with follow-up (%)
Landers and Sweet[6]	217	175 (81)	8/58 (13.8)
Franklin et al[10,a]	120	110 (92)	10/108 (9.3)
Ginsberg et al[12]	110	76 (69)	9/95 (9.5)
Edelman and Berger[13]	318	175 (55)	NS
Scott[47]	33	24 (73)	NS
Manara[18]	26	11 (42)	1/26 (3.8)
Hager[8]	32	5 (16)	4/8 (50)
Hemsell et al[82]	41	39 (95)	6/41 (15)
Reed et al[83]	119	90 (75)	NS
McNeeley et al[33]	74	52 (70)	NS
Total	1090	757 (69.4)	38/336 (11.3)

[a]Includes some patients treated with colpotomy drainage.

Reprinted with permission from Sweet RL, Gibbs RS. Infectious Diseases of the Female Genital Tract. Philadelphia: Lippincott, Williams and Wilkins, 2002: 194.

120 patients treated with an initial conservative approach.[10] In this study, 85 patients were treated with antibiotics alone, and 35 patients were treated with antibiotics plus colpotomy drainage. An initial clinical response was noted in 110 (92%) of patients. Ultimately, 16.5% of patients required additional treatment, resulting in an overall response rate of nearly 75%, with a failure rate of 26.5%, of which 10% were early failures. One hundred and eight patients were followed between 2.5 and 8 years after discharge, with a subsequent intrauterine pregnancy rate of 9.3%.[10] In 1980, Ginsberg et al reported a series of 110 patients with TOAs who were initially treated with antibiotics alone.[12] Initial clinical response to antibiotics alone was reported for 76 (69%) of TOA patients. During the follow-up period, 35% of patients were noted to be late failures.[12] These authors reported on long-term follow-up, ranging from 1 month to 10 years, in 95 of the patients, with a subsequent intrauterine pregnancy rate of 9.5%.[12] Landers and Sweet reported a series of 232 patients with TOAs, 217 of whom were treated initially with antibiotics alone.[6] Early clinical response was reported in 175 (81%) of patients, with early failure occurring in 19.4% and late failure in an additional 31% of patients.[6] Long-term follow-up of greater than 2 years was available in 58 patients, with a subsequent intrauterine pregnancy rate of 13.8%. Hemsell et al reported that 39 of 41 (95%) of patients with TOAs responded initially to antibiotic therapy alone.[82] Readmission for surgery was subsequently necessary in 4 (12%) of patients, and 6 (15%) of the 41 patients subsequently had intrauterine pregnancies.[82] Reed et al reported the results of a study comparing cefoxitin plus doxycycline with clindamycin plus gentamicin for the initial treatment of unruptured TOAs.[83] These authors demonstrated that 90 (75%) of 119 TOAs responded initially to medical therapy alone, with equivalent results noted for both antimicrobial regimens.[90] They also demonstrated that the initial clinical response to antibiotic therapy was, to a large extent, related to the size of the TOA, as determined on ultrasound imaging (Figure 7.8).[83] Whereas surgery was required in only 15% of patients with TOAs in the 4–6 cm size range, this rose to 35% and nearly 60%

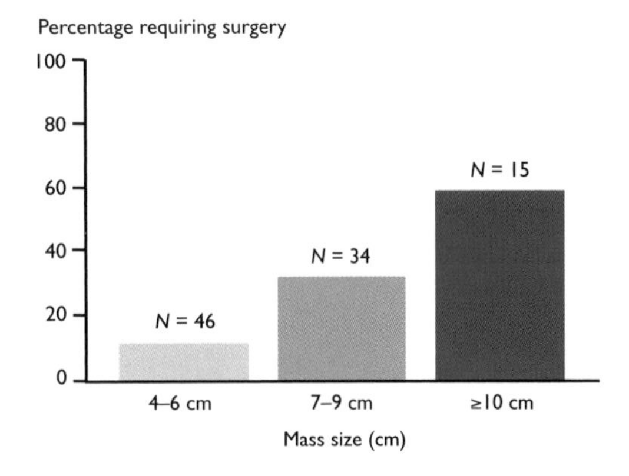

Figure 7.8 The response to antimicrobial therapy is inversely proportional to the size of tubo-ovarian abscesses. An additional two patients had surgery recommended but left without further follow-up. Reprinted with permission from Reed SD, Landers DV, Sweet RL. Antibiotic treatment of tubo-ovarian absecess: comparison of clindamycia-containing regimens. Am J Obstet Gynecol 1991;164:1556–62.

for TOAs in the 7–9 cm and ≥10 cm size ranges, respectively.[83] Recently, McNeeley and co-workers reported their results from a study comparing cefotetan plus doxycycline, clindamycin plus gentamicin, or ampicillin plus clindamycin plus gentamicin in the treatment of TOAs.[33] Overall, they noted that 52 (70%) of 74 TOAs responded to antibiotic therapy alone. However, unlike Reed et al, they reported that triple therapy (clindamycin plus gentamicin plus ampicillin) was significantly more effective (87.5%) than cefotetan plus doxycycline (34%) or clindamycin plus gentamicin (47%) ($p = 0.001$). Neither Reed et al nor McNeeley et al provided follow-up information on pregnancy rates. In contradistinction to the bulk of such studies, Manara[18] reported that 60% of TOA patients initially treated with antibiotics alone failed to respond. Hager also reported less favorable results with medical therapy alone in a series of 32 TOA patients, of whom only 5 (16%) had an initial clinical response.[8] However, Hager used a much more restrictive definition of clinical improvement – afebrile and a documented decrease in abscess size.[8] Taken together, these studies demonstrate a response to medical therapy in 69.4%, with a range of 16–95%. The rate of subsequent intrauterine pregnancy ranged from 9.5% to 15%, with an 11.3% rate overall. This is a minimum and overly pessimistic estimate of fertility chances, because those women using contraception and/or not attempting to get pregnant are not excluded. For example, Hager reported a substantially better 50% pregnancy rate among patients with TOAs treated medically who actually attempted to become pregnant.[8]

Clinically, and at times even with ultrasound imaging, it may be difficult to distinguish a TOA from a pyosalpinx, ovarian abscess, or some other inflammatory complex. This becomes somewhat less crucial among those patients treated with an initial conservative antibiotic-only approach, because such initial therapy is appropriate therapy for any of these pelvic inflammatory masses. In addition, future reproductive capability is an important concern for most patients with TOAs and this concern plays a major role in the desire for pursuing a more conservative approach to therapy.

A variety of antibiotic regimens have been employed in the series of TOAs listed in Table 7.2 and for which the therapeutic regimens were stated. In the series by Franklin et al,[10] patients were treated primarily with penicillin and streptomycin. Concomitant colpotomy drainage was performed in some patients. Ginsberg et al,[12] while not specifically stating which antibiotic regimens were used, did note that patients were treated with "broad spectrum antibiotics, with multiple agents being employed frequently". In the Manara series, patients were treated with intravenous penicillin plus an aminoglycoside.[18] In Hager's study, patients were treated initially with parenteral penicillin or a first-generation cephalosporin in combination with an aminoglycoside.[8] In most patients anaerobe coverage (unspecified, but presumably clindamycin or chloramphenicol) was added. From the summary of the conservative antibiotic therapy for TOAs, there appears to be a tremendous variation in response rates to antimicrobial therapy alone. This variation is due in part to the variety of definitions used for response and the degree of aggressiveness in using surgical intervention. A major omission in most of these studies is the lack of detailed analysis comparing responses to particular antibiotic regimens. If one accepts that these abscesses contain high concentrations of resistant Gram-negative anaerobes such as *B. fragilis*, *P. bivia*, and *P. disiens*, then improved results should be noted in patients treated aggressively with antibiotics that are effective against these resistant Gram-negative anaerobes, such as clindamycin, metronidazole, cefoxitin, third-generation cephalosporins, extended-spectrum pencillins, the β-lactamase inhibition combinations, and carbapenems such as Primaxin (imipenem with cilastatin) and meropenem.

In the Landers and Sweet series of 232 TOAs treated from 1970 to 1980, the various treatment regimens that were employed were delineated.[6] Patients treated in the earlier years received high-dose penicillin.[6] Subsequently, an aminoglycoside was added, and the dose of penicillin was reduced. In the later years of the study, patients were treated primarily with combination therapy including clindamycin and an aminoglycoside. Determination of response to therapy was based on improvement in symptoms, absence of fever, reduction of pelvic tenderness, and decrease in size of the abscess. Since all patients not requiring surgery during the initial hospitalization became afebrile with symptomatic improvement, evaluation of the mass was used to assess differences in therapeutic response.

Among the patients treated with antibiotics alone, a total of 167 had examinations documented prior to discharge. Reduction in abscess size was noted in 25% of patients treated with penicillin alone, 49% of patients treated with penicillin and an aminoglycoside, and 68% of patients treated with regimens that included clindamycin ($p < 0.01$).[6] Among the 104 patients who had been treated with antibiotic regimens that did not include clindamycin and were available for follow-up, the response rate was 36.5%, compared with a 68% response rate in the 63 patients treated with regimens that included clindamycin.[6] The opposite trend was noted among patients whose abscess increased in size. Forty-two patients required surgical extirpation of an abscess during the initial hospitalization because of failure to respond to initial antimicrobial therapy.[6] Of these, 64% had been treated with regimens not containing clindamycin, compared with 36% who had received a clindamycin-containing regimen. Among the patients treated with antibiotics alone, 134 returned for follow-up 2–4 weeks after discharge.[6] In 46% of the patients treated with nonclindamycin regimens, the abscesses were decreased in size or absent, whereas 86% of clindamycin-treated patients showed a similar response.[6] The excellent results obtained by Hemsell et al,[82] Reed et al,[83] and McNeeley et al[33] provide additional evidence that utilizing an agent effective against Gram-negative anaerobic rods such as *B. fragilis*, *P. bivia*, and *P. disiens* optimizes the clinical response to antimicrobial therapy.

An abscess is a unique environment characterized by a low level of oxygen tension that allows anaerobes to proliferate.[1,2] In turn, this leads to tissue destruction and circulatory compromise, which prevents or makes it difficult for many antibiotics to reach the abscess area. The combination of these factors and the poor phagocytosis of neutrophils in this environment are all important contributors to the resistance of abscesses to antimicrobial therapy. There are 10^7–10^9 bacteria/ml in an abscess. Thus, an inoculum effect occurs in which the laboratory standard of 10^5 organisms is sensitive to an antibiotic, but tremendous numbers of organisms in the abscess are resistant. In addition, the high levels of enzymes produced by bacteria within the abscess lead to the destruction of many antibiotics such as penicillin, ampicillin, first-generation cephalosporins, ticarcillin, carbenicillin, and chloramphenicol. In addition, many anaerobic bacteria, in particular *B. fragilis*, are often resistant to the penicillins and many cephalosporins. Similarly, *P. disiens* and *P. bivia*, which are especially prevalent in the female genital tract, are often resistant to the penicillins and cephalosporins. The role of *B. fragilis* as an important pathogen in abscesses is evident from recovery of this organism in abscess aspirates,[6,20] serologic studies demonstrating an antigenic response in patients with abscesses,[84] and experimental work in animals showing that *B. fragilis* promotes abscess formation.[85]

The microenvironment of abscesses results in a variety of adverse effects upon host immune function.[97] Low oxygen tension leads to hypoxia, which impairs neutrophil function and decreases aminoglycoside activity. The low pH impairs both neutrophil migration and killing. Within the abscess there are large numbers of bacteria in the stationary phase, resulting in decreased antibiotic efficacy secondary to an inoculum effect and the absence of bacterial proliferation. A high concentration of bacterial byproducts, components, or toxins diminishes phagocytic cell function, causes local tissue damage, and depletes complement. Necrotic debris within the abscess deactivates neutrophils and depletes complement. Whereas fibrin production protects the abdominal cavity from infection, fibrin reduces access of phagocytic cells to bacteria in the abscess and impairs microbicidal killing.

The characteristics of clindamycin and other antibiotics, such as cefoxitin, metronidazole, and third-generation cephalosporins, which are active against resistant Gram-negative anaerobes, provide some explanation for the improved response of TOAs to antimicrobial treatment regimens incorporating those antimicrobial agents. The extracellular antimicrobial activity of clindamycin may further explain the favorable results seen with this agent, which may reach especially high concentrations within the abscesses as a result of active transport into the abscess by polymorphonuclear leukocytes.[87,88] In addition, clindamycin (in an animal model) has been shown to enter infected encapsulated subcutaneous abscesses in mice in a higher concentration (43–63% of peak serum levels) than other antimicrobial agents, including metronidazole and cefoxitin.[89] However, these other antimicrobials also entered the abscesses in significant amounts. When the activity of 10 antimicrobial agents was measured in subcutaneous abscesses by reduction in bacterial counts, it was found that the most active antimicrobials in order of decreasing activity were metronidazole, clindamycin, and cefoxitin.[89]

The introduction of newer β-lactam agents offers additional treatment options. However, the in-vitro ability of the extended-spectrum penicillins, piperacillin and mezlocillin, other third-generation cephalosporins, and the β-lactamase inhibition combinations to penetrate into abscesses and/or to reduce bacterial counts in abscesses has not been extensively studied. Nor have these agents been widely studied in clinical practice.

At present, we consider the combination of metronidazole or clindamycin with an aminoglycoside to be the most effective regimen available for the treatment of TOAs. The recent pattern of increased resistance by the *B. fragilis* group to clindamycin has led many clinicians to prefer metronidazole. In addition, many clinicians add ampicillin to their regimen for TOAs.[33] Cefoxitin or possibly cefotetan plus doxycycline are also active against anaerobes, including *B. fragilis*, *P. bivia*, and *P. disiens*, and have generally provided comparable results vs clindamycin or metronidazole regimens.[83] The major disadvantage of this approach is the lack of an oral form of cefoxitin or cefotetan for continued therapy after discontinuation of parenteral therapy. Unfortunately, the *B. fragilis* group of bacteria have demonstrated increasing levels of resistance to these cephamycins.

SURGICAL MANAGEMENT OF TUBO-OVARIAN ABSCESS

In the preantibiotic era, the treatment for pelvic infections in general and TOA specifically consisted of bed rest, fluids, and heat. The semifowler position was encouraged to promote purulent material collecting, via gravity, in the region of the cul-de-sac, where it would be accessible to colpotomy drainage. The first surgical drainage of a pelvic abscess was performed in the 1800s.[9] This remained the only available option until the mid 20th century, when antimicrobial preparations, beginning with sulfa drugs and eventually penicillin, became available. In spite of the addition of antibiotics to our armamentarium, surgical removal of infected pelvic organs remained the predominant mode of therapy. In 1959, Collins and Jansen[90] summarized the current approach to the treatment of pelvic abscesses as follows:

> In the therapy of acute pelvic infections, one operates immediately in case of ruptured abscesses or abscesses pointing into the cul de sac or in the region of Poupart's ligament. Otherwise, medical therapy is employed. Failure to respond to these measures is a definite indication for surgery.

These authors went on to suggest that while most pelvic abscesses eventually require surgical drainage or removal, delaying the surgery until the infection had "cooled" was preferable.[90] In recent years, with the improvement in available antibiotics and the enhanced concern about infertility, an increasing number of investigators, as discussed above, have encouraged conservative management of the unruptured TOA.[6,10,12,83]

As a result, the current general consensus is that surgical intervention should be reserved for patients with TOAs who do not show prompt clinical improvement or in whom rupture of the abscess is suspected.[1,2] Even following this more conservative approach, a significant number of patients continue to require surgical intervention secondary to failure of the initial antimicrobial therapy.[6,12,21] Landers and Sweet demonstrated that while initially only 20% of TOA patients required surgical intervention, during follow-up an additional 31% required subsequent surgery.[6,21] Similarly, Ginsburg et al reported early failure in 31% and late failure in an additional 35% of TOA patients initially receiving antimicrobial therapy.[12]

The approach we currently recommend for the management of suspected TOAs is presented in the algorithm in Figure 7.9. If a ruptured TOA is suspected, the patient is stabilized, antibiotics are begun, and immediate surgical intervention is undertaken. The only other indication for immediate surgery is when the diagnosis is in question and there is the strong possibility of a surgical emergency. Otherwise, the patient is begun on intravenous antibiotics that include an agent effective against resistant Gram-negative anaerobes such as *B. fragilis* and *B. bivius* (see previous section on medical treatment). Despite appropriate antimicrobial therapy, if the patient fails to demonstrate evidence of a favorable response in a reasonable amount of time (i.e. 48–72 hours), we would then proceed with surgical intervention. This does not mean that complete cure occurs, but rather that there is evidence of response such as decreased temperature, decreased WBC count, or subjective improvement in the patient's symptoms. During the initial antibiotic therapy, the clinician must be cognizant that the abscess may rupture and become a surgical emergency. Once the decision to operate has been made, there should be no delay. However,

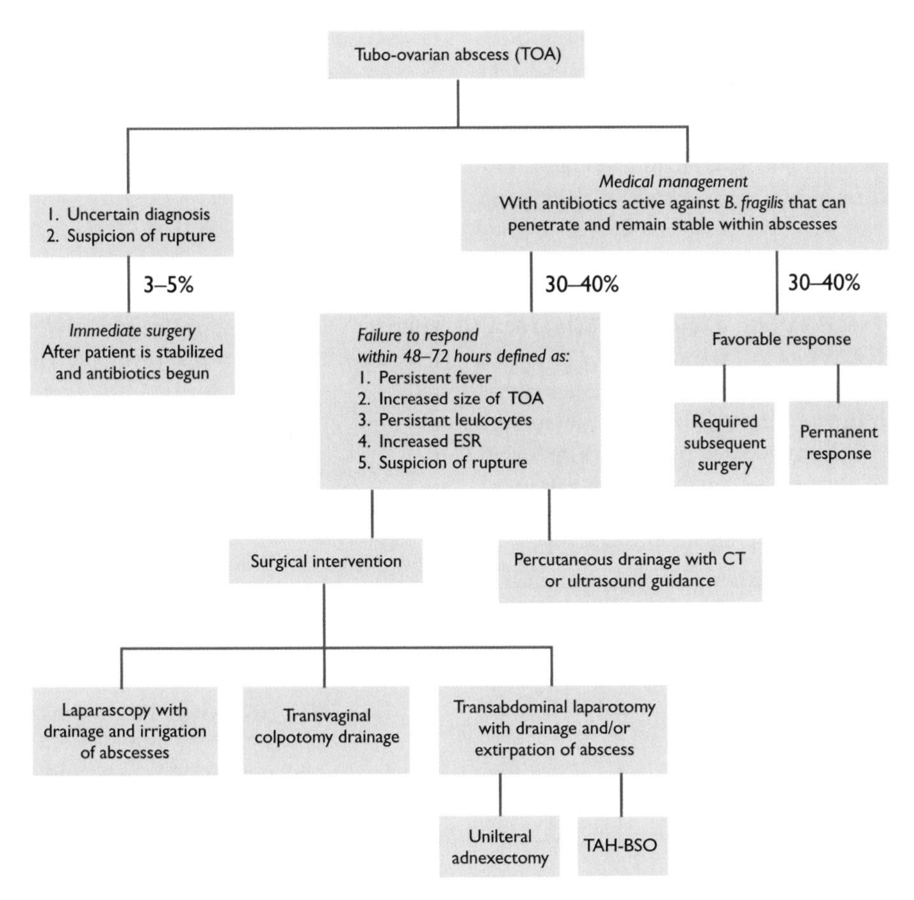

Figure 7.9 Algorithm for the management of tubo-ovarian abscesses. ESR = erythrocyte sedimentation rate; CT = computed tomography; TAH-BSO = total abdominal hysterectomy with bilateral salpingo-oophorectomy.

each case must be individualized and clinical judgment is crucial. For example, in young, nulliparous patients an additional 24–48 hours is often allowed in hopes that a response will be forthcoming.

A number of factors seem to have some predictive value in determining which patients are more likely to fail antibiotic therapy alone. Ginsberg and associates noted that adnexal masses larger than 8 cm and/or bilateral adnexal involvement were predictive of failure to respond to medial therapy.[12] Reed et al demonstrated that response to antimicrobial therapy was inversely proportional to the size of the abscess (see Figure 7.8).[83] Surprisingly, the presence of fever, the degree of leukocytosis, or a past history of PID are not predictive of the clinical response to initial antibiotic therapy.[1,2] However, persistent fever and/or rising WBC count, despite appropriate antimicrobial therapy, identify patients who are likely to require surgical intervention.

RUPTURED TUBO-OVARIAN ABSCESSES

The most serious complication associated with TOAs is intra-abdominal rupture, which is an acute surgical emergency in which the mortality rate rapidly increases with unnecessary delay. In 1964, Pedowitz and Bloomfield reported a series of 143 cases of ruptured adnexal abscesses.[4] In the 16 cases of ruptured TOAs treated prior to 1947, there was a 100% mortality rate. From 1947 to 1959, 127 ruptured TOAs were treated with a more aggressive surgical approach combined with available antimicrobial therapy, resulting in an improved mortality rate of 3.1%.[4] In their report, Pedowitz and Bloomfield reviewed an additional 235 published cases of ruptured TOAs managed after 1948 by centers using an operative approach; in analyzing the 14 deaths that occurred, they noted that 10 may have been preventable.[4] Physician delay in establishing the diagnosis was cited as the most common cause of preventable death. Collins and Jansen similarly reported an 85% mortality rate prior to 1952.[90] However, after adopting an aggressive surgical approach in addition to antibiotic therapy for ruptured TOAs from 1953 to 1959, they reported only 1 death among 58 patients with ruptured TOAs.[90] They estimated an expected recovery rate of 10–15% utilizing a medical regimen, and an 85–90% recovery rate with the surgical approach.[90] Subsequent investigators have continued to show improved survival with aggressive surgical management of ruptured TOAs. In 1969, Mickal and Sellmann reported a mortality rate of 11.1% from 1951 to 1959, compared with a rate of 3.7% from 1959 to 1966.[19] On the other hand, in 1977, Rivlin and Hunt reported a 71% mortality rate in 113 patients with ruptured TOAs.[91] The major difference in their series was the more limited extent of surgery performed at the time of laparotomy. In the Rivlin and Hunt series, hysterectomy was performed in only 3% of the patients, with hormonal and menstrual function being retained in 73.5%.[91] This finding is surprising, considering the 70% hysterectomy rate reported by Pedowitz and Bloomfield, as well as the 80% rate in the Mickal and Sellmann series.[4,19] In addition, only 17.5% of patients in the Rivlin and Hunt report required further surgery at a later date in the 1- to 5-year follow-up period.[91] Landers and Sweet reported on four patients with ruptured TOAs who underwent unilateral adnexectomy, and none required further surgery in the 2–10 year follow-up.[6] One of these patients carried a subsequent intrauterine pregnancy to term. It appears that when aggressive surgical intervention is combined with appropriate antibiotic therapy in the treatment of ruptured unilateral TOAs, a conservative surgical approach utilizing unilateral adnexectomy and aimed at preserving hormonal and reproductive function can be safely employed.

UNRUPTURED TUBO-OVARIAN ABSCESS

Whereas surgical intervention is recommended for patients with unruptured TOAs who do not respond to initial antimicrobial therapies, there is no general consensus as to the appropriate surgical approach that should be utilized. Multiple surgical techniques have been advocated, including:

- extraperitoneal drainage
- posterior colpotomy drainage
- transabdominal drainage
- unilateral adnexectomy
- total abdominal hysterectomy with bilateral salpingo-oophorectomy (TAH with BSO).

Extraperitoneal drainage of TOAs was used in the preantibiotic era to drain abscesses accessible to an incision just above Poupart's ligament. The rationale for this approach was concern that a transabdominal approach would result in contamination of the peritoneal cavity and subsequent peritonitis with a high likelihood of mortality in the preantibiotic era. This procedure unfortunately requires adherence of the parietal and visceral peritoneum. This procedure will not be described in detail, as its place in the treatment of TOAs is very limited and it has been replaced with better results by imaging directed percutaneous or laparoscopic directed drainage.

POSTERIOR COLPOTOMY

Posterior colpotomy drainage of TOAs has been used for many years. This procedure is an effective mode of treatment when combined with antimicrobial therapy and restricted to patients with fluctuant abscesses in the midline that dissect the rectovaginal septum and are firmly attached to the parietal peritoneum. Adherence to these requirements markedly reduces the number of TOAs that can be safely drained by posterior colpotomy. The morbidity associated with colpotomy is significantly greater when these requirements are not met. Rubenstein et al reported a series of 65 patients with pelvic abscesses that were drained by posterior colpotomy or rectal incision.[92] One-third of the patients required a subsequent major operation due to persistent pain or infection.[92] In 1982, Rivlin and associates reported a combined series of 348 cases in which colpotomy drainage of abscesses was used.[93] They noted that in 23 (6.5%) cases, diffuse peritoneal sepsis developed post attempted colpotomy drainage. Among these 23 cases, 6 (26%) deaths occurred.[93] In 1983, Rivlin described an additional 59 patients treated over a 20-year span with colpotomy drainage for pelvic abscesses in which there were 2 deaths, both related to diffuse peritonitis.[94] During the same admission, subsequent surgery was required in 13 patients. Additional surgery at a later date was performed in 11 patients. In 14 (58%) of these 24 patients, the repeat surgical procedure was performed as an emergency operation.[94] Colpotomy drainage, in appropriate circumstances, is ideally performed under general anesthesia, with the patient in the dorsal lithotomy position. After the bladder is emptied, an examination under anesthesia is performed to verify that the abscess is adherent to the peritoneum (i.e. cannot be moved out of the cul-de-sac) and appropriate for colpotomy drainage. Following Betadine (povidone-iodine) preparation of the vagina, a tenaculum is attached to the posterior lip of the cervix for countertraction. The vaginal mucosa is incised in a transverse manner at the junction of the posterior vaginal fornix with the cervix. A Kelly clamp is used to enter the abscess cavity and then to enlarge the incision. Appropriate cultures should be obtained (anaerobic techniques), and the abscess cavity explored, usually with the surgeon's finger, to break down any adhesions or loculation(s) present within the abscess. Intraoperative real-time sonography greatly facilitates and insures drainage of the entire abscess, especially when it is multiloculated. At completion of the procedure, a closed-suction catheter is inserted into the cavity for drainage. In approximately 48–72 hours, the catheter is removed if drainage has stopped. Colpotomy drainage can be a useful adjuvant in the treatment of those TOAs, especially unilocular, that meet the requirements for vaginal drainage and are resistant to treatment with antibiotics alone. There still exists some danger of diffuse peritoneal sepsis and death, but this can be minimized by carefully selecting the patients who would benefit from posterior colpotomy drainage and by using real-time ultrasound guidance.

At the present time, vaginal colpotomy drainage is rarely performed. It was designed for and was appropriate for use in the preantibiotic era when extraperitoneal drainage of abscesses was a paramount need. Without concurrent antibiotic therapy, a transabdominal approach to an acute abscess would most likely result in peritonitis and high mortality rates. Our lack of enthusiasm for vaginal colpotomy drainage is based on the following:

- there is a high rate of complications and, subsequently, more definitive surgery following colpotomy drainage[92–94]
- most TOAs in the antibiotic era do not meet the requisite requirements for the vaginal approach (i.e. a midline mass that adheres to pelvic peritoneum and dissects the upper one-third of rectovaginal septum)
- with the high incidence of unilateral abscesses being reported, it is our belief that unilateral adnexectomy with extirpation of infected tissue offers a better chance for preservation of future fertility and/or hormonal production from the contralateral adnexa.

Similarly, ultrasound-, CT scan-, or laparoscopy-directed drainage have become the preferred alternatives for drainage of TOAs unresponsive to antimicrobial therapy.

CONSERVATIVE SURGERY VS TOTAL HYSTERECTOMY WITH BILATERAL ADNEXECTOMY

There exists some controversy over the extent of surgery that is indicated for those patients requiring surgical intervention for the treatment of TOA. Extirpation of all reproductive organs by TAH with BSO has been advocated by some for the management of unruptured TOAs unresponsive to antimicrobial therapy.[4,59,81,90] This approach was fostered largely by the report of Pedowitz and

Bloomfield that in patients with only unilateral TOAs seen grossly, one-third had microscopic abscesses in the contralateral ovary.[4]

With the introduction of more potent and broad-spectrum antimicrobial agents, especially those that have substantial activity in abscess environments and that are effective against Gram-negative anaerobes (e.g. the *B. fragilis* group and *Prevotella* species), concern over such microabscesses is probably not warranted. As an alternative approach, unilateral salpingo-oophorectomy for unilateral TOAs has been more recently recommended, with BSO being limited to patients with bilateral disease. Although complete removal of reproductive organs (TAH with BSO) is most often curative, unilateral adnexectomy offers the advantage of a hope for future fertility, maintenance of hormonal (and menstrual) function, and the avoidance of potential adverse psychologic effects associated with hysterectomy and gonadectomy. The major issue is whether or not these benefits outweigh the risk of requiring further surgical therapy. As antibiotic regimens continue to improve and more data accumulate on the patients treated with conservative surgery, it appears that such a conservative approach is appropriate in patients with unilateral TOA. Clearly, patients need to be involved in this decision-making process, thus allowing individualization according to patient needs and desires.

Several investigators have reported excellent results with conservative surgical management of patients with unilateral TOAs.[4,6,8,12,18,19,20,91] These data, as summarized in Table 7.3, demonstrate that 17% of patients treated with unilateral adnexectomy will require additional surgery at a later date, whereas 14% will achieve subsequent intrauterine pregnancy. Unfortunately, the data on conservative surgical treatment of TOAs are retrospective and suffer from poor long-term follow-up. A unique series was reported by Rivlin and Hunt in which they combined conservative surgery with intra- and postoperative antibiotic peritoneal lavage for the treatment of 113 patients with ruptured TOAs.[91] They found that only 4 patients (3%) required hysterectomy during initial treatment. In the 83 patients treated with adnexal procedures (unilateral or bilateral) without removal of the uterus, 16 (19%) required further surgical intervention. In the series by Landers and Sweet, 19 patients were treated with unilateral adnexectomy, and only 2 required subsequent surgery, whereas 3 had subsequent pregnancies.[6] Thus, it appears that although there is a risk that further surgery will be required, the conservative surgical approach does offer the TOA patient who fails initial antibiotic therapy another alternative to that of permanent sterilization and castration. Perhaps patients with unilateral TOAs that do respond to antibiotic initially but have persistence of their mass could also benefit from unilateral adnexectomy in terms of preserving future fertility and preventing flare-ups. There is likely to be a continued demand for the

Table 7.3 Summary of treatment with unilateral adnexectomy

Study	No. treated with unilateral adnexectomy	No. requiring subsequent surgery (%)	No with subsequent pregnancy (%)
Pedowitz and Bloomfield[4]	14	6 (43)	NS
Landers and Sweet[6]	19	2 (10.5)	3 (15.8)
Hager[8,a]	6	0 (0)	4 (80)[a]
Ginsberg et al[12]	5	1 (20)	NS
Mickal and Sellmann[19]	8	1 (12.5)	NS
Golde et al[20]	12	0 (0)	1 (8.3)
Manara[18]	10	0 (0)	NS
Rivlin and Hunt[93,b]	27	7 (26)	1 (3.7)
Total	101	17 (16.8)	9/64 (14.1)

[a]Only five of the six patients treated with unilateral adnexectomy attempted to conceive.
[b]All patients had ruptured TOAs, and 10 were treated with incomplete unilateral adnexectomy.
Reprinted with permission from Sweet RL, Gibbs RS. Infectious Diseases of the Female Genital Tract, 4th edn. Philadelphia: Lippincott, Williams and Wilkins, 2002: 200.

conservative surgical approach, especially with techniques such as in-vitro fertilization and donor embryo transplantation becoming more widely available. Conservative surgery, in which the uterus is left in place and any normal ovarian tissue is preserved, may be an acceptable procedure in selected cases where future fertility is desired. Drainage guided by ultrasound, CT scan, or laparoscopy probably accomplishes the same goals (see discussion below).

NEWER APPROACHES TO THE MANAGEMENT OF TUBO-OVARIAN ABSCESSES

PERCUTANEOUS DRAINAGE

Percutaneous drainage guided by CT or real-time ultrasound has, in many institutions, revolutionized the approach to management of intra-abdominal and pelvic abscesses and is now commonly utilized for the treatment of intra-abdominal abscesses and, more recently, pelvic abscesses. Ultrasound- or CT-guided drainage has been reported to be successful in 75–89% of intra-abdominal abscesses.[95–98] In these early studies, the majority of abscesses successfully drained by this technique were unilocular abscesses. More recently, percutaneous drainage has been performed on multilocular abscesses.[95,99] Mandel et al reported success with placement of more than one drainage tube for multilocular abscesses.[95] Interest in less-invasive techniques in an attempt to decrease morbidity, decrease hospital stay, and decrease cost, in combination with improved imaging technology and the advent of interventional radiologic techniques, has led to increasing interest in the use of percutaneous approaches to drainage of pelvic abscesses. Worthen and Gunning reported excellent results with a 95% (18/19) success rate with transabdominal ultrasonographically guided percutaneous aspiration drainage of small pelvic abscesses and a 78% (7/9) rate with catheter drainage of larger abscesses.[100] Of note was their difficulty draining abscesses in the retrouterine location or where bowel or vascular structures intervened. Tyrrel and coworkers utilized CT-guided drainage in 8 patients with TOAs and reported success in 7 (87.5%).[101] These authors also noted technical difficulties in accessing retrouterine abscesses, which were addressed by utilizing a transgluteal approach. However, the increased cost of CT relative to ultrasound and the discomfort associated with the transgluteal approach has limited the usefulness of CT-directed drainage of tubo-ovarian and pelvic abscesses.[59] In an alternative approach, Nosher et al reported success using abdominal ultrasound to monitor transvaginal drainage of abscesses in the cul-de-sac.[102]

Subsequently, attention was focused on the use of endovaginal ultrasound guidance and transvaginal drainage of pelvic abscesses.[59,102–109] Endovaginal ultrasound-directed transvaginal drainage of pelvic abscesses has been successful in approximately 85% of reported cases.[59,102–109]

The initial report utilizing the endovaginal technique was by Abbitt et al, who used endovaginal ultrasonography in the operating room with the patient under general anesthesia to guide placement of a guidewire transvaginally to facilitate placement of an indwelling catheter.[103] Shortly thereafter, a small series of four cases of catheter drainage of small pelvic abscesses under endovaginal ultrasound guidance was reported by Van Der Kolk.[104] van Sonnenberg and associates reported success in 12 (86%) of 14 patients, who had failed antibiotic therapy, with endovaginal ultrasonographically guided transvaginal drainage and catheter placement.[105] Teisala et al demonstrated successful drainage of 10 TOAs without complications using transvaginal ultrasound guidance.[106] Similarly, Aboulghar and colleagues reported successful transvaginal drainage under transvaginal ultrasonography guidance in 15 patients with TOA; all patients improved and were afebrile within 24–72 hours.[109] In addition, at the 6-month follow-up, all patients were symptom-free. Picker et al described 12 cases of ultrasound-directed transvaginal fine-needle aspiration of pelvic abscesses.[110] All patients had multiple pelvic abscesses; 6 patients developed their abscesses following transvaginal oocyte retrieval during in-vitro fertilization.[110] Clinical cure was noted in all 12 patients at 2 months, with 3 patients requiring a single aspiration, 3 patients two aspirations, and 6 patients three to six aspirations.[110] Nelson and coworkers reported successful drainage in 26 (84%) of 31 patients with endovaginal ultrasonographically guided transvaginal drainage of pelvic abscesses.[59] However, in the 6- to 21-month follow-up, 8 women had sequelae related to pelvic infection, 8 were lost to follow-up, and only 10 women remained symptom-free.[59] Most recently, Corsi et al retrospectively analyzed 27 pelvic abscesses in 22 women: 13 TOAs and 14 postoperative abscesses.[111] In this series, transvaginal drainage was successful in 25 (92.5%) of 27 abscesses.[111] No complications were noted in any of the cases.

As noted by Nelson et al,[65] endovaginal ultrasonographically guided transvaginal drainage for treatment of pelvic abscesses has distinct advantages. It avoids the morbidity and the rare mortality associated with major pelvic surgery. In young women, it preserves the potential for future fertility and hormonal production. The endovaginal approach provides better visualization of the intervening structures and avoids the ureters, sciatic nerves, and major blood vessels. In addition, transvaginal ultrasonographically guided transvaginal drainage of abscesses can be performed without general anesthesia, at a lower cost than CT and without fluoroscopic guidance.[59]

Transrectal ultrasonographically guided drainage of gynecologic pelvic abscesses has also been attempted.[112–119] Nelson et al reported excellent results utilizing this approach for retrouterine abscesses.[112] These authors successfully drained 14 (93%) of 15 pelvic abscesses using transrectal ultrasonographic guidance.

In addition to localization and percutaneous insertion of catheters for drainage of abscesses, the CT scan and real-time ultrasound can also be used to assess the response of these abscesses to the drainage procedure. Repeat scans are generally performed within 48 hours after drainage to evaluate response. These catheters may also be used to irrigate the abscess cavities, as well as to inject contrast material to assure reduction of cavity size on repeat scans. The evaluation of this technique in the treatment of TOAs in significant numbers has yet to be reported.

LAPAROSCOPIC DRAINAGE

Laparoscopy has been instrumental in our approach to the diagnosis and management of salpingitis and has revolutionized current thought on the etiology and pathogenesis of PID. It has been suggested that the laparoscope may also be extremely useful in the management of TOAs. This technique offers the advantage of direct visualization of the abscess being drained, as well as confirmation of the diagnosis. The laparoscopic approach is associated with less morbidity and cost than laparotomy with either drainage or surgical extirpation of abscesses. The laparoscopic approach to the management of adnexal abscesses was first proposed by Dellenbach et al in 1972.[120] Other investigators have subsequently published results demonstrating the effectiveness of this approach.[121–125] Adducci described his experience with successful colpotomy drainage under laparoscopy guidance in 9 patients with PID-associated pelvic abscesses.[121] Henry-Suchet et al also noted excellent results with laparoscopic treatment of TOAs.[122] These authors reported complete and rapid recovery in 45 (90%) of 50 cases.[122] Among the 32 recent TOAs, 31 (97%) responded to laparoscopic drainage compared with 14 (78%) of 18 long-standing abscesses. However, a word of caution seems appropriate because it appears that what were described as recent TOAs may well have been acute PID with early adhesive disease. Reich and McGlynn reported a series of 25 patients with TOA and/or pelvic abscess in which 24 (96%) responded to laparoscopic drainage, whereas only 1 (4%) failed, requiring a TAH with BSO 1 month later.[123] In the 5 women in this series who underwent second-look laparoscopy, only minimal adhesions were seen.[123] In an updated report, Reich noted that he had treated 40 pelvic abscesses laparoscopically between 1976 and 1989.[126] Only a single patient required TAH with BSO, whereas 39 (97.5%) showed long-term resolution of TOA.[126] In 10 patients undergoing second-look laparoscopies, only minimal filmy adhesions were seen.[126] In a study from Finland, Teisala and coworkers[124] diagnosed acute pyosalpinx in 8 patients with laparoscopy. In 5 cases, the pus was aspirated through the laparoscope, with an uncomplicated short-term clinical response.[124] Raiga et al also reported excellent results with the laparoscopy-guided drainage approach.[125] These authors treated 39 patients with adnexal abscesses by laparoscopic drainage.[125] An immediate clinical response was noted in all 39 patients. In 35 patients, a second-look laparoscopy at 3–6 months was performed; lysis of adhesions was necessary in all 35, and a distal tuboplasty was performed in 17 patients.[136] Twelve (63%) of 19 patients not using any contraception obtained a spontaneous intrauterine pregnancy.

Whereas laparoscopy-directed drainage of TOAs and pelvic abscesses appears to be a useful alternative, additional evaluation is required. To date, there have not been any prospective randomized controlled studies comparing laparoscopic draining with ultrasonographic/CT scan-directed percutaneous drainage or medical treatment alone. Of most importance is the need not only to assess early clinical response but also to determine long-term outcomes (e.g. fertility and ectopic pregnancy) between antimicrobial therapy alone and antimicrobial therapy in combination with drainage procedures.

FERTILITY FOLLOWING TUBO-OVARIAN ABSCESSES

Although preservation of reproductive organs in the management of TOAs is a laudatory goal, it in no way guarantees future fertility, especially in patients who may well have tubal damage from previous episodes of upper genital tract infection. Several investigators have reported the incidence of subsequent pregnancy following TOAs.[6,8,10,12,20,91,93] However, the follow-up was very limited, making it impossible to assess the number of patients attempting to conceive and their success rate. The pregnancy rates reported in these studies were 9.5–15% following conservative medical management,[6,8,10,12,18] 3.7–16% following unilateral adnexal procedures with preoperative antibiotics,[6,12,20,91] and 10–15% following antibiotics plus colpotomy drainage.[91,93] In a more meaningful approach, Hager published a series in which 50 patients treated for TOAs were evaluated;[8] whereas 11 of these patients had reproductive potential following treatment, only 8 attempted to conceive. Four of the 8 (50%) conceived a total of five intrauterine pregnancies. There were no ectopic pregnancies. Included in this group were 5 patients who underwent a unilateral salpingo-oophorectomy and attempted to conceive, of whom 4 were successful (80%) Although these numbers are small, we must recognize that there may be a dramatic underestimation of reproductive potential following TOAs, unless we consider the number of patients attempting to conceive following conservative medical or surgical management.

SUMMARY: PELVIC ABSCESS

TOAs remain a common sequela of acute PID and are associated with significant reproductive morbidity. Patients with TOAs most commonly present with lower abdominal pain associated with adnexal mass(es). It is important to recognize that fever and leukocytosis may be absent. Ultrasound, CT scans, or laparoscopy may be necessary to confirm the diagnosis. TOAs may be unilateral or bilateral, regardless of IUD usage. The microbiology of TOAs is polymicrobial, with a preponderance of anaerobic organisms.

An initial conservative antimicrobial approach to the management of the unruptured TOA is appropriate. Antimicrobial agents that can penetrate abscesses, remain active within the abscess environment, and are active against the major pathogens in TOAs, including the resistant Gram-negative anaerobes such as *B. fragilis* and *P. bivia*, should be used. However, if the patient does not begin to show a response within a reasonable amount of time (i.e. 48–72 hours), surgical intervention should be undertaken. Suspicion of rupture remains an indication for immediate surgery. Once surgery is undertaken, a conservative approach with unilateral adnexectomy for unilateral TOA is appropriate if future fertility or hormone production is desired. The surgery may be difficult, requiring careful dissection and postoperative intraperitoneal drainage. Delayed primary closure can be used to decrease postoperative infectious complications. Percutaneous drainage guided by ultrasound or CT scan or laparoscopic drainage are increasingly used alternative approaches for patients not responding to antimicrobial therapy alone.

REFERENCES

1. Sweet RL, Gibbs RS. Pelvic inflammatory disease. In: Infectious Diseases of the Female Genital Tract, 4th edn. Philadelphia: Lippincott, Williams and Wilkins, 2002: 368–412.
2. Landers DV. Tubo-ovarian abscess complicating pelvic inflammatory disease. In: Sweet RL, Landers DV, eds. Pelvic Inflammatory Disease. New York: Springer-Verlag, 1997: 94–106.
3. Eschenbach DA. Acute pelvic inflammatory disease; etiology, risk factors and pathogenesis. Clin Obstet Gynecol 1976;19:147–69.
4. Pedowitz P, Bloomfield RD. Ruptured adnexal abscess (tuboovarian) with generalized peritonitis. Am J Obstet Gynecol 1964;88:721–9.
5. Nebel WA, Lucas WE. Management of tubo-ovarian abscess. Obstet Gynecol 1968;32:382–6.
6. Landers DV, Sweet RL. Tubo-ovarian abscess: contemporary approach to management. Rev Infect Dis 1983;5:876–84.
7. Burkman R, Schlesselman S, McCaffrey L, et al. The relationship of genital tract actinomycetes and the development of pelvic inflammatory disease. Am J Obstet Gynecol 1982;143:585–9.
8. Hager WD. Follow-up of patients with tubo-ovarian abscess(es) in association with salpingitis. Obstet Gynecol 1983;61:680–4.
9. Benigno BB. Medical and surgical management of the pelvic abscess. Clin Obstet Gynecol 1981;224:1187–97.
10. Franklin EW 3rd, Hevron JE Jr, Thompson JD. Management of the pelvic abscess. Clin Obstet Gynecol 1973;16:66–79.
11. Brunham RC, Binns B, Guijon F, et al. Etiology and outcome of acute pelvic inflammatory disease. J Infect Dis 1988;158:510–17.
12. Ginsberg DS, Stern JL, Hamod KA, et al. Tubo-ovarian abscess: a retrospective review. Am J Obstet Gynecol 1980;138:1055.
13. Edelman DA, Berger GS. Contraceptive practice and tuboovarian abscess. Am J Obstet Gynecol 1980;138:541–4.
14. Chow AW, Malkasian KL, Marshall JR, Guze LB. Acute pelvic inflammatory disease and clinical response to parenteral doxycycline. Antimicrob Agents Chemothr 1975;7:133–8.
15. Dawood MY, Birnbaum SJ. Unilateral tubo-ovarian abscess and intrauterine contraceptive devices. Obstet Gynecol 1975;46,429–32.
16. Golditch IM, Huston JE. Serious pelvic infections associated with intrauterine contraceptive devices. Int J Fertil 1973;18:156–60.
17. Taylor ES, McMillan JH, Greer BE, et al. The intrauterine device and tubo-ovarian abscess. Am J Obstet Gynecol 1975;123:338–48.
18. Manara LR. Management of tubo-ovarian abscess. J Am Osteopath Assoc 1982;81:476–80.
19. Mickal A, Sellmann AH. Management of tubo-ovarian abscess. Clin Obstet Gynecol 1969;12:252–64.
20. Golde SH, Israel R, Ledger WJ. Unilateral tuboovarian abscess: a distinct entity. Am J Obstet Gynecol 1977;127:807–10.
21. Landers DV, Sweet RL. Current trends in the diagnosis and treatment of tubo-ovarian abscess. Am J Obstet Gynecol 1985;151:1098–1110.
22. Sweet RL, Gibbs RS. Mixed anaerobic-aerobic pelvic infection and pelvic abscess. In: Infectious Diseases of the Female Genital Tract, 4th edn. Philadelphia: Lippincott, Williams and Wilkins, 2002: 176–206.
23. Swenson RM, Michaelson TC, Daly MJ, Spaulding EH. Anaerobic bacterial infections of the female genital tract. Obstet Gynecol 1973;42:538–41.
24. Thadepalli H, Gorbach SL, Keith L. Anaerobic infections of the female genital tract: bacteriologic and therapeutic aspects. Am J Obstet Gynecol 1973;117:1034–40.
25. Altemeier WA. The anaerobic streptococci in tuboovarian abscess. Am J Obstet Gynecol 1940;39:1038.
26. Ledger WJ, Campbell C, Willson JR. Postoperative adnexal infections. Obstet Gynecol 1968;31:83–9.
27. Pearson HE, Anderson GV. Genital bacteroidal abscesses in women. Am J Obstet Gynecol 1970;107:1264–5.
28. Weinstein WM, Onderdonk AB, Bartlett JG, Gorbach SL. Experimental intra-abdominal abscess in rats: development of an experimental model. Infect Immun 1974;10:1250–5.
29. Onderdonk AB, Kasper DL, Cizneros RL, Bartlett JG. The capsular polysaccharide of *Bacteroides fragilis* as a virulence factor: comparison of the pathogenic potential of encapsulated and unencapsulated strains. J Infect Dis 1977;136:82–9.
30. Bjornson AB, Bjornson HS. Participation of immunoglobulin and the alternative complement pathway in opsonization of *Bacteroides fragilis* and *Bacteroides thetaiotaomicorn*. Rev Infect Dis 1979;1(2):347.
31. Tzianabos AU, Kasper DL, Onderdonk AB. Structure and function of *Bacteroides fragilis* capsular polysaccharides: relationship to induction and prevention of abscesses. Clin Infect Dis 1995;20(Suppl 2):S132–40.
32. Zaleznik DF, Kasper DL. The role of anaerobic bacteria in abscess formation. Ann Rev Med 1982;38:217.
33. McNeeley SG, Hendrix SL, Mazzoni MM, et al. Medically sound, cost-effective treatment for pelvic inflammatory disease and tuboovarian abscess. Am J Obstet Gynecol 1998;178:1272–8.
34. Cox SM, Faro S, Doddon MG, et al. Role of *Neisseria gonorrhoeae* and *Chlamydia trachomatis* in intraabdominal abscess formation in the rat. J Reprod Med 1991;36:202–5.
35. Chow AW, Malkasian KL, Marshall JR, Guze, LB. The bacteriology of acute pelvic inflammatory disease. Am J Obstet Gynecol 1975;122:876–9.
36. Monif GRC, Welkos SL, Baer H, Thompson RJ. Cul-de-sac isolates from patients with endometritis–salpingitis–peritonitis and gonococcal endocervicitis. Am J Obstet Gynecol 1976;126:158–61.
37. Holmes KK, Eschenbach DA, Knapp JS. Salpingitis: overview of etiology and epidemiology. Am J Obstet Gynecol 1980;138:893–900.
38. Schiffer MA, Elguezabal A, Sultana M, Allen AC. Actinomycosis infections associated with intrauterine contraceptive devices. Obstet Gynecol 1975;45:67–72.
39. Lomax CW, Harbert GM Jr, Thornton WN Jr. Actinomycosis of the female genital tract. Obstet Gynecol 1976;48:341–6.
40. Gupta PK, Erozan YS, Frost JK. *Actinomyces* and the IUD: an update. Acta Cytol 1978;22:281–2.
41. Piepert JF. *Actinomyces*: normal flora or pathogen? Obstet Gynecol 2004;104:1132–3.
42. Carney FE, Taylor-Robinson D. Growth and effect of *Neisseria gonorrhoeae* in organ cultures. Br J Vener Dis 1973;49:435–40.
43. Patton DL, Cosgrove Sweeney TY, Kuo CC. Demonstration of delayed hypersensitivity in *Chlamydia trachomatis* salpingitis in monkeys. A pathogenic mechanism of tubal damage. J Infect Dis 1994;169:680–3.
44. Hare MJ, Barnes CFJ. Fallopian-tube organ culture in the investigation of *Bacteroides* as a cause of pelvic inflammatory disease. In: Philips I, Collier J, eds. Proceedings of the 2nd International Symposium on Metronidazole. London: The Royal Society of Medicine, 1979: 191–8.

45. Bieluch VM, Tally FP. Pathophysiology of abscess formation. Clin Obstet Gynecol 1983;10:93–103.
46. Sweet RL. Pelvic inflammatory disease and tubo-ovarian abscess. In: Gorbach SL, Bartlett JG, Blacklow NR, eds. Infectious Diseases. Philadelphia: WB Saunders, 1998: 1025–36.
47. Scott WC. Pelvic abscess in association with intrauterine contraceptive device. Am J Obstet Gynecol 1978;131:149–56.
48. Burnhill MS. Syndrome of progressive endometritis associated with intrauterine contraceptive devices. Adv Planned Parent 1973;8:144–50.
49. Mishell DR Jr, Bell JH, Good RG, Moyer DL. The intrauterine device: a bacteriologic study of the endometrial cavity. Am J Obstet Gynecol 1966;96:119–26.
50. Sparks RA, Purrier BG, Watt PJ, Elstein M. Bacteriological colonisation of uterine cavity: role of tailed intrauterine contraceptive devices. BMJ 1981;282:1189–91.
51. Canas AM, Holloran-Schwartz B, Myles T. Tuboovarian abscess 12 years after total abdominal hysterectomy. Obstet Gynecol 2004;104:1039–41.
52. Roth TM, Rivlin ME. Tuboovarian abscess: a postoperative complication of endometrial ablation. Obstet Gynecol 2004;104:1198–9.
53. Das S, Kirwan J, Drakeley AJ, Kingsland CR. Pelvic abscess following microwave endometrial ablation. Br J Obstet Gynaecol 2005;112:118–19.
54. Heaton FC, Ledger WJ. Postmenopausal tuboovarian abscess. Obstet Gynecol 1976;47:90–4.
55. Clark JR, Moore-Hines S. A study of tubo-ovarian abscess at Howard University Hospital (1965 through 1975). J Natl Med Assoc 1979;71:1109.
56. Vermereen J, Te Linde RW. Intraabdominal rupture of pelvic abscess. Am J Obstet Gynaecol 1954;68:402–9.
57. Lehtinen M, Laine S, Heinonen PK, et al. Serum C-reactive protein determination in acute pelvic inflammatory disease. Am J Obstet Gynecol 1986;154:158–9.
58. Mercer LJ, Hajj SM, Ismail MA, Block BS. Use of C-reactive protein to predict the outcome of medical management of tuboovarian abscesses. J Reprod Med 1988;33:164–7.
59. Nelson AL, Sinow RM, Renslo R, et al. Endovaginal ultrasonography guided transvaginal drainage for treatment of pelvic abscesses. Am J Obstet Gynecol 1995;172:1926–35.
60. Filly RA. Detection of abdominal abscesses: a combined approach employing ultrasonography, computed tomography and gallium-67 scanning. J Assoc Can Radiol 1979;30:202.
61. Norton L, Eule J, Burdick D. Accuracy of techniques to detect intraperitoneal abscess. Surgery 1978;84:370–8.
62. Hopkins GB, Kan M, Mende CW. Gallium-67 scintography and intraabdominal sepsis. Clinical experience in 140 patients with suspected intraabdominal abscess. West J Med 1976;125:425–30.
63. Carroll B, Silverman PM, Goodwin DA, McDougall R. Ultrasonography and indium 111 white blood cell scanning for the detection of intraabdominal abscesses. Radiology 1981;140:155–60.
64. Coleman RE, Black RE, Welch DM, Maxwell JG. Indium-111 labeled leukocytes in the evaluation of suspected abdominal abscesses. Am J Surg 1980;139:99–104.
65. Bicknell TA, Kohatsu S, Goodwin DA. Use of indium-111-labeled autologous leukocytes in differentiating pancreatic abscess from pseudocyst. Am J Surg 1981;142:312–16.
66. Taylor KJW, Wasson JF, De Graaff C, et al. Accuracy of grey-scale ultrasound diagnosis of abdominal and pelvic abscesses in 220 patients. Lancet 1978;i:83–4.
67. Spirtos NJ, Bernstine EL, Crawford WL, Fayle J. Sonography in acute pelvic inflammatory disease. J Reprod Med 1982;27:312–20.
68. Uhrich PC, Sanders RC. Ultrasonic characteristics of pelvic inflammatory masses. J Clin Ultrasound 1976;4:199–204.
69. Moir C, Robins RE. Role of ultrasonography, gallium scanning, and computed tomography in the diagnosis of intraabdominal abscess. Am J Surg 1982;143:582–5.
70. Peters AM, Danpure HJ, Osoman S, et al. Clinical experience with ^{99m}Tc-hexamethylpropylene-amineoxime for labeling leukocytes and imaging inflammation. Lancet 1986;2:946–9.
71. Mountford PJ, Kettle AG, O'Doherty MN, Coakley AJ. Comparison of technetium-99m-HM-PAO leukocytes with indium-111-oxine leukocytes for localizing intraabdominal sepsis. J Nucl Med 1990;31:311–15.
72. Fischman AJ, Rubin RH, Khaw BA, et al. Detection of acute inflammation with ^{111}In-labelled nonspecific polyclonal IgG. Semin Nucl Med 1988;18:335–44.
73. Rubin RH, Fischman AJ, Callahan RJ, et al. ^{111}In-labelled nonspecific immunoglobulins scanning in the detection of focal infection. N Engl J Med 1989;321:935–40.
74. Oyen WJ, Claessens RA, van der Meer JW, Corstens FH. Detection of subacute infectious foci and indium-111-labeled human nonspecific immunoglobulin G: a prospective comparative study. J Nucl Med 1991;32:1854–60.
75. Gerzof SG, Robbins AH, Johnson WC, et al. Percutaneous catheter drainage of abdominal abscesses: a five-year experience. N Engl J Med 1981;305:653–7.
76. Ferrucci JT Jr, van Sonnenberg E. Intraabdominal abscess. Radiological diagnosis and treatment. JAMA 1981;246:2728–33.
77. Jasinski RW, Glazer GM, Francis IR, Harkness RL. CT and ultrasound in abscess detection at specific anatomic sites: a study of 198 patients. Comput Radiol 1987;11:41–7.
78. McClean KL, Sheehan GJ, Harding GKM. Intraabdominal infection: a review. Clin Infect Dis 1994;19:100–16.
79. Gagliardi PD, Hoffer PB, Rosenfield AT. Correlative imaging in abdominal infection: an algorithmic approach using nuclear medicine, ultrasound, and computed tomography. Semin Nucl Med 1988;18:320–34.
80. Saini S, Kellum JM, O'Leary MP, et al. Improved localization and survival in patients with intraabdominal abscesses. Am J Surg 1983;154:136–42.
81. Kaplan AL, Jacobs WM, Ehresman JB. Aggressive management of pelvic abscess. Am J Obstet Gynecol 1967;98:482–7.
82. Hemsell DL, Santos-Ramos R, Cunningham FG, et al. Cefotaxime treatment for women with community acquired pelvic abscesses. Am J Obstet Gynecol 1985;151:771–7.
83. Reed SD, Landers DV, Sweet RL. Antibiotic treatment of tubo-ovarian abscess: comparison of broad-spectrum beta-lactam agents versus clindamycin-containing regimens. Am J Obstet Gynecol 1991;164:1556–62.
84. Kasper DL, Onderdonk AB, Polk BF, Bartlett JG. Surface antigens as virulence factors in infection with *Bacteroides fragilis*. Rev Infect Dis 1979;1:278–90.
85. Bartlett JG, Onderdonk AB, Louie TJ, et al. A review. Lessons from an animal model of intra-abdominal sepsis. Arch Surg 1978;113:853–7.
86. Nathans AB, Ahrenholz DH, Simmons RL, Rotstein O. Peritonitis and other intra-abdominal infections. In: Howard RJ, Simmons RL, eds. Surgical Infectious Diseases. East Norwalk, CT: Appleton and Lange, 1995: 959–1009.
87. Klempner MS, Styrt B. Clindamycin uptake by human neutrophils. J Infect Dis 1981;144:472–9.
88. Prokesch RC, Hand WL. Antibiotic entry into human polymorphonuclear leukocytes. Antimicrob Agents Chemother 1982;21:373–80.

89. Joiner KA, Lowe BR, Dzink JL, Bartlett JG. Antibiotic levels in infected and sterile subcutaneous abscesses in mice. J Infect Dis 1981;143:487–4.
90. Collins CG, Jansen FW. Treatment of pelvic abscess. Clin Obstet Gynecol 1959;2:512.
91. Rivlin ME, Hunt JA. Ruptured tubo-ovarian abscess. Is hysterectomy necessary? Obstet Gynecol 1977;50(5):518–22.
92. Rubenstein PR, Mishell DR, Ledger WJ. Colpotomy drainage of pelvic abscess. Obstet Gynecol 1976;48(2):142–5.
93. Rivlin ME, Golan A, Darling MR. Diffuse peritoneal sepsis associated with colpotomy drainage of pelvic abscess. J Reprod Med 1982;27(7):406–10.
94. Rivlin ME. Clinical outcome following vaginal drainage of pelvic abscess. Obstet Gynecol 1983;61(2):169–73.
95. Mandel SR, Body D, Jacques PF, et al. Drainage of hepatic, intraabdominal and mediastinal abscesses guided by computerized axial tomography. Am J Surg 1983;145:120.
96. van Sonnenberg E, Ferrucci JT, Mueller PR, et al. Percutaneous radiographically guided catheter drainage of abdominal abscesses. JAMA 1982;247(2):190.
97. Gerzof SG, Robbins AH, Johnson WC, et al. Percutaneous catheter drainage of abdominal abscesses: a five-year experience. N Engl J Med 1981;305(12):653–7.
98. Gronvall S, Gammelgaard J, Haubek A, Holm HH. Drainage of abdominal abscesses guided by sonography. Am J Radiol 1982;138:527–9.
99. Gerzof SG, Johnson WC, Robbins AH, Nabseth DC. Expanded criteria for percutaneous abscess drainage. Arch Surg 1985;120:227–32.
100. Worthen NJ, Gunning JE. Percutaneous drainage of pelvic abscesses: management of tuboovarian abscesses. J Ultrasound Med 1986;5:551–6.
101. Tyrrel T, Murphy FB, Bernardino ME. Tuboovarian abscesses: CT-guided percutaneous drainage. Radiology 1990;175:87–9.
102. Nosher JL, Winchman HK, Needell CS. Transvaginal pelvic abscess drainage with US guidance. Radiology 1987;165:872–3.
103. Abbitt PL, Goldwag S, Urbanski S. Endovaginal sonography for guidance in draining pelvic fluid collections. AJR Am J Roentgenol 1990;154:849–50.
104. Van Der Kolk HL. Small, deep pelvic abscesses: definition and drainage guided with an endovaginal probe. Radiology 1991;181:283–4.
105. van Sonnenberg E, D'Agostino HB, Casola G, et al. US-guided transvaginal drainage of pelvic abscesses and fluid collections. Radiology 1991;181:53–6.
106. Teisala K, Heinonen PK, Punnonen R. Transvaginal ultrasound in the diagnosis and treatment of tuboovarian abscess. Br J Obstet Gynaecol 1990;97:178–9.
107. Loy RA, Galup DG, Hill JA, et al. Pelvic abscess: examination and transvaginal drainage guided by real-time ultrasonography. South Med J 1989;82:788–90.
108. Sinow R, Nelson A, Renslo R, et al. Ultrasound guided transvaginal aspiration of pelvic abscesses. Surg Forum 1992;43:520–2.
109. Aboulghar MA, Mansur RT, Serour GI. Ultrasonographically guided transvaginal aspiration of tuboovarian abscesses and pyosalpinges: an optional treatment for acute pelvic inflammatory disease. Am J Obstet Gynecol 1995;172:1501–3.
110. Picker RH, McLennan AC, Robertson RD, Porter RN. Conservative management of pelvic abscess in recurrent pelvic inflammatory disease. Ultrasound Obstet Gynecol 1991;1:60–2.
111. Corsi PJ, Johnson SC, Gonik B, et al. Transvaginal ultrasound-guided aspiration of pelvic abscesses. Infect Dis Obstet Gynecol 1999;7:216–21.
112. Nelson AL, Sinow RM, Oliak D. Transrectal ultrasonographically guided drainage of gynecologic pelvic abscesses. Am J Obstet Gynecol 2000;182:1283–8.
113. Kuligowska E, Keller E, Ferrucci JT. Treatment of pelvic abscesses: value of one-step sonographically guided transrectal needle aspiration and lavage. AJR Am J Roentgenol 1995;164:2061–6.
114. Bennett JD, Kozak RI, Taylor BM, Jory TA. Deep pelvic abscesses: transrectal drainage with radiologic guidance. Radiology 1992;185:825–8.
115. Feld R, Eschelman DJ, Sagerman JE, et al. Treatment of pelvic abscesses and other fluid collections: efficacy of transvaginal sonographically guided aspiration and drainage. AJR Am J Roentgenol 1994;163:1141–5.
116. Chung T, Hoffer, FA, Lund DP. Transrectal drainage of deep pelvic abscesses in children using a combined transrectal sonographic and fluoroscopic guidance. Pediatr Radiol 1996;26:874–8.
117. Kastan DJ, Nelsen KM, Shetty PC, et al. Combined transrectal sonographic and fluoroscopic guidance for deep pelvic abscess drainage. J Ultrasound Med 1996;15:235–9.
118. Hovsepian DM. Transrectal and transvaginal abscess drainage. Radiology 1997;8:501–15.
119. Hovsepian DM, Steele JR, Skinner CS, Malden ES. Transrectal versus transvaginal abscess drainage: survey of patient tolerance and effect on activities of daily living. Radiology 1999;212:159–63.
120. Dellenbach P, Muller P, Philippe E. Infections utero annexielles aigues. Encyl Med Chir Gynecol 1972;470:A10.
121. Adducci JE. Laparoscopy in the diagnosis and treatment of pelvic inflammatory disease with abscess formation. Int Surg 1981;66:359–60.
122. Henry-Suchet J, Soler A, Laffredo V. Laparoscopic treatment of tuboovarian abscesses. J Reprod Med 1984;29:579–82.
123. Reich H, McGlynn F. Laparoscopic treatment of tuboovarian and pelvic abscess. J Reprod Med 1987;32:747–52.
124. Teisala K, Heinonen PK, Punnonen R. Laparoscopic treatment of acute pyosalpinx. J Reprod Med 1990;35:19–21.
125. Raiga J, Canis M. LeBouedec G, et al. Laparoscopic management of adnexal abscesses: consequences for fertility. Fertil Steril 1996;66:712–17.
126. Reich H. Role of laparoscopy in treating TOA and pelvic abscess. Contemp OB/Gyn 1989;34:91–102.
127. Sweet RL, Gibbs RS. Atlas of Infectious Diseases of the Female Genital Tract. Philadelphia: Lippincott, Williams and Wilkins 2005.

8. Post-Procedural Upper Genital Tract Infection

Matthew F. Reeves and Mitchell D. Creinin

INTRODUCTION

Any gynecologic procedure in which instruments or devices are passed through the cervix into the uterine cavity has the potential to seed infection of the upper genital tract. For most minor procedures, this risk is quite small; however, it is important to understand what the risks are and how they may be minimized.

This chapter will examine the risks, identifiable risk factors, prophylactic measures, and treatment for the most common minor gynecologic procedures such as elective abortion, hysteroscopy, intrauterine device (IUD) placement, and endometrial biopsy. Because surgical abortions are one of the most common surgical procedures in the United States, the majority of data come from studies of these procedures. The microbiology and epidemiology is similar for the group of procedures discussed here, as the vagina and cervix are the portal through which all are performed.

In general, preoperative antibiotic therapy has been shown to decrease the rate of postoperative infection.[1] However, for most minor gynecologic procedures, the risk of infection is quite low. Therefore, for each procedure, it is important to carefully weigh the risks of universal prophylaxis with the prevention of a relatively rare complication. The seemingly cautious provider who supplies antibiotics unnecessarily for all procedures puts patients at risk for adverse reactions without predictably obtaining any benefit. Furthermore, overuse of antibiotics needs to be avoided to prevent the development of resistance and to preserve the utility of these drugs for treatment of infection.

Procedures to be examined are the following:

- surgical abortion
- medical abortion
- dilation and curettage (D & C) in the non-pregnant state
- hysteroscopy
- IUD insertion
- hysterosalpingography.

ELECTIVE SURGICAL ABORTION

Elective abortion is one of the most common surgical procedures in the United States, with over 1.3 million performed in 2000.[2] In the United States, the annual abortion rate is 21 per 1000 women (2.1%).[3] In the United States, the proportion of abortions performed before 12 weeks gestation has remained stable over the past decade at approximately 88%.[4] Following surgical abortion, the rate of infection ranges widely between sites and by diagnostic criteria and ascertainment method. When objective measures are used, such as temperature ≥38°C, the infection rate ranges from 0.01% to 2.44%.[5–7] When the diagnosis is based on physician concern, the rate ranges from 0.5% to 4.7%.[8–11] Some studies have reported higher rates of infection. Most of these studies have various degrees of ascertainment and diagnostic biases that result in more infection being diagnosed.[12] For unclear reasons, the reported rates of infection are uniformly highly in Scandinavian countries in comparison with North America. In randomized trials of antibiotic prophylaxis, the infection rates in the placebo groups show similar variability, depending on the definition of infection and the ascertainment method. The risk remains low for dilation and evacuation (D & E) procedures.[13,14] The rate of upper genital tract infection after abortion is under 1% in most clinical settings.[5,15] Because abortion is so common, small improvements in post-procedural infection rates can have profound impacts on the absolute number of post-procedure infections.

Surgical abortions can be divided into two main types: suction (D & C) and D & E. Suction D & C entails dilation of the cervix sufficient to pass a suction curette through which the uterine contents may be removed. This procedure is generally used for abortions up to 13–14 weeks' gestation. Sharp curettage alone is rarely used in developed countries for termination of pregnancy, as the complication rate is more than double that for suction abortion (relative risk (RR) = 2.3).[16] In the developing world, however, sharp curettage is often still used when suction equipment is not available.

D & E involves more cervical dilation and the use of forceps to remove the products of conception. The dilation of the cervix often involves the use of osmotic dilators for 2–48 hours prior to the procedure. A combination of suction curettage and a forceps are then used to remove the uterine contents. The most widely available osmotic dilator used in the United States is Laminaria, a natural osmotic dilator made from the stalks of *Laminaria japonica*, a type of seaweed. Two synthetic osmotic dilators, Lamicel and Dilapan, are also commonly used. None of these three types of osmotic dilators has been shown to increase the risk of infection when left in place for up to 24 hours before a D & E.[17–20] Although misoprostol use has been reported to prepare the cervix prior to D & E, controlled studies are not available.[21]

Second-trimester abortion can also be accomplished by induction of labor using intra-amniotic injection or prostaglandin. However, data from the Joint Program for the Study of Abortion indicate that these forms of abortion have twice the mortality rate of D & E (RR=1.9, 95% confidence interval (CI) 1.2–3.1).[13] Consequently, labor induction abortion is recommended only when D & E is not available.

RISK FACTORS

Although there are numerous risk factors discussed below, many post-abortal infections occur in women without any risk factors. The vast majority of the data below come from studies of patients undergoing suction D & C abortions.

NEISSERIA GONORRHOEAE *AND* CHLAMYDIA TRACHOMATIS

Untreated cervical gonorrhea increases the rate of post-abortal endometritis three-fold.[22] Multiple studies have identified the presence of *Chlamydia trachomatis* at the time of procedure with increased risk of infection afterwards.[23–25]

In a cohort study of 1032 women in Sweden, the presence of chlamydia prior to first-trimester abortion increased the risk of laparoscopically confirmed salpingitis by 30-fold (RR=29.9, 95% CI 10.5–85.1, p <0.0001).[25] The rate of endometritis (without salpingitis) was increased by four-fold if chlamydia was present (RR=4.1, 95% CI 2.5–6.7, p <0.0001).[25] In a study of 85 patients undergoing D & C for missed or incomplete abortion, the presence of chlamydia increased the risk of PID by 32-fold (RR=32, 95% CI 3.5–296).[26] Levallois and Rioux[27] found that the presence of chlamydia increased the risk of PID by nine-fold in a randomized trial of prophylactic antibiotics. This increase in RR occurred regardless of whether antibiotics were given, but the absolute risk with antibiotic prophylaxis was significantly lower.[27]

Because of both the high risk of post-abortal infection and the public health implications, screening for chlamydia and gonorrhea prior to abortion is essential.

PRIOR PELVIC INFLAMMATORY DISEASE

A history of pelvic inflammatory disease (PID) has been identified as a risk factor for post-abortal infection.[28, 29] Although the association between past PID and risk after abortion is probably confounded by many other factors, such as risk of chlamydia, it is a clinically useful marker of increased risk.

BACTERIAL VAGINOSIS

Limited epidemiologic data exist on bacterial vaginosis (BV) as a risk factor for post-abortal upper genital tract infection.[30] The magnitude of the association is not well defined. Three studies have shown that prophylactic antibiotics with good anaerobic coverage such as metronidazole or clindamycin can decrease the risk of PID in women with bacterial vaginosis.[31–33] However, in one of these studies,[31] the results did not reach statistical significance. A recent study showed that metronidazole does not appear to add benefit when doxycycline is used routinely.[34]

ANTIBIOTIC PROPHYLAXIS FOR SURGICAL ABORTION

The issue of antibiotic prophylaxis for surgical abortion was controversial until a meta-analysis was published by Sawaya et al[35] in 1996. This meta-analysis showed that a variety of antibiotics are effective for women of all risk strata. Based primarily upon this meta-analysis, the World Health Organization (WHO), the American College of Obstetricians and Gynecologists, the Royal College of Obstetricians and Gynecologists, and the National Abortion Federation recommend antibiotic prophylaxis for all elective abortion as standard practice.[36–39] Members of the nitroimidazole (metronidazole and tinidazole) and tetracycline families were shown to be effective in multiple studies.[35]

Doxycycline is commonly recommended for prophylaxis and is used by over 80% of abortion providers who use prophylactic antibiotics.[40] It has been shown to reduce the risk of post-abortion infection substantially in several randomized placebo-controlled trials when used as a short course at the time of abortion.[27,28,41] Doxycycline also has the advantages of being cheap and equally effective orally as parenterally.[42] In longer courses, it is an effective treatment against chlamydia, the microorganism most associated with post-abortion infection.[27,43]

The meta-analysis by Sawaya et al[35] strictly included only randomized blinded placebo-controlled trials. The authors concluded that no further placebo-controlled trials should ethically be performed given that there are effective regimens for prophylaxis.[35] Based on the studies included in the meta-analysis, the protective effect of antibiotics was easily demonstrable regardless of what subgroup was analyzed.[35]

However, because multiple antibiotics were used and multiple regimens for each antibiotic, the implications for clinical practice are unclear. Meta-analysis methodology does not provide insight into the best regimen for use in clinical practice. Moreover, the authors' methodology excludes several instructive studies and includes several studies of questionable value to current practice. Nine of the 12 studies in this meta-analysis, primarily from Scandinavia, reported infection rates over 10% in the control group. Four studies reported infections rate of 10% or greater in the treatment group.

These infection rates are significantly greater than those reported in clinical practice. None of the studies of clinic practice have reported infection rates above 5%, even in Scandinavia (Table 8.1).[5–11] Most clinical sites that use a strict definition of infection report infection rates well below 1%.[5,8,10] Although there is probably some degree of under-reporting in the reports of infection in clinical practice, the true infection rate is unlikely to be as high as reported in many of the antibiotic studies. The high rates reported in antibiotic trials probably represent a combination of ascertainment and diagnostic biases.

Two of the studies[27,28] included in the meta-analysis by Sawaya et al[35] and one study[41] excluded from that meta-analysis give strong support to the use of single-dose doxycycline. The first of these studies was published by Brewer in 1980.[41] In a high-volume British clinic, he gave 500 mg of doxycycline (or placebo) to 2950 women at the time of abortion. The study was randomized by using drug or placebo for calendar blocks in a blinded fashion. Patients were asked to report any subsequent infections. Although the methodology is suboptimal for a study setting, it closely mimics the setting of most clinics. He reported an 88% reduction in the risk of PID after abortion (RR=0.12, 95% CI 0.015–0.94).

A study conducted by Darj et al[28] was a large randomized placebo-controlled trial of single-dose preoperative antibiotic prophylaxis for first-trimester abortion. The investigators gave women 400 mg of doxycycline (or placebo) the night before the abortion procedure. Using standardized study criteria, 2.1% of women who received doxycycline and 6.2% of women who received placebo were diagnosed with PID (RR=0.33, 95% CI 0.15–0.73, p <0.005*). This study is the only clinical trial that

*RR, CI, and p-value were recalculated based on information provided in the orginal article by Darj et al.[28]

Table 8.1 Summary of infectious rates after abortion by suction D & C in cohort studies

Study	Number of abortions	Years	Diagnostic criteria for infection	Number of infections	Infection rate (%)	Gestational age (weeks)	Facility type (location)	Antibiotic prophylaxis	Ascertainment method
Hakim-Elahi et al[5]	170 000	1971–1987	Physician concern, tenderness, fever not required	784	0.46%	≤14	Three free-standing clinics New York City	None	Retrospective
			≥2 days of fever <40°C	6	0.004%				
Hodgson[8]	20 248	1972–1973	Bleeding, fever, and/or pain, with or without reaspiration	135	0.67%	≤12	Free-standing clnic Washington, DC	"As indicated"	Prospective
			Bleeding, fever, and/or pain, without reaspiration	45	0.22%				
Heisterberg and Kringelbach[6]	5 851	1980–1985	Readmission, fever ≥38°C	143	2.4%		Hospital Copenhagen, Denmark	None	Retrospective
			Readmission, antibiotic	190	3.2%	≥12			
Fried et al[7]	1 000	1987	"Infection"	47	4.7%		Hospital Stockholm, Sweden	Doxycycline if chlamydia (+)	Prospective
			Fever ≥38°C	16	1.6%	≥15			
Wadhera[9]	351 789	1975–1980	"Infection"	633	0.18%	≥15	Canada (national data)	Uncertain	Retrospective
Joint Study of RCGP & RCOG[11]	6 105	1976–1979	"Infection"	218	3.6%		Hospital Great Britain (national data)	Uncertain	Prospective
			"PID"	100	1.6%	≤15			
Wulff & Freiman[10]	16 410	1973–1976	Infection, JPSA criteria	16	0.10%	≤14	Free-standing clinic St Louis, Missouri	All patients	Retrospective

gave antibiotics so far in advance (10-12 hours). In many institutions where patients must be nil by mouth after midnight, this regimen may be a good alternative to having women take doxycycline on the morning of the procedure on an empty stomach. Despite allowing women to take the 400 mg of doxycycline with food on the night prior to operation, there was still a surprisingly high rate of nausea and emesis. The rate among women who took doxycycline was five-fold higher than placebo controls (26% vs 5 %, RR=5.1, 95% CI 3.2–8.0, p <0.001).[28] This may be due to the large dose (400 mg) of doxycycline.

Levallois and Rioux[27] showed in a randomized double-blind placebo-controlled trial of 1074 subjects that an abbreviated regimen of doxycycline was highly effective in reducing the risk of post-abortion infection in a low-risk population. The study included all women presenting to a hospital-based family planning clinic in Quebec but excluded women with positive gonorrhea cultures. This study then divided women into those with and without chlamydia. Their regimen consisted of 100 mg 1 hour before and 200 mg 30 min after the abortion. This regimen reduced the risk of the diagnosis of infection by 87% (RR=0.132, 95% CI 0.030–0.574) both in women with chlamydia (RR=0.12, 95% CI 0.02–0.85) and in those without chlamydia (RR=0.12 95% CI 0.04–0.38).[27] The absolute risk, however, was much higher among the women with chlamydia (Table 8.2). Twelve of the 29 cases of PID were in the 75 women with chlamydia. By removing women with gonorrhea and separating out women with chlamydia, this study was able to demonstrate that an abbreviated course of doxycycline is very effective in a low-risk population.

Several factors make this study particularly compelling. The follow-up rate was exceptionally high; only three subjects did not return for a follow-up examination. Despite the fact that subjects were examined shortly after the abortion, infection was only diagnosed in 29 of the 1074 women (2.7%, 95% CI 1.8–3.9%). This rate of infection is consistent with the observed infection rates in clinical practice.

A fourth study published by Henriques et al.[44] in 1994 examined the use of ceftriaxone administered by the anesthesiologist after induction of anesthesia. Although we discuss this study here, it was excluded from the meta-analysis by Sawaya et al[35] because a placebo was not used. This study divided women into high and low risk based on a history of any sexually transmitted infection (STI) or PID. The high-risk women were all given antibiotics, whereas the low-risk women were randomized to 1 g of ceftriaxone or no antibiotics. Among the low-risk women, ceftriaxone reduced the risk of post-abortal PID by 76% (RR=0.24, 95% CI 0.06–0.93). This regimen may be useful in some settings where parenteral antibiotics are needed and doxycycline is not available. It is important to remember that ceftriaxone is not an effective treatment for chlamydia.

One option that has been adopted by some institutions is to give doxycycline after the procedure only. However, perioperative antibiotic prophylaxis has been shown to be most effective when given at least 30 minutes *before* surgery.[1] There are no studies to support the idea that *single-dose post-abortion* antibiotics are effective, whereas there are several studies showing that single-dose pre-abortion antibiotics are very effective.

Because single-dose post-abortion prophylaxis has never been examined in clinical trials, many institutions give a full treatment course of doxycycline. Two studies suggest that no more than 3 days of doxycycline are needed.[45,46] Reedy et al[46] demonstrated that a 3-day course of doxycycline (100 mg twice daily) is equivalent to a 7-day course in the treatment of chlamydia cervicitis in the outpatient setting (RR=1.0, 95% CI 0.71–1.40). Lichtenberg and Shott[45] then showed that post-abortion prophylaxis using a 3-day course of doxycycline (100 mg twice daily) is not statistically different from a 7-day course. Despite enrolling 800 subjects, this study did not have enough power to detect a small difference due to only one infection (in the 7-day group) among all subjects.

Although risk-based strategies for the use of prophylactic antibiotics (as opposed to universal usage) have been proposed, there is little evidence to support this strategy. In a relatively low-risk setting, Levallois and Rioux[27] suggest that a risk-based strategy would use 71% less antibiotic while preventing 62% of the cases of PID compared with universal prophylaxis. By their analysis,[27] high-risk

Table 8.2 Summary of randomized trials of antibiotic prophylaxis using short courses of antibiotics with infection rates in controls less than 5%

Author	Year	Antibiotic	Dosing method[a]	Population[b]	Total *N*	Antibiotic group			Placebo group			Relative risk	NNT[c]
						Infection	No infection	Rate	Infection	No infection	Rate		
Levallois and Rioux[27]	1988	Doxycycline	100 mg pre, 200 mg post	Chl neg	999	2	500	0.4%	15	482	3.0%	0.13	38
				Chl pos	75	1	32	3.0%	11	31	26.2%	0.12	4
				All patients (GC neg)	1074	3	532	0.6%	26	513	4.8%	0.12	23
Darj et al[28]	1987	Doxycycline	400 mg 10–12 h pre	All 1st trimester	769	8	378	2.1%	24	359	6.3%	0.33	24
Brewer[41]	1980	Doxycycline	500 mg pre	All patients	2950	1	1518	0.1%	8	1423	0.6%	0.12	203
Henriques et al[44]	1994	Ceftriaxone	1 g pre i.v.	Low risk[d]	549	2	273	0.7%	10	264	3.6%	0.20	34
Total					**5342**	**14**	**2701**	**0.5%**	**68**	**2559**	**2.6%**	**0.20**	**48**

[a]pre = immediately pre-procedure; post = post-procedure (within hours); i.v. = intravenous.
[b]Chl = chlamydia; GC = *Neisseria gonorrhoeae*.
[c]Number need to treat (to prevent 1 infection)
[d]No history of pelvic inflammatory disease or sexually transmitted infections.

patients were found to be nulliparous patients with two or more sex partners or women with a history of gonorrhea. They appear to favor this strategy as a way to increase efficiency. However, given the marginal improvement in efficiency at the cost of increasing the number of cases of a preventable disease with long-term sequelae, this strategy would only be acceptable in settings where there is an insufficient supply of antibiotics to provide universal prophylaxis.[39]

Although multiple studies have shown prophylactic antibiotics to be effective, all the studies (including the ones with the lowest infection rates) report rates higher than the cohort series from abortion clinics in North America (see Table 8.1). The benefits of antibiotic prophylaxis are not clear in a population at very low risk (e.g. 0.5% infection risk without antibiotics). As the chlamydia prevalence and infection risk decrease, the number of women who need to get antibiotics to prevent one infection increases dramatically (Table 8.3). It is possible that the side effects and risks of universal prophylaxis may outweigh the benefit when large numbers of women receive antibiotics to prevent relatively few infections.

Universal antibiotic prophylaxis for abortion is recommended by all organizations involved in abortion provision, based on the available evidence. However, it is not clear that universal antibiotic prophylaxis is warranted in low-risk settings common in clinic practice. Given that antibiotics are being used as prophylaxis in most practices, it would be most logical to use them in the manner shown to be best for surgical prophylaxis, as opposed to full-treatment regimens. Thus, preoperative administration of doxycycline appears to be the best option for the prevention of infection after abortion. Preoperative regimens are the simplest to administer and are highly effective in preventing post-abortal PID.

Table 8.3 Number needed to treat (NNT) to prevent post-abortal infection

Infection risk without antibiotics	Relative risk	Infection risk with universal antibiotics[a]	NNT[b]
5.0%	0.20	1.0%	25
4.0%	0.20	0.8%	31
3.0%	0.20	0.6%	42
2.0%	0.20	0.4%	63
1.0%	0.20	0.2%	125
0.5%	0.20	0.1%	250
0.2%	0.20	0.04%	625
0.1%	0.20	0.02%	1250
0.05%	0.20	0.01%	2500

[a]Infection rate calculated using a constant RR of 0.20.
[b]NNT= 1/[risk(no antibiotics)–risk(antibiotics)].

SEQUELAE OF POST-ABORTION PELVIC INFLAMMATORY DISEASE

In a follow-up survey of women who did and did not have post-abortion PID, Heisterberg et al[47] found that women who developed PID after abortion were significantly more likely to have secondary infertility, dyspareunia, pelvic pain, and future spontaneous abortions (Table 8.4). These

Table 8.4 Sequelae of post-abortal pelvic inflammatory disease (PID)[a]

	Post-abortal PID				No post-abortal PID						95% CI	
Sequelae[b]	Total	(+)	(–)	Rate	Total	(+)	(–)	Rate	p^c	RR[d]	Lower	Upper
Recurrent PID	27	11	16	40.7%	299	15	284	5.0%	<0.0001	8.12	4.15	15.89
Infertility	31	3	28	9.7%	323	6	317	1.9%	0.0082	5.21	1.37	19.82
Chronic pelvic pain	29	4	25	13.8%	323	7	316	2.2%	0.006	6.36	1.98	20.47
Dyspareunia	30	6	24	20.5%	308	15	293	4.9%	0.001	4.11	1.72	9.80
Ectopic pregnancy	38	0	38	0.0%	323	5	318	1.5%	0.44	–	–	–
Spontaneous abortion	32	7	25	21.9%	293	15	278	5.1%	0.003	4.27	1.88	9.70

[a]The rates of each sequela are compared for women who developed post-abortal PID and those who did not. For the columns (+), this indicates that the sequela was present and (–) indicates that the sequela was absent.
[b]As reported in Heisterberg et al.[47]
[c]For difference between PID and no PID groups, by chi-square.
[d]Of having sequelae if post-abortal PID.
Adapted from Heisterberg et al[47] with additional statistical analysis.

sequelae are similar to those found in women who develop PID unrelated to a surgical procedure. Prevention of post-abortal PID is essential to prevent the sequelae of PID.

MEDICAL ABORTION

An increasing number of abortions are being performed medically, using a combination of mifepristone and misoprostol. In some parts of Europe, the proportion of induced abortions performed using mifepristone and a prostaglandin analogue is approaching 50%.[48,49] The percentage of abortions performed using mifepristone and prostaglandins is much lower in the United States, but has been increasing since the approval of mifepristone by the US Food and Drug Administration (FDA) in September 2000. The risk of infection following medical abortion appears to be very low (Table 8.5). In the largest trial reported in the United States,[50] there were 10 cases of infection attributed to medical abortion among 2121 women receiving mifepristone and misoprostol for medical abortion (0.47%, 95% CI 0.23–0.86%). In a large trial comparing different timing of mifepristone and misoprostol, Creinin et al.[51] reported 3 cases of infection among 1080 patients (0.28%, 95% CI 0.06–0.81%). Similarly, Schaff et al[52] reported 2 cases of endometritis treated with oral antibiotics in their study of 933 women receiving medical abortion (0.21%, 95% CI 0.026–0.77%). All of these patients were treated as outpatients.

In the first 18 months since mifepristone became available in the United States, there were approximately 80 000 medical abortions.[53] Only 10 cases of infection were reported to the manufacturer, Danco Laboratories LLC, but this probably represents incomplete ascertainment. A single case report has detailed a case of *Clostridium sordellii* infection that resulted in death.[54] Two other such cases have been reported to the FDA. Still, although there have not been any large clinical trials of antibiotic prophylaxis for medical abortion, the rate of infection is so low that prophylactic antibiotics are probably not warranted.

INTRAUTERINE DEVICE INSERTION

The IUD is an extremely effective method of contraception that has fallen out of common use in the United States. Results of the 2002 National Survey of Family Growth show that approximately 2% of American women use IUDs as their contraceptive method.[55] In large part, the lack of interest in the IUD is a result of misperceptions of risk and the negative press that resulted from several cases of septic abortion associated with the Dalkon Shield in the 1970s.

Currently in the United States, there are only two intrauterine devices available: the copper T380A (ParaGard, CuT380A) and the levonorgestrel-releasing intrauterine system (Mirena, LNG-IUS). These intrauterine devices provide safe and effective contraception. The CuT380A has a cumulative pregnancy rate of 1.9% over 12 years.[56]

Table 8.5 Summary of infection rates after medical abortion using mifepristone and prostaglandin analogues from prospective studies. None of the studies used antibiotic prophylaxis

Study	Infections[a]	Number receiving medical abortion	Percentage	95% confidence interval	
				Lower	Upper
Ulmann et al[89]	43	16 173	0.27%	0.19%	0.36%
Spitz et al[50]	10	2 121	0.47%	0.23%	0.87%
Schaff et al[52]	2	933	0.21%	0.03%	0.77%
Silvestre et al[90]	2	2 115	0.09%	0.01%	0.34%
Creinin et al[51]	3	1 080	0.28%	0.06%	0.81%
Total	**60**	**22 422**	**0.27%**	**0.20%**	**0.34%**

[a]Defined as any evidence of infection beyond an isolated fever, a known side effect of prostaglandin analogs.

The LNG-IUS has a cumulative pregnancy rate of 0.5% over 5 years.[57]

Mishell et al[58] showed that transient introduction of bacteria is a normal part of IUD placement. They studied the presence of bacteria within the endometrial cavity in which IUDs (Lippes loop) were placed shortly before hysterectomy in 59 women (Table 8.6). Endometrial cultures were positive in all 5 women who had a hysterectomy within 24 hours of IUD placement. One of 5 cultures was positive from 24 to 48 hours after IUD placement. There were 4 other positive endometrial cultures at 6, 10, 18, and 30 days after placement, for a total of 10 positive endometrial cultures. The remaining 49 cultures after the initial 48 hours up to 7 months later were negative. In 8 of the 10 cases of positive endometrial cultures, the same species was identified in cultures of the cervical mucus. Only 1 of the 10 cases showed evidence of chronic endometritis on histology. This patient's cultures grew *N. gonorrhoeae*. It is important to note that all of the women were healthy at the time of hysterectomy; none had symptoms of infection.

These microbiologic data agree with epidemiologic data. However, the effect seen clinically is much smaller than might be expected from the microbiology studies. In an American case–control study of 622 women hospitalized with PID compared with 2369 women hospitalized with no history of PID, the increased risk of PID was limited to the initial 4 months after IUD insertion.[59] A decade later, an analysis of 22 908 plastic and copper IUD insertions performed as part of WHO clinical trials showed that the risk of PID is 9.7 per 1000 woman-years during the first 20 days after insertion but thereafter the risk of PID is six-fold lower, at 1.4 per 1000 women-years.[60]

The rate after the initial few weeks is substantially lower than the rate of PID in the general population of 2% per year. Physician selection of low-risk patients probably explains why the rate of PID is lower with an IUD in place. PID in women with an IUD is more probably related to sexual exposures than to the presence of the IUD.[60–62] Older data showing an association between IUDs and PID were confounded by sexual exposure status and falsely elevated by inclusion of women who used the Dalkon Shield.[59,62] In addition, biases such as the over-diagnosis of PID in women with an IUD and inappropriate control groups led early research to conclude that IUDs caused tubal disease. In one study, correction of some of these biases eliminated the relationship between copper IUDs and PID.[63]

The risk of infection after IUD placement does not appear to be any greater in nulligravid women, and recent evidence shows that there is little risk of infectious or reproductive sequelae. Using a case–control design with two sets of controls, Hubacher et al[64] found that women with primary infertility did not have a higher chance of previous IUD use compared with either primigravid controls or women with primary infertility but without tubal disease. Rather, it was found that positive antibody titers for chlamydia were associated with tubal infertility compared with the control groups. Prior use of an IUD was not associated with the presence of chlamydial antibodies, reinforcing the

Table 8.6 Rate of positive endometrial cultures at hysterectomy by time from Lippes loop insertion

		Endometrial culture			95% confidence interval	
Time	Women	Negative	Positive	Percent positive	Lower	Upper
0–24 hours	5	0	5	100.0%	47.8%	100.0%
24–48 hours	5	4	1	20.0%	0.5%	71.6%
2–7 days	5	4	1	20.0%	0.5%	71.6%
7-14 days	12	11	1	8.3%	0.2%	38.5%
14–45 days	24	22	2	8.3%	1.0%	27.0%
45–201 days	8	8	0	0.0%	0.0%	31.2%
Total	**59**	**49**	**10**	**16.9%**		

Adapted from Mishell et al.[58]

concept that sexual exposure is the primary risk factor, whether an IUD is present or not.

In comparison with copper IUDs, the levonorgestrel-releasing IUS may have a lower rate of pelvic infection. Theoretically, thickened cervical mucus and an atrophic endometrium should protect the upper genital tract from ascending infection. A randomized trial of the LNG-IUS compared with the Nova-T, a copper IUD on the same polyethylene frame as the LNG-IUS, showed a significantly lower PID rate.[57] The cumulative PID rate was 0.8% over 5 years, compared with 2.2% for the Nova-T ($p < 0.01$).[57] A randomized comparison of the CuT380A and LNG-IUS, however, showed that both have equally low rates of PID over the course of 7 years, with the majority of cases occurring shortly after insertion.[65] The cumulative rate of PID over 7 years was 3.6% (standard error 0.8%) for both groups.[65] Although there is no convincing evidence of a protective effect in these conflicting trials, there is clearly not an increased risk of ascending infection.

Antibiotic prophylaxis with doxycycline or azithromycin has not been shown to reduce the incidence of post-insertion infection.[66–69] A Cochrane meta-analysis[70] analyzed the data from four large randomized placebo-controlled trials with a total of more than 5600 women. The rate of PID was not lower after receiving antibiotics ($p = 0.43$) and there was no difference in the rate of IUD removal before 90 days ($p = 0.80$). A marginal effect was seen in decreasing unscheduled clinic visits, with a combined odds ratio (OR) of 0.82 (95% CI 0.70–0.98).

The largest of these trials examined the effect of 500 mg of azithromycin compared with placebo on the rate of IUD removal for all indications other than expulsion at 90 days in over 1800 women in southern California.[67] This surrogate outcome was chosen as the primary outcome because PID is so rare. At 90 days, the removal rates were not different and there were only two cases of PID, one case in each group. This rate for first 90 days is roughly 1 per 1000 women (4.4 cases per 1000 woman-years), which agrees with epidemiologic data.

Since post-insertion infection is rare, a study would require several thousand subjects to have sufficient power to detect a difference in infection rates. Even if an effect were to be identified in a study of such size, however, the risk of adverse events in the thousands of women exposed to the antibiotic would probably outweigh the benefits of reduced infection. Thus, even without larger studies, it is reasonable to conclude that routine antibiotic prophylaxis is not indicated for IUD insertion.

Although testing for gonorrhea and chlamydia are often routinely performed prior to IUD placement, the results are not needed before IUD placement as long as the woman is at relatively low risk. The insertion of an IUD through a cervix infected with gonorrhea and chlamydia does not appear to substantially increase the risk of PID above the risk of simply having gonorrhea or chlamydia in the absence of an IUD.[61] Although there are no direct trials, the rates of PID after IUD insertion in women with cervical gonorrhea or chlamydia are the same as or lower than the rates of PID in women with these infections but without an IUD.[61] As with women without an IUD, gonorrhea and chlamydial cervicitis should be treated as soon as possible. Removal of the IUD is not necessary. With acute upper genital tract infection, there is limited evidence to suggest that removal of the IUD is not necessary. A small randomized trial of IUD removal showed no increase in treatment response – as measured by normalization of the erythrocyte sedimentation rate (ESR) – in comparison with allowing the IUD to remain in place.[71]

INTRAUTERINE USE IN WOMEN WITH HUMAN IMMUNODEFICIENCY VIRUS

Although it may seem unlikely that pre-existing human immunodeficiency virus (HIV) infection would not make infection more likely after IUD insertion, there is evidence to contest this assumption. In a prospective cohort study, 156 women with and 493 without HIV were followed for 4 months after insertion of a CuT380A.[72] There was no difference in infection rates (adjusted OR=1.02, 95% CI 0.46–2.3) or overall complications (adjusted OR=0.80, 95% CI 0.38–1.68).[72] Notably, all physicians involved were blinded to the subjects' HIV status.

POST-ABORTAL INSERTION OF INTRAUTERINE DEVICES

Immediate insertion of an IUD after abortion is a safe way to provide effective contraception.[73–75] Despite concerns about leaving a foreign body within the uterine cavity after abortion, there is no evidence that post-abortion IUD insertion increases the risk of infection.[73–75] In the study of prophylactic doxycycline before abortion by Darj et al,[28] one-third of subjects elected to receive an IUD after their abortion; doxycycline reduced the risk of infection with concurrent IUD placement as well. Certainly, the most controversial group to provide IUDs would be nulliparous adolescents seeking abortion. Goldman et al[76] randomized 162 nulliparous adolescents to one of three plastic or copper IUDs and found 3 cases of "mild pelvic inflammation" (1.8%).

DILATION AND CURETTAGE IN THE NON-PREGNANT STATE

There is insufficient evidence on the risk of infection after D & C in the non-pregnant state to make specific recommendations. The American College of Obstetricians and Gynecologists currently advises the use of single-dose preoperative antibiotic prophylaxis based on extrapolation of data from suction D & C for termination of pregnancy.[36] However, the age and sexual practices of women having a D&C for menorrhagia or postmenopausal bleeding are likely to place women having such procedures at a significantly different risk level. As such, in the absence of data, each case must be approached individually.

HYSTEROSCOPY

Hysteroscopy presents a low risk of infection. A randomized trial of no antibiotics vs preoperative intravenous amoxicillin and clavulanate showed that bacteremia is markedly decreased from 16% to 2% ($p < 0.02$).[77] Blood culture isolates involved 8 cases of coagulase-negative staphylococcus (1 case in the Augmentin group), 1 case of *Aerococcus viridans*, 1 case of corynebacterium, and 1 case of *Prevotella bivia*. The absolute risk reduction with antibiotic usage was 14.6% (95% CI 4.6–24.5%), with a risk ratio of 0.11 (96% CI 015–0.84). This study was stopped early after these findings with 116 patients enrolled. No evidence of a difference between the two groups was identified clinically despite the large difference in rates of bacteremia. In addition, the bacteria isolated are of dubious clinical significance. Similar to the study of endometrial cultures after IUD placement by Mishell et al,[58] this study indicated that transient bacteremia may be a normal finding immediately after hysteroscopy.

There are no randomized trials of hysteroscopy powered to examine clinical infection. A review of operative hysteroscopy at one institution in France over a 10-year period showed a rate of endomyometritis of 0.85%.[78] In a large survey of German hysteroscopists, the incidence of endomyometritis was reported at 0.01%.[79] Based on the low incidence of infection, prophylactic antibiotics are not generally warranted.

HYSTEROSALPINGOGRAPHY

Hysterosalpingography (HSG) is used to confirm patency of the fallopian tubes by passage of X-ray-opaque contrast media through the fallopian tubes via a catheter placed within the cervix. Oil-based contrast media have been shown to result in better rates of subsequent pregnancy in comparison with no intervention or to water-based contrast media.[80] Oil-based contrast media may lower the risk of infection.[81] The incidence of infection after HSG varies with the population being studied. In most published studies, the incidence is between 1 and 4%.[81–83]

Dilated fallopian tubes have been found to be a strong risk factor for infection following HSG. In two cohort studies, all cases of post-HSG infection were in women found to have tubal disease.[82,83] In one of these studies, doxycycline (100 mg twice daily for 5 days) significantly decreased the risk of infection when given once tubal dilation was identified (0% vs 11%, $p < 0.02$).[83]

VAGINAL PREPARATION WITH BACTERICIDAL SOLUTIONS FOR MINOR GYNECOLOGIC SURGERY

It is usually assumed that vaginal preparation (prep) with antibacterial solutions is beneficial, but data to support this conclusion are lacking. Povidone–iodine is one of the most commonly used solutions to prepare the cervix and vagina before transcervical procedures. Although povidone–iodine decreases vaginal bacterial counts substantially within 10 minutes, this effect does not persist.[84] With 30 minutes after application of povidone–iodine solution, the vaginal bacterial counts are not significantly different from prior to its application.[84]

Perhaps more important is evidence that povidone–iodine fails to eliminate bacteria from the endocervix, a location from which bacteria can easily be passed upward into the uterus. Osborne and Wright[85] examined the ability of povidone–iodine surgical prep to eliminate bacteria from the vagina compared with the endocervix: 50 premenopausal women received a 3-minute wash with povidone–iodine soap followed by a 2-minute wash with povidone–iodine solution. Although the average number of recoverable bacterial species in the vagina went from 5.6 to 0.1 per patient, the number of species in the endocervix decreased only from 3.9 to 1.7 per patient. The reduction in vaginal bacterial species was not correlated with the change in the number of endocervical bacterial species. Notably, of 2 patients with *N. gonorrhoeae* before the prep, both still had this pathogen within the endocervix after the povidone–iodine vaginal prep.

A recent randomized study compared povidone–iodine with chlorhexidine for vaginal prep prior to vaginal hysterectomy.[86] At 30 minutes, 17 of 27 vaginal cultures (63%) showed growth in the povidone–iodine group compared with 5 of 23 (22%) in the chlorhexidine group ($p < 0.005$). All subjects received prophylactic antibiotics and no infections were seen clinically.

Two clinical studies have examined the use of antibacterial vaginal prep.[87,88] Both showed that antibacterial vaginal prep did not decrease post-procedural infection rates. Moreover, there was a trend towards increased rates of infection with antibacterial vaginal prep in both studies.

A large double-blind randomized controlled trial of chlorhexidine (0.5% chlorhexidine digluconate) for vaginal prep prior to first-trimester elective abortion was performed in Sweden.[87] Subjects were randomized to routine chlorhexidine vaginal prep ($N = 372$) or a vaginal prep with a single pad moistened with saline ($N = 350$). Subjects with positive gonorrhea cultures or signs of active infection were excluded. Chlamydia testing was not performed. The authors did not specify if perioperative antibiotics were used. Additionally, 40% of subjects had immediate post-abortal IUD placement. In the full chlorhexidine prep, 21 (5.6%) had evidence of post-procedural upper genital infections compared with 16 (4.6%) in the brief saline prep.

A small nonrandomized controlled trial examined the usage of povidone–iodine surgical prep compared with saline prior to vaginal hysterectomy.[88] In this study, all patients received a douche of 10% povidone–iodine or saline on the night prior and morning of surgery followed by routine preoperative prep with povidone–iodine or saline. All patients received perioperative antibiotic prophylaxis for 24 hours. Cervicovaginal culture was performed preoperatively, postoperatively, and if fever occurred. Preoperatively, there were fewer organisms per subject in the povidone–iodine group than in the saline group (2.9 vs 1.7 organisms per subject isolated on culture). Postoperatively, the same number of organisms was cultured in each group (0.9 organisms per subject). Interestingly, there was a trend towards more postoperative infectious morbidity in the povidone–iodine prep group. There were 6 cases of cuff cellulitis in the povidone–iodine prep group compared with 3 cases in the saline prep group. This finding, however, did not reach statistical significance ($p > 0.05$) and cannot be reliably interpreted due to lack of power.

CONCLUSION

The studies of vaginal prep[87,88] provide reasonable evidence that neither chlorhexidine nor povidone–iodine vaginal preps are superior to saline alone. The failure of povidone–iodine vaginal prep to sterilize the endocervix[85] may explain how transcervical surgical procedures such as dilation and curettage seed the upper genital tract. The success of systemic preoperative antibiotic prophylaxis may lie in its ability to eliminate bacteria from the endocervix or to prevent seeded bacteria from forming a nidus of infection in the upper genital tract.

Despite knowledge that many gynecologic procedures result in seeding of the upper genital tract, infections remain rare. For most minor gynecologic procedures, the risk of infection can only be estimated by retrospective cohort reviews. With the exception of elective abortion, prospective trials to evaluate infectious morbidity are lacking. Further study of methods to safely decrease post-procedural infections is warranted.

REFERENCES

1. Classen DC, Evans RS, Pestotnik SL, et al. The timing of prophylactic administration of antibiotics and the risk of surgical-wound infection. N Engl J Med 1992;326(5):281–6.
2. Finer LB, Henshaw SK. Abortion incidence and services in the United States in 2000. Perspect Sex Reprod Health 2003;35(1):6–15.
3. Jones RK, Darroch JE, Henshaw SK. Patterns in the socioeconomic characteristics of women obtaining abortions in 2000–2001. Perspect Sex Reprod Health 2002;34(5):226–35.
4. Strauss LT, Herndon J, Chang J, et al. Abortion surveillance – United States, 2001. MMWR Surveill Summ 2004;53(9):1–32.
5. Hakim-Elahi E, Tovell HM, Burnhill MS. Complications of first-trimester abortion: a report of 170,000 cases. Obstet Gynecol 1990;76(1):129–35.
6. Heisterberg L, Kringelbach M. Early complications after induced first-trimester abortion. Acta Obstet Gynecol Scand 1987;66(3):201–4.
7. Fried G, Ostlund E, Ullberg C, Bygdeman M. Somatic complications and contraceptive techniques following legal abortion. Acta Obstet Gynecol Scand 1989;68(6):515–21.
8. Hodgson JE. Major complications of 20,248 consecutive first trimester abortions: problems of fragmented care. Adv Plan Parent 1975;9(3–4):52–9.
9. Wadhera S. Early complication risks of legal abortions, Canada, 1975–1980. Can J Public Health 1982;73(6):396–400.
10. Wulff GJ Jr, Freiman SM. Elective abortion. Complications seen in a free-standing clinic. Obstet Gynecol 1977;49(3):351–7.
11. Frank PI, Kay CR, Wingrave BA, et al. Induced abortion operations and their early sequelae. J R Coll Gen Pract 1985;35:175–80.
12. Jensen JT, Astley SJ, Morgan E, Nichols MD. Outcomes of suction curettage and mifepristone abortion in the United States. A prospective comparison study. Contraception 1999;59(3):153–9.
13. Grimes DA, Schulz KF. Morbidity and mortality from second-trimester abortions. J Reprod Med 1985;30(7):505–14.
14. Jacot FR, Poulin C, Bilodeau AP, et al. A five-year experience with second-trimester induced abortions: no increase in complication rate as compared to the first trimester. Am J Obstet Gynecol 1993;168(2):633–7.
15. Paul M, Lichtenberg ES, Borgatta L, et al. A Clinician's Guide to Medical and Surgical Abortion. New York: Churchill Livingstone, 1999.
16. Grimes DA, Cates W Jr. Complications from legally-induced abortion: a review. Obstet Gynecol Surv 1979;34(3):177–91.
17. Hern WM. Laminaria versus Dilapan osmotic cervical dilators for outpatient dilation and evacuation abortion: randomized cohort comparison of 1001 patients. Am J Obstet Gynecol 1994;171(5):1324–8.
18. Jonasson A, Larsson B, Bygdeman S, Forsum U. The influence of cervical dilatation by laminaria tent and with Hegar dilators on the intrauterine microflora and the rate of postabortal pelvic inflammatory disease. Acta Obstet Gynecol Scand 1989;68(5):405–10.
19. Skjeldestad FE, Tuveng J. Cervical dilatation with Lamicel in first trimester therapeutic abortion. Intl J Gynaecol Obstet 1990;33(2):153–7.
20. Wells EC, Hulka JF. Cervical dilation: a comparison of Lamicel and Dilapan. Am J Obstet Gynecol 1989;161(5):1124–6.
21. Todd CS, Soler M, Castleman L, et al. Buccal misoprostol as cervical preparation for second trimester pregnancy termination. Contraception 2002;65(6):415–8.
22. Burkman RT, Tonascia JA, Atienza MF, King TM. Untreated endocervical gonorrhea and endometritis following elective abortion. Am J Obstet Gynecol 1976;126(6):648–51.
23. Wein P, Kloss M, Garland SM. Postabortal pelvic sepsis in association with *Chlamydia trachomatis*. Aust N Z J Obstet Gynaecol 1990;30(4):347–50.
24. Barbacci MB, Spence MR, Kappus EW, et al. Postabortal endometritis and isolation of *Chlamydia trachomatis*. Obstet Gynecol 1986;68(5):686–90.
25. Osser S, Persson K. Postabortal pelvic infection associated with *Chlamydia trachomatis* and the influence of humoral immunity. Am J Obstet Gynecol 1984;150(6):699-703.
26. Knudsen A, Junge O, Kjaergaard B, et al. The clinical significance of the genital microbiologic flora at vacuum aspiration following miscarriage. Acta Obstet Gynecol Scand 1989;68(2):153–5.
27. Levallois P, Rioux JE. Prophylactic antibiotics for suction curettage abortion: results of a clinical controlled trial. Am J Obstet Gynecol 1988;158(1):100–5.
28. Darj E, Stralin EB, Nilsson S. The prophylactic effect of doxycycline on postoperative infection rate after first-trimester abortion. Obstet Gynecol 1987;70(5):755–8.
29. Heisterberg L, Branebjerg PE, Bremmelgaard A, et al. The role of vaginal secretory immunoglobulin A, *Gardnerella vaginalis*, anaerobes, and *Chlamydia trachomatis* in postabortal pelvic inflammatory disease. Acta Obstet Gynecol Scand 1987;66(2):99–102.
30. Bjornerem A, Aghajani E, Maltau JM, Moi H. [Occurrence of bacterial vaginosis among abortion seekers]. Tidsskr Nor Laegeforen 1997;117(9):1282–4 [in Norwegian]
31. Crowley T, Low N, Turner A, et al. Antibiotic prophylaxis to prevent post-abortal upper genital tract infection in women with bacterial vaginosis: randomised controlled trial. BJOG 2001;108(4):396–402.
32. Larsson PG, Platz-Christensen JJ, Dalaker K, et al. Treatment with 2% clindamycin vaginal cream prior to first trimester surgical abortion to reduce signs of postoperative infection: a prospective, double-blinded, placebo-controlled, multicenter study. Acta Obstet Gynecol Scand 2000;79(5):390–6.
33. Larsson PG, Platz-Christensen JJ, Thejls H, et al. Incidence of pelvic inflammatory disease after first-trimester legal abortion in women with bacterial vaginosis after treatment with metronidazole: a double-blind, randomized study. Am J Obstet Gynecol 1992;166(1 Pt 1):100-3.
34. Miller L, Thomas K, Hughes JP, et al. Randomised treatment trial of bacterial vaginosis to prevent post-abortion complication. BJOG 2004;111(9):982–8.

35. Sawaya GF, Grady D, Kerlikowske K, Grimes DA. Antibiotics at the time of induced abortion: the case for universal prophylaxis based on a meta-analysis. Obstet Gynecol 1996;87(5 Pt 2):884–90.
36. Antibiotics Prophylaxis for Gynecologic Procedures. Washington: American College of Obstetricians and Gynecologists; January 2001. Report No. 23.
37. 2003 Clinical Policy Guidelines. Washington: National Abortion Federation; 2003.
38. Bidgood K, Furedi A, Jones I, et al. The Care of Women Requesting Induced Abortion. London: Royal College of Obstetricians & Gynaecologists, March 2000.
39. Safe Abortion: Technical and Policy Guidance for Health Systems. Geneva: World Health Organization, 2003.
40. Lichtenberg ES, Paul M, Jones H. First trimester surgical abortion practices: a survey of National Abortion Federation members. Contraception 2001;64(6):345–52.
41. Brewer C. Prevention of infection after abortion with a supervised single dose of oral doxycycline. BMJ 1980; 281(6243):780–1.
42. Saivin S, Houin G. Clinical pharmacokinetics of doxycycline and minocycline. Clin Pharmacokinet 1988;15(6):355–66.
43. Qvigstad E, Skaug K, Jerve F, et al. Pelvic inflammatory disease associated with *Chlamydia trachomatis* infection after therapeutic abortion. A prospective study. B J Vener Dis 1983;59(3):189–92.
44. Henriques CU, Wilken-Jensen C, Thorsen P, Moller BR. A randomised controlled trial of prophylaxis of post-abortal infection: ceftriaxone versus placebo. Br J Obstet Gynaecol 1994;101(7):610–14.
45. Lichtenberg ES, Shott S. A randomized clinical trial of prophylaxis for vacuum abortion: 3 versus 7 days of doxycycline. Obstet Gynecol 2003;101(4):726–31.
46. Reedy MB, Sulak PJ, Miller SL, et al. Evaluation of 3-day course of doxycycline for the treatment of uncomplicated *Chlamydia trachomatis* cervicitis. Infect Dis Obstet Gynecol 1997;5(1):18–22.
47. Heisterberg L, Hebjorn S, Andersen LF, Petersen H. Sequelae of induced first-trimester abortion. A prospective study assessing the role of postabortal pelvic inflammatory disease and prophylactic antibiotics. Am J Obstet Gynecol 1986;155(1):76–80.
48. Bygdeman M, Danielsson KG, Marions L. Medical termination of early pregnancy: the Swedish experience. J Am Med Womens Assoc 2000;55(3 Suppl):195–6.
49. Jones RK, Henshaw SK. Mifepristone for early medical abortion: experiences in France, Great Britain and Sweden. Perspect Sex Reprod Health 2002;34(3):154–61.
50. Spitz IM, Bardin CW, Benton L, Robbins A. Early pregnancy termination with mifepristone and misoprostol in the United States. N Eng J Med 1998;338(18):1241–7.
51. Creinin MD, Fox MC, Teal S, et al. A randomized comparison of misoprostol 6 to 8 hours versus 24 hours after mifepristone for abortion. Obstet Gynecol 2004;103(5 Pt 1):851–9.
52. Schaff EA, Eisinger SH, Stadalius LS, et al. Low-dose mifepristone 200 mg and vaginal misoprostol for abortion. Contraception 1999;59(1):1–6.
53. Hausknecht R. Mifepristone and misoprostol for early medical abortion: 18 months experience in the United States. Contraception 2003;67(6):463–5.
54. Wiebe E, Guilbert E, Jacot F, et al. A fatal case of *Clostridium sordellii* septic shock syndrome associated with medical abortion. Obstet Gynecol 2004;104(5 Pt 2):1142–4.
54. Mosher WD, Martinez GM, Chandra A, et al. Use of contraception and use of family planning services in the United States, 1982–2002. Hyattsville, Maryland: National Center for Health Statistics, December 10, 2004.
56. Long-term reversible contraception. Twelve years of experience with the TCu380A and TCu220C. Contraception 1997;56(6):341–52.
57. Andersson K, Odlind V, Rybo G. Levonorgestrel-releasing and copper-releasing (Nova T) IUDs during five years of use: a randomized comparative trial. Contraception 1994;49(1):56–72.
58. Mishell DR Jr, Bell JH, Good RG, Moyer DL. The intrauterine device: a bacteriologic study of the endometrial cavity. Am J Obstet Gynecol 1966;96(1):119–26.
59. Lee NC, Rubin GL, Ory HW, Burkman RT. Type of intrauterine device and the risk of pelvic inflammatory disease. Obstet Gynecol 1983;62(1):1–6.
60. Farley TM, Rosenberg MJ, Rowe PJ, et al. Intrauterine devices and pelvic inflammatory disease: an international perspective. Lancet 1992;339(8796):785–8.
61. Grimes DA. Intrauterine device and upper-genital-tract infection. Lancet 2000;356(9234):1013–19.
62. Lee NC, Rubin GL, Borucki R. The intrauterine device and pelvic inflammatory disease revisited: new results from the Women's Health Study. Obstet Gynecol 1988;72(1):1–6.
63. Buchan H, Villard-Mackintosh L, Vessey M, et al. Epidemiology of pelvic inflammatory disease in parous women with special reference to intrauterine device use. Br J Obstet Gynaecol 1990;97(9):780–8.
64. Hubacher D, Lara-Ricalde R, Taylor DJ, et al. Use of copper intrauterine devices and the risk of tubal infertility among nulligravid women. N Engl J Med 2001;345(8):561–7.
65. Sivin I, Stern J, Coutinho E, et al. Prolonged intrauterine contraception: a seven-year randomized study of the levonorgestrel 20 mcg/day (LNg 20) and the copper T380 Ag IUDS. Contraception 1991;44(5):473–80.
66. Walsh TL, Bernstein GS, Grimes DA, et al. Effect of prophylactic antibiotics on morbidity associated with IUD insertion: results of a pilot randomized controlled trial. IUD Study Group. Contraception 1994;50(4):319–27.
67. Walsh T, Grimes D, Frezieres R, et al. Randomised controlled trial of prophylactic antibiotics before insertion of intrauterine devices. IUD Study Group. Lancet 1998;351(9108):1005–8.
68. Ladipo OA, Farr G, Otolorin E, et al. Prevention of IUD-related pelvic infection: the efficacy of prophylactic doxycycline at IUD insertion. Adv Contraception 1991;7(1):43–54.
69. Grimes DA, Schulz KF. Antibiotic prophylaxis for intrauterine contraceptive device insertion. Cochrane Database Syst Rev 2001(1):CD001327.
70. Grimes D, Schulz K, Van Vliet H, Stanwood N. Immediate post-partum insertion of intrauterine devices. Cochrane Database Syst Rev 2003(1):CD003036.
71. Soderberg G, Lindgren S. Influence of an intrauterine device on the course of an acute salpingitis. Contraception 1981;24(2):137–43.
72. Sinei SK, Morrison CS, Sekadde-Kigondu C, et al. Complications of use of intrauterine devices among HIV-1-infected women. Lancet 1998;351(9111):1238–41.
73. Grimes D, Schulz K, Stanwood N. Immediate postabortal insertion of intrauterine devices. Cochrane Database Syst Rev 2002(3):CD001777.
74. IUD insertion following termination of pregnancy: a clinical trial of the TCu 220C, Lippes loop D, and copper 7. Stud Fam Plann 1983;14(4):99–108.
75. Pakarinen P, Toivonen J, Luukkainen T. Randomized comparison of levonorgestrel- and copper-releasing intrauterine systems immediately after abortion, with 5 years' follow-up. Contraception 2003;68(1):31–4.
76. Goldman JA, Dekel A, Reichman J. Immediate postabortion intrauterine contraception in nulliparous adolescents. Israel J Med Sci 1979;15(6):522–5.
77. Bhattacharya S, Parkin DE, Reid TM, et al. A prospective randomised study of the effects of prophylactic antibiotics on the incidence of bacteraemia following hysteroscopic surgery. Eur J Obstet Gynecol Reprod Biol 1995;63(1):37–40.

78. Agostini A, Cravello L, Shojai R, et al. Postoperative infection and surgical hysteroscopy. Fertil Steril 2002;77(4):766–8.
79. Aydeniz B, Gruber IV, Schauf B, et al. A multicenter survey of complications associated with 21,676 operative hysteroscopies. Eur J Obstet Gynecol Reprod Biol 2002;104(2):160–4.
80. Vandekerckhove P, Watson A, Lilford R, et al. Oil-soluble versus water-soluble media for assessing tubal patency with hysterosalpingography or laparoscopy in subfertile women. Cochrane Database Syst Rev 2000(2):CD000092.
81. Lindequist S, Justesen P, Larsen C, Rasmussen F. Diagnostic quality and complications of hysterosalpingography: oil- versus water-soluble contrast media – a randomized prospective study. Radiology 1991;179(1):69–74.
82. Forsey JP, Caul EO, Paul ID, Hull MG. Chlamydia trachomatis, tubal disease and the incidence of symptomatic and asymptomatic infection following hysterosalpingography. Hum Reprod 1990;5(4):444–7.
83. Pittaway DE, Winfield AC, Maxson W, et al. Prevention of acute pelvic inflammatory disease after hysterosalpingography: efficacy of doxycycline prophylaxis. Am J Obstet Gynecol 1983;147(6):623–6.
84. Monif GR, Thompson JL, Stephens HD, Baer H. Quantitative and qualitative effects of povidone–iodine liquid and gel on the aerobic and anaerobic flora of the female genital tract. Am J Obstet Gynecol 1980;137(4):432–8.
85. Osborne NG, Wright RC. Effect of preoperative scrub on the bacterial flora of the endocervix and vagina. Obstet Gynecol 1977;50(2):148–51.
86. Culligan PJ, Kubik K, Murphy M, et al. A randomized trial that compared povidone iodine and chlorhexidine as antiseptics for vaginal hysterectomy. Am J Obstet Gynecol 2005;192(2):422–5.
87. Lundh C, Meirik O, Nygren KG. Vaginal cleansing at vacuum aspiration abortion does not reduce the risk of postoperative infection. Acta Obstet Gynecol Scand 1983;62(3):275–7.
88. Amstey MS, Jones AP. Preparation of the vagina for surgery. A comparison of povidone–iodine and saline solution. JAMA 1981;245(8):839–41.
89. Ulmann A, Silvestre L, Chemama L, et al Medical termination of early pregnancy with mifepristone (RU 486) followed by a prostaglandin analogue. Study in 16,369 women. Acta Obstet Gynecol Scand 1992;71(4):278–83.
90. Silvestre L, Dubois C, Renault M, et al. Voluntary interruption of pregnancy with mifepristone (RU 486) and a prostaglandin analogue. A large-scale French experience. N Engl J Med 1990;322(10):645–8.

9. Management

Cheryl K. Walker and Richard L. Sweet

INTRODUCTION

Fifty years ago, we understood very little about pelvic inflammatory disease (PID) and had little to offer afflicted patients except for supportive care. Even without antimicrobial interventions, approximately 85% of women with PID recovered spontaneously, although it is not clear whether those women were cured or had long-term complications.[1] Many of the remaining 15% of women had prolonged or progressive symptoms that required surgery. We now have a more sophisticated understanding of the clinical spectrum and microbiology of PID, but still struggle to reduce long-term complications.

Clinicians acknowledge a wide breadth of presentations for PID, with symptoms and objective findings ranging from non-existent to severe life-threatening sepsis. Classically, women with PID present with pelvic pain, abnormal vaginal discharge, fever, and other symptoms of systemic infection; findings include fever, elevated concentrations of white blood cells, erythrocyte sedimentation rate, C-reactive protein, and tenderness of the cervix, uterus, and bilateral adnexae.[2,3] Experts also recognize a category of PID that is not easily discerned either by the patient herself or by healthcare providers. Affected women may be asymptomatic; more often, however, they experience mild symptoms such as mild discomfort, pain with sexual intercourse, and abnormal vaginal bleeding or discharge, and most have tenderness when examined.[4] Alternately known as "atypical", "subacute", "subclinical", or "silent" PID, this mild version of the infectious process has been shown to have the potential to cause the same long-term complications as are found in women with more clinically profound PID; these include infertility, ectopic pregnancy, and pelvic pain.[5–7]

The difficulty in pinning down a clear simple set of diagnostic criteria that are both sensitive and specific for the wide range of presentations in women with PID has made the design and implementation of treatment trials complicated. Great progress has been made over the last few decades in our understanding of the microbiology of PID. There is broad consensus that PID is a polymicrobial upper genital tract infection that may include sexually transmitted microbes such as *Neisseria gonorrhoeae* and/or *Chlamydia trachomatis* as well as a host of vaginal aerobes and anaerobes most commonly associated with bacterial vaginosis. Data regarding short-term clinical and microbiologic cure are excellent and guide therapeutic interventions. Thus, current treatment focuses on administration of anti-infective regimens aimed at this broad spectrum of putative microorganisms.

TARGET SPECTRUM OF ACTIVITY

PID is a polymicrobial infection. There are excellent data supporting the contributions of *C. trachomatis*, *N. gonorrhoeae*, facultative Gram-negative bacteria, and anaerobic bacteria to symptoms and signs of the infection itself as well as the damage that often results.[8–14] Investigators have suspected for a long time that other specific agents might function prominently in the pathogenic process, although consistent reproducible evidence to support this contention has been lacking.

N. gonorrhoeae and *C. trachomatis* are commonly identified from the upper genital tracts of women with PID.[8–14] Further, a large body of evidence supports the etiologic role of each pathogen in promoting tubal damage.[15–23] It is important to choose regimens effective against those organisms, even in women whose lower genital tract laboratory testing fails to identify them because results may correlate poorly with presence of the pathogens in the upper genital tract. Although some anti-infective drug regimens without adequate coverage against these sexually transmitted pathogens have been studied and found to have excellent clinical cure rates, long-term outcome data are lacking. Despite their clinical success, official treatment recommendations continue to suggest that all regimens used to treat women with PID should provide adequate coverage against these organisms, given their ability to cause tubal factor infertility.

More contentious is the extent to which anaerobes participate in upper genital tract pathogenesis and whether regimens should necessarily cover these bacteria. Some believe that anaerobic coverage is needed only for the most severely ill patients with PID. The proportion of women with anaerobic bacteria isolated from genital tract specimens of women with PID ranges from 13% to 78%.[9–13,24–33] A wide variety of explanations have been put forward to account for this discrepancy, including differences in patient population, clinical severity, study enrollment biases, and microbiologic isolation methods. A recent multicenter study of women with mild-to-moderate PID appears to offer data that transcend many prior study flaws.[34] The clinical sites for patient recruitment are wide-ranging, including hospital emergency departments, outpatient clinics, and private practices of 13 sites scattered through the eastern, southern, and central regions of the United States. Perhaps most importantly, the microbiologic techniques used were superb. In a study of 278 women drawn from the PID Evaluation and Clinical Health (PEACH) study, women with acute endometritis and mild-to-moderate clinical signs and symptoms of PID had a high likelihood of being infected with *Gardnerella vaginalis* (30.5%), anaerobic Gram-negative rods (which include many *Prevotella* and *Bacteroides* species) (31.7%), and anaerobic Gram-positive cocci (22%). In addition, 67.6% had bacterial vaginosis (BV). The authors conclude that BV-associated organisms are extremely common among women with mild-to-moderately severe PID, and recommend that treatment regimens for all women with PID include agents effective against anaerobes.

A paper by Walker and colleagues examined the role of anaerobes in PID in an effort to guide the development of PID treatment recommendations.[35] Their conclusions expressed concern over the lack of availability of long-term outcomes in women treated with various treatment regimens. Initial clinical and microbiologic cure may not correlate well with the prevention of long-term adverse outcomes. Thirty years ago, Chow and colleagues showed that tubo-ovarian complexes develop when PID is treated with tetracycline alone,[27] and Sweet and colleagues showed over 20 years ago that incompletely treated upper tract chlamydial infections can fester and result in ongoing tubal damage despite supposed clinical cure in patients receiving single-agent cephalosporins.[36] Finally, Crombleholme and colleagues reported persistence of anaerobes in the endometrial cavities of hospitalized women with acute PID who were treated with single-agent quinolones and deemed clinically cured at the end of the study period.[37] In a recent proof of concept study, Eckert and colleagues demonstrated that women at high risk for PID but without a clinical diagnosis of PID benefited from antimicrobial therapy that included anaerobic coverage with clinical improvement and resolution of histologic endometritis.[38]

Given that there is ample evidence that anaerobes are highly prevalent among women with all levels of clinical severity of PID and that failure to eradicate them can allow damage to the upper genital tract to continue, it seems prudent that all treatment regimens cover anaerobes. Whereas the 2002 Centers for Disease Control and Prevention (CDC) sexually tansmitted disease (STD) treatment guidelines[3] hesitate to advocate this strongly, the new data described above may allow for a less ambiguous recommendation in the future. Until regimens that do not adequately cover anaerobes have been demonstrated to prevent sequelae as successfully as those do, clinicians should choose regimens that provide adequate anaerobic coverage. Finally, the fact that up to 70% of women with PID also have BV provides another compelling argument for inclusion of anaerobic coverage for PID treatment regimens.[39]

ANTI-INFECTIVE TREATMENT REGIMENS

Logically, management of PID is directed at the containment of this infection. Although this may seem a simple concept, it has broadened considerably over the last few decades to include not only the resolution of clinical symptoms and signs but also the eradication of pathogens from the upper genital tract and abdomen and the prevention of subsequent complications, including infertility, ectopic pregnancy, and chronic pelvic pain. Only a few prospective studies have examined long-term outcomes in women treated for PID.

Whereas modern management relies heavily on antimicrobial intervention, early observational studies recorded high rates of clinical resolution without any antibiotics whatsoever.[1] Crude post-PID fertility rates were reasonable also, with one large study of 1262 women measuring a 23% fertility rate.[40] These data provide a backdrop against which to compare modern management schemes.

Early regimens were penicillin-based and appeared moderately effective, particularly in women with gonococcal PID. Early treatment trials were non-comparative, failed to define carefully inclusion and outcome criteria, and did not have the technical capacity to measure microbiologic eradication or long-term outcomes. Most trials noted considerable improvement in treated women, reducing the mortality rate to nearly zero, reducing the rate of persistent or ruptured tubo-ovarian abscesses (TOAs) requiring surgery dramatically, and improving fertility.[40–43] Although better than in the pre-antibiotic era, these fertility rates were far from ideal.

The largest study to date regarding treatment of women with PID was published over a decade ago from Westrom and colleagues in Sweden.[44] These investigators performed a retrospective study of 1732 cases and 601 controls identified over the course of 24 years. These women were subjected to laparoscopy to determine case or control status, treated with antibiotic regimens that changed over the years as new efficacy data were generated, and followed to determine fertility status. The primary findings of the study were that tubal factor infertility was associated with number and severity of PID episodes and that ectopic pregnancy was associated with case status.

An extensive body of literature has investigated the efficacy of modern antimicrobial regimens used to treat PID, and serves as the basis for recent PID treatment guidelines. A meta-analysis published in 1993 evaluated treatment trials published between 1966 and 1992.[45] This work has been updated by surveying all the English-language treatment trials published through 2004 using the same methodology as was used in the original paper, and the tables from the original articles have been amended to include newer data.

Treatment studies published between 1966 and 2004 were identified using Medline and bibliographies, and evaluated qualitatively and quantitatively in a meta-analysis. Twenty-nine studies met the criteria for inclusion in this evaluation. These criteria were an appropriate system for making the diagnosis of PID, standardized assessment of clinical outcome, and entry and follow-up evaluation for lower genital tract infection with *N. gonorrhoeae* and *C. trachomatis*. A number of antimicrobial regimens appear to have very good short-term clinical and microbiologic efficacy (Table 9.1). Pooled clinical cure rates and pooled microbiologic cure rates both range from 70% to 100%. As can be seen from Table 9.2, antimicrobial activity profiles are similar, although costs differ.

PARENTERAL CHOICES

A number of antimicrobial regimens appear to have very good short-term clinical and microbiologic efficacy. The combinations with the broadest support in the literature are cefoxitin or cefotetan plus doxycycline and gentamicin plus clindamycin; these two regimens constitute the current recommended treatment regimens established by the CDC. Fewer studies have established high efficacy rates also for ofloxacin with or without metronidazole, and ampicillin–sulbactam plus doxycycline; these two are considered alternative parenteral regimens in the 2002 CDC STD treatment guidelines.[3]

A multicenter US single-arm trial used ofloxacin in 70 hospitalized women with laparoscopically proven PID.[46] Its clinical efficacy of 98% and

Table 9.1 Clinical and microbiologic cure rates for pelvic inflammatory disease treatment regimens

	Clinical cure			Microbiologic cure		
Regimen	No. of studies	No. of patients	Percent	No. of studies	No. of patients	Percent
Parenteral						
Clindamycin/aminoglycoside	11	470	92	8	143	97
Cefoxitin/doxycycline	9	836	95	7	581	96
Cefotetan/doxycycline	3	174	94	2	71	100
Ceftizoxime/tetracycline	1	18	88	1	–	100
Cefotaxime/tetracycline	1	19	94	1	–	100
Ciprofloxacin	4	90	94	4	72	96
Ofloxacin	2	86	99	2	50	98
Sulbactam–ampicillin/doxycycline	1	37	95	1	33	100
Metronidazole/doxycycline	2	36	75	1	7	71
Azithromycin	1	30	100	1	30	100
Azithromycin/metronidazole	1	30	97	1	30	97
Oral						
Ceftriaxone/probenecid/doxycycline	1	64	95	1	8	100
Cefoxitin/probenecid/doxycycline	3	212	90	3	71	93
Cefoxitin/doxycycline	4	634	94	4	493	95
Amoxicillin-clavulanic acid	2	35	100	2	35+	100
Sulbactam–ampicillin/doxycycline	1	38	70	1	36	70
Ciprofloxacin/clindamycin	1	67	97	1	10	90
Ofloxacin	2	165	95	2	42+	100
Levofloxacin	1	41	85	1	9	89

microbiologic efficacy of 100% were similar to prior data gleaned from comparative trials. The primary contribution of this study was that cases were more accurately diagnosed than is common for routine PID clinical trials. Ofloxacin is already a recommended parenteral regimen for PID. Of note, parenteral ofloxacin is not available currently in the United States, and thus it is likely to be dropped from the next CDC STD treatment guidelines.

There are no published trials using parenteral levofloxacin in women with PID at this time. However, this drug is an optical isomer of ofloxacin and has been well studied in several well-designed clinical trials for other major abdominal infections. Its broad-spectrum activity against Gram-positive and Gram-negative microorganisms, including *N. gonorrhoeae* and *C. trachomatis*, and especially its expanded coverage of anaerobes, and daily dosing make it a reasonable choice. For these reasons, levofloxacin 500 mg IV (intravenous) once a day was added to the recommended choices in the 2002 CDC STD treatment guidelines.[3] Levofloxacin is the only drug with broad-enough coverage against the spectrum of bacteria believed to be involved in PID to be considered appropriate as a single agent for the duration of therapy; its once-daily dosing makes it attractive from an adherence perspective.

Given the widespread use of azithromycin in the treatment of chlamydial infections and other sexually transmitted infections (STIs), some clinicians have used it to treat PID. Recent research into its immunomodulatory properties implies that azithromycin may enhance host defense mechanisms shortly after initial administration and then restrict local infection/inflammation subsequently.[47] New data from two European studies suggest that it may be an excellent addition to existing parenteral regimens.[48] Both studies were performed by the same investigators, and results are published in a single article describing 309 women with PID and comparing azithromycin, either alone or with metronidazole, with two standard oral PID therapies. The authors report clinical cure rates of 97% for azithromycin alone and 98% for the drug in combination with metronidazole. Microbiologic cure rates were 100% for azithromycin alone and 97% when used in combination with metronidazole. Given these data and its once-daily dosing, it

Table 9.2 Cost and antimicrobial activity of pelvic inflammatory disease treatment regimens

Drug regimen	Average daily cost[ab]	*Neisseria gonorrhoeae*		*Chlamydia trachomatis*	Anaerobic bacteria		Facultative bacteria			
		Non-PP	PP		Non-BL[c]	BL[c]	Gram-negative enterics	Streptococci	Staphylococci	Enterococci
Inpatient[d]										
Cefoxitin–doxycycline	$25.19	+++	+++	+++	+++	+++	+++	+++	++	NA
Cefotetan–doxycycline	$18.24	+++	+++	+++	+++	+++	+++	+++	++	NA
Ceftizoxime–doxycycline	$20.59	+++	+++	+++	+++	+++	+++	+++	++	NA
Cefotaxime–doxycycline	$20.75	+++	+++	+++	+++	+++	+++	+++	++	NA
Clindamycin–gentamicin	$25.00	++	++	++	+++	+++	+++	++	++	NA
Clindamycin–tobramycin	$39.95	++	++	++	+++	+++	+++	++	++	NA
Clindamycin–amikacin	$61.60	++	++	++	+++	+++	+++	++	++	NA
Metronidazole–doxycycline	$12.78	+	+	+++	+++	+++	+	+	+	NA
Ciprofloxacin	$13.10	+++	+++	+	+	+	+++	+	++	NA
Ofloxacin	[e]	+++	+++	+	+	+	+++	+	++	NA
Levofloxacin	$17.77	+++	+++	+	+++	+++	+++	+	++	NA
Sulbactam–ampicillin–doxycycline	$20.46	+++	++	+++	++	++	++	++	++	+
Azithromycin	$13.51	++	++	+++	++	++	++	++	++	++
Azithromycin–metronidazole	$20.26	++	++	+++	+++	+++	++	++	++	++
Outpatient[f]										
Ofloxacin	$12.57	+++	+++	+	+	+	+++	+	++	NA
Levofloxacin	$12.00	+++	+++	+	++	++	+++	+	++	NA
Ciprofloxacin–clindamycin	$24.60	+++	+++	+	+	+	+++	+	++	NA
Amoxicillin–clavulanic acid–doxycycline	$17.21	+++	++	+++	++	++	++	++	++	+
Sulbactam–ampicillin–doxycycline	$2.92	+++	++	+++	++	++	++	++	++	+
Ceftriaxone–doxycycline–metronidazole	$28.58	+++	+++	+++	+++	+++	+++	+++	++	NA
Cefoxitin–probenecid–doxycycline	$34.59	+++	+++	+++	+++	+++	+++	+++	++	NA

Note: +++ = excellent activity, ++ = good activity, + = some activity, PP = penicillinase-producing.
[a]Cost based on average wholesale drug price drawn from 2005 Cardinal Distribution. It includes pharmacy costs.
[b]Based on a 14-day course.
[c]BL = beta-lactamase.
[d]Assumption of 48 hours of parenteral dosing in a 65 kg woman.
[e]Parenteral ofloxacin is not available currently in the United States.
[f]May include a single parenteral dose at treatment initiation, followed by oral treatment for the remainder of the course.

is possible that the CDC will consider adding this regimen to coming recommendations as an alternative parenteral option.

Antimicrobial choice must always be a dynamic process, however, and should be guided by a number of sources of information, including efficacy data and surveillance of both microbiology and susceptibility patterns. New data from a multicenter survey of changing in-vitro antimicrobial susceptibilities of 556 clinical isolates of anaerobes of the type commonly identified in women with PID revealed the following:

- piperacillin–tazobactam was the only agent to which all isolates were sensitive
- imipenem, meropenem, and metronidazole were highly active
- the lowest susceptibility rates were noted for penicillin G, ciprofloxacin, and clindamycin.[49]

This raises concern that resistance to clindamycin appears to be increasing among members of the *Bacteroides fragilis* group, and renews our search for new data on PID treatment.

Thus, the current list of parenteral treatment options with excellent data to support their efficacy, which were included in the 2002 CDC STD treatment guidelines,[3] are listed in Table 9.3. Of note is the fact that the language regarding the use of metronidazole with certain regimens was softened for the sake of consistency, in recognition of the fact that other recommended regimens with theoretically suboptimal anaerobic coverage appear to have excellent short-term clinical and microbiologic efficacy. The newly published multicenter data showing the high prevalence of BV-associated flora infecting the upper genital tracts of women with PID[34] and the high frequency of coexistent BV among women with PID (up to 70%)[39] strengthens the need to provide coverage against anaerobic bacteria and may prompt the CDC to strengthen its recommendations for anaerobic coverage once again for the next guidelines.

Table 9.3 Parenteral regimens for pelvic inflammatory disease[3]

Regimen A
Cefotetan 2 g IV every 12 hours
OR
Cefoxitin 2 g IV every 6 hours
PLUS
Doxycycline 100 mg orally or IV every 12 hours
After response, continue doxycycline 100 mg orally every 12 hours to complete a 14-day course
Regimen B
Clindamycin 900 mg IV every 8 hours
PLUS
Gentamicin loading dose IV or IM (2 mg/kg of body weight) followed by a maintenance dose (1.5 mg/kg) every 8 hours. Single daily dosing may be substituted
After response, continue clindamycin 450 mg orally 4 times a day to complete a 14-day course
Alternatives
Ofloxacin[a] 400 mg IV every 12 hours
OR
Levofloxacin 500 mg IV once daily
WITH OR WITHOUT
Metronidazole 500 mg IV or orally every 8 hours
After response, continue ofloxacin 400 mg orally twice a day or levofloxacin 500 mg orally once a day to complete a 14-day course
Ampicillin–sulbactam 3 g IV every 6 hours
PLUS
Doxycycline 100 mg orally or IV every 12 hours
After response, continue doxycycline 100 mg orally every 12 hours to complete a 14-day course

[a]Parenteral ofloxacin is not available currently in the United States.

ORAL CHOICES

It is ironic that oral regimens, which are used far more broadly than parenteral choices in the United States, have been poorly studied. The CDC 2002 STD treatment guidelines[3] recommended the use of a single dose of ceftriaxone or cefoxitin or other parenteral third-generagion cephalosporin plus doxycycline or ofloxacin with or without metronidazole for the treatment of PID.

A non-comparative study using oral levofloxacin in 41 women with PID was conducted in Japan.[50] Diagnostic criteria and outcome measures are carefully described. Clinical efficacy was assessed using a four-category rating system and judged both by doctors-in-charge and by committee, and ranged from 85.4% to 87.8%; bacteriologic efficacy was 88.9%. Levofloxacin is the only drug with broad enough coverage against the spectrum of bacteria believed to be involved in PID to be considered appropriate as a single agent for the duration of therapy; its once-daily dosing makes it attractive from an adherence perspective.

It took until 1997 for the first study on outpatient management of PID using ceftriaxone plus doxycycline to be published.[51] The study of women with laparoscopically proven PID reported an excellent clinical response (95%) despite rather poor in-vivo ability to eradicate anaerobes. For theoretical reasons, the CDC guidelines[3] recommended that metronidazole be used with this regimen to enhance anaerobic coverage.

There are no published data using azithromycin, either alone or with metronidazole, as an oral regimen for the treatment of PID.

Concern regarding the contribution of anaerobes to the pathogenesis of PID prompted the 2002 guidelines[3] to continue to recommend that all regimens include adequate anaerobic coverage, irrespective of published data showing excellent clinical and microbiologic cure rates in studies using short-term clinical outcomes. To this end, limited new data suggest that use of the combination of oral metronidazole plus doxycycline after primary parenteral therapy for PID is safe and effective. Bevan et al[48] provided data on 69 women treated with cefoxitin plus probenecid plus metronidazole plus doxycycline as part of a comparative open-label trial against azithromycin. There were no concerns raised regarding adverse events in these women.

Table 9.4 Oral regimens for pelvic inflammatory disease[3]

Regimen A
Ofloxacin 400 mg orally twice a day for 14 days or levofloxacin 500 mg orally once a day for 14 days
WITH OR WITHOUT
Metronidazole 500 mg orally twice a day for 14 days

Regimen B
Ceftriaxone 250 mg IM once
OR
Cefoxitin 2 g IM plus probenecid, 1 g orally in a single dose concurrently once
OR
Other parenteral third-generation cephalosporin (e.g. ceftizoxime or cefotaxime)
PLUS
Doxycycline 100 mg orally twice a day for 14 days
WITH OR WITHOUT
Metronidazole 500 mg orally twice a day for 14 days

The revised list of oral treatment options for PID with excellent data to support their efficacy, which were included in the 2002 CDC STD treatment guidelines,[3] are listed in Table 9.4. As with parenteral regimens, recommendations regarding the use of metronidazole with certain regimens were softened in 2002 in recognition of the fact that other recommended regimens with theoretically suboptimal anaerobic coverage appear to have excellent efficacy. Based on the high prevalence of BV among women with PID[39] and the newly published multicenter data showing the high prevalence of BV-associated flora infecting the upper genital tracts of women with PID,[34] this recommendation may be strengthened once again in the next guidelines.

ADHERENCE TO PELVIC INFLAMMATORY DISEASE TREATMENT REGIMENS

Many studies have shown that treatment trials done under controlled circumstances with optimal patient selection may not reflect common practices and probably overestimate success rates in the general population. A disturbing study was published recently from data drawn from the PEACH study.[52] It showed that, irrespective of whether the study subject had been hospitalized at the time of treatment initiation, women took an average of 70% of prescribed oral medication doses, took them for less than half of their outpatient days recommended, took an unscheduled drug holiday for nearly 25% of their outpatient days, and took only 17% of their doses within the optimal timing interval. These data underscore the need to enhance patient education and motivation and to identify effective regimens involving shorter courses and longer dosing intervals.

Adherence problems also exist among healthcare providers. Many studies show that clinicians find it difficult to make the diagnosis of PID and treat women appropriately. One recent study examined emergency room chart documentation by clinicians evaluating patients diagnosed with a variety of STIs, including 121 women with PID.[53] This study reported that only 14% of women with

PID had documentation of proper historical criteria, 22% had requisite physical examination findings noted, 71% had appropriate diagnostic testing, 32% were treated with a CDC-approved regimen, and only 15% received information on safe sex. There were no women diagnosed with PID whose clinicians achieved compliance in all five areas. Although some of these reponses might be the result of suboptimal documentation, this suggests major problems in the diagnosis and treatment of women with PID. Of note is that a study like this fails to capture those women with PID who fail to be properly diagnosed in such settings.

Similarly, only 18% of clinicians using the International Classification of Diseases (ICD-9) billing code for PID (614.9) had actually documented appropriate diagnostic criteria.[54] The study has no way of knowing whether women who carried that ICD-9 code actually had the infection, and how many women with PID were assigned non-PID diagnostic codes.

SITE AND ROUTE OF TREATMENT ADMINISTRATION

Nearly 1 million women are diagnosed with PID each year according to an analysis based on a national survey of hospital discharges and visits to emergency rooms and outpatient settings.[55] The incidence of PID treated in both inpatient and outpatient settings appears to have declined, however, and the decline appears most prominent among inpatients, whose numbers fell 69% during this time interval. Even with only 11% of women with PID being treated in hospital settings, it represents the leading cause for hospital admission among non-pregnant women of reproductive age in the United States, with a rate of 49.3 per 10 000 hospital discharges.

Prior to 1998, the CDC categorized their recommendations for hospitalization based on the assumption that parenteral regimens would be administered in inpatient settings and oral ones would be provided to outpatients. But it is no longer necessary to hospitalize women to treat parenterally. The last two decades and the revolution in the US healthcare economy have seen an amazing trend away from inpatient care.[56,57] This has fostered development of a broad infrastructure designed to enhance delivery of many sophisticated healthcare services, including the administration of most parenteral antibiotics, outside of the acute-care setting. This has broadened treatment options, allowing for outpatient parenteral therapy in selected women with PID.

For this reason, a new distinction has been drawn between the route of antibiotic administration (parenteral or oral) and setting for treatment (inpatient or outpatient). Antibiotic regimens for PID are categorized currently by the route of administration during the first days of treatment. Thus, drugs that require more than a single dose of intravenous or intramuscular antibiotic in the initial stages of treatment are considered "parenteral", despite the fact that nearly all of the women treated are weaned within a few days to oral antibiotics to complete their treatment courses once the acute phase of illness has passed. Parenteral regimens may be administered in an acute-care facility or at home, depending on the conclusiveness of the diagnosis, the severity of the clinical presentation, and associated clinical factors. Alternatively, those regimens that are primarily oral, with or without an initial parenteral dose, are designated as "oral" and are most commonly administered to outpatients.

Hospitalization with intravenous administration of antibiotics has long been considered the gold standard for treatment of women with PID in light of the capacity to monitor patients closely and to maximize bed rest, and the theoretical ability to achieve higher tissue levels of parenteral drugs. In the absence of compelling data, the criteria initially proposed by the CDC for hospitalization of women with PID for parenteral therapy were based largely on anecdotal information and consensus opinion of clinical experts. These criteria included:

- uncertain diagnosis in which surgical emergencies have not been excluded
- pregnancy
- failure of outpatient management
- inability to tolerate or follow an oral regimen
- severe illness

- presence of a TOA
- inability to follow-up after a 72-hour trial of an outpatient regimen
- being an adolescent
- co-existent HIV infection.

The CDC hospitalization criteria were re-evaluated for the 1998 and 2002 guidelines process in an effort to become more evidence-based. High rates of fetal wastage and preterm delivery have been reported in pregnant women with PID, and make hospitalization appropriate.[58,59] In addition, there are ample data available suggesting that women with TOAs should be hospitalized to maximize antimicrobial dosing and allow for early recognition of serious complications such as leaking or rupture.[60–62]

For the other criteria, specific data were not available and decisions regarding site of treatment administration were less obvious. Diagnostic uncertainty, particularly when the differential diagnosis includes an illness that might require surgical intervention, makes sense even in the absence of explicit evidence. Similarly, women who are severely ill typically require intravenous hydration and a high level of supportive care.

In women with mild signs and symptoms of PID who require parenteral therapy, individual circumstances should guide treatment setting. Women who have failed oral treatment require parenteral therapy and may benefit from hospitalization to achieve careful observation in a monitored environment. Women who cannot follow an oral regimen, or who may not physically tolerate one, require parenteral therapy, although the need for hospitalization may not be immediately obvious. Finally, it has long been held that women who are candidates for oral therapy but who cannot follow-up within 72 hours after treatment initiation should be hospitalized because assessment of treatment response would be compromised and transition to appropriate parenteral intervention delayed. It would seem that creative outpatient support solutions might prevail once a woman understood the gravity of this requirement and its implications for her own long-term health and well-being.

Perhaps the most important contribution to this discussion in decades was published by Ness and colleagues.[39] The PEACH study was a multicenter randomized controlled trial comparing parenteral antibiotic therapy with cefoxitin and doxycycline delivered in a hospital setting with outpatient treatment using a single dose of parenteral cefoxitin and an oral course of doxycycline in women with mild-to-moderate PID. These investigators found no significant differences in the short-term clinical and microbiologic response rates. Further, long-term outcomes, including pregnancy, time to pregnancy, recurrence of PID, chronic pelvic pain, and ectopic pregnancy, were similar as well. Pregnancy rates calculated after a mean follow-up of 35 months were 42.0% for women treated as outpatients and 41.7% for hospitalized women. These data suggest that neither site nor route of treatment administration affect the short- and long-term major outcomes of women with mild and moderate clinical presentation. The only benefit for hospitalized patients receiving parenteral antibiotics was lower rates of post-treatment histologic endometritis. Given data supporting the potential for smoldering infection, ongoing tubal damage, and increased rates for fertility among such women in previous studies,[27,36] this may be an important observation.

ADOLESCENTS

There are no data to support the practice of hospitalization of adolescent women with PID. For this reason, this criterion was removed from the 1998 and 2002 treatment guidelines.[3,63] That change prompted a strong critique from Hemsel and colleagues representing the International Infectious Disease Society for Obstetrics and Gynecology – USA.[64] In their article, the authors adamantly advocated that all adolescents and nulligravid young women be hospitalized for treatment and education based on theoretical concerns. They referred to a paper published in 1987 opining that adolescence be considered a proxy for poor adherence, high-risk sexual behavior, delayed presentation for medical care, and high antimicrobial failure rates.[65] They also suggested that the fertility of adolescents should be protected to a degree greater than that of more mature women. Thus, many adolescent care providers continue to hospitalize their patients, despite the lack of data to suggest that their patients benefit from inpatient PID treatment. If there were data to suggest that hospitalization improved outcome either of the immediate infection or in terms of fewer complications, then hospitalization would be recommended for all women, irrespective of age or parity. Such is not the case, however. The data described in detail above from Ness and colleagues[39] provide strong evidence that there is no compelling benefit to hospitalization and parenteral therapy in women with mild or moderate PID. There is no reason to expect that adolescent women would respond differently than adults.

WOMEN OVER AGE 35

An interesting recent finding is that women 35 years of age or older who are hospitalized with PID appear to be at increased risk for complications, including surgical intervention, readmission for PID, or having a hospital stay $\geq$14 days: odds ratio (OR) = 3.9; 95% confidence interval (CI) 1.3, 11.6.[66] Although this question is different from whether or not women in this age group require hospitalization in the first place, these findings suggest the possibility that older women may have a more complicated course of PID.

In another study that raised a concern for older women with PID, women with sonographically diagnosed TOAs who fail to respond to broad-spectrum antibiotic regimens were older than those who were cured (45.3 ± 6.6 vs 39.6 ± 8.3, p = 0.02).[67] Postmenopausal women with TOAs are more likely to harbor a genital tract malignancy (47%) than premenopausal controls (1.3%), according to a recent retrospective case–control study of 93 women.[68] In both cases, the women with TOAs would probably be admitted for treatment based on the finding of a TOA.

WOMEN WITH HUMAN IMMUNODEFICIENCY VIRUS (HIV) INFECTION

It has long been suspected that when HIV-1-infected women develop PID, they have a more serious clinical presentation. An early retrospective case–control study found that HIV-infected women exhibited a diminished immune response and poorer response to antimicrobial therapy, resulting in an increased incidence of surgical intervention (OR = 5.5; 95% CI 1.0, 29.3).[69] New data suggest that HIV infection appears to increase the risk of TOA, but seropositive women respond equally well to oral and parenteral therapy. There are no data to suggest that immunosuppressed women benefit from hospitalization or parenteral therapy for PID.

In a group of Kenyan women with laparoscopically proven PID, risk of TOA was elevated among those coinfected with HIV-1 (OR = 2.8; 95% CI 1.2, 6.5), but was not significantly associated with immunosuppression (OR = 3.1; 95% CI 0.6, 15.3).[70] HIV-infected women responded as well to standard parenteral antibiotic regimens and had similar hospital stays compared with their uninfected counterparts. Immunosuppressed women (CD4 <14%) had prolongation of their hospital stay. In a subsequent study, 162 Kenyan women with new onset of pelvic pain underwent endometrial biopsy to screen for PID.[71] Endometritis was more frequent among HIV-1-infected women (OR = 3.0; 95% CI 1.5, 5.9). Clinical improvement or cure after outpatient oral therapy was documented in 81% of those with HIV and 86% of HIV-seronegative women, which was not statistically different.

A US study of women with clinically diagnosed PID compared 44 HIV-positive with 163 HIV-negative women.[72] Symptoms prior to medical evaluation were similar between the two groups, although more of the former group had received antibiotics already. HIV-infected women were more likely to have a TOA, although this did not achieve statistical significance (45.8% vs 27.1%, p = 0.08). Clinical response to antibiotic regimens recommended by the CDC STD treatment guidelines did not differ by serostatus. In addition, rates of sexually transmitted and other bacteria do not differ appreciably by serostatus, although mycoplasmas and streptococci were isolated more frequently from HIV-seropositive women.

Table 9.5 Criteria for pelvic inflammatory disease treatment site and route

Hospitalization/parenteral[a]
- Surgical emergencies (e.g. appendicitis) not excluded
- Pregnancy
- Clinical failure of oral antimicrobial regimen
- Inability to follow or tolerate a parenteral outpatient regimen
- Severe illness, nausea, vomiting, or high fever
- Tubo-ovarian abscess

Outpatient/parenteral (possible)
- Mild-to-moderate presentation and:
  - Clinical failure of an oral antimicrobial regimen
  - Intolerance of oral medications
  - Inability to follow-up within 72 hours of treatment initiation

Outpatient/oral
- Mild presentation and able to tolerate oral medications

[a]Adapted, with changes, from the 2002 CDC STD treatment guidelines[3]

Thus, the current 2002 CDC STD treatment guidelines[3] recommend hospitalization and parenteral PID therapy for women who have uncertain diagnoses that may require surgery, concurrent pregnancy, failed oral therapy, inability to tolerate or follow an oral regimen, severe presentations including high fever, nausea and/or vomiting, or a TOA (Table 9.5). Although not advocated by the CDC, women with mild presentation who cannot tolerate oral medications or who have failed a trial of oral medication may receive parenteral therapy at home under close supervision. For the vast majority of women who have a mild uncomplicated presentation and can tolerate oral medications, home oral therapy is warranted.

ANTI-INFECTIVE TIMING ISSUES

Rapidity of treatment initiation appears critical to prevention of long-term sequelae in both animal models and human treatment trials. Mouse chlamydial PID models have shown that antibiotic treatment initiated within 6 days of onset of clinically apparent infection results in good fertility outcome.[73] Hillis and colleagues reported that women treated within 3 days of symptom onset had significantly higher fertility rates than those whose antibiotic treatment began later (92.7% vs 81.3%).[74] The best data have used follow-up laparoscopy or hysterosalpingogram (HSG) to assess tubal patency following treatment. Viberg and colleagues[75] reported 0% involuntary infertility and 100% tubal patency on HSG when treatment was initiated within 2 days of clinical onset vs only 70% tubal patency among women whose treatment did not commence until day 7 or later after symptom onset.

Most parenteral regimens involve continuation of parenteral therapy for 48 hours before transitioning to oral therapy. The rationale for this appears arbitrary, and it may be shortened at the discretion of the provider, based on clinical response.

Recommendations for treatment duration of 14 days have been maintained due to concern about the long half-life of *C. trachomatis* and potential delay in antimicrobial access to the upper genital tract. Although evidence evaluating shorter treatment durations is scant, several investigators have suggested shortening treatment duration to 7 or 10 days on theoretical grounds to enhance adherence. Now open-label comparative trials, which have compared 7-day regimens using azithromycin either alone or with metronidazole (1 or 2 days of parenteral followed by 5 or 6 days of oral) with standard longer regimens, show equivalence in both instances. One caveat in the above-mentioned study is that if anaerobic microorganisms are suspected, addition of a 12-day course of metronidazole is recommended; the criteria that should lead one to suspect anaerobes are not elucidated. Given that it is reasonable to assume that anaerobes are always present, treatment duration should not be shortened from the standard 14 days. More data are needed to resolve this issue. Clinical experience should guide all decisions regarding overall length of treatment course and timing of transition from parenteral to oral therapy.

Traditional recommendations rely on maintenance of adequate dosing for 72 hours before considering non-response to therapy a failure. At that time, consensus suggests initiation of triple therapy in the form of an aminoglycoside, clindamycin, and ampicillin. If this fails over a 72-hour course, or if clinical deterioration ensues, surgical treatment is warranted.

MANAGEMENT OF SEX PARTNERS

Although specific data on reinfection rates in women with gonococcal or chlamydial PID are scant, Eschenbach and Holmes reported 30 years ago that 25% of women with gonococcal PID were readmitted with recurrent PID within 10 weeks despite adequate treatment and negative post-treatment test-of-cure.[76] Two potential partner treatment strategies – diagnosis and treatment of the female sex partners of men infected with *C. trachomatis* (strategy 1) and diagnosis and treatment of the male sex partners of women with lower genital tract chlamydial infection (strategy 2) – were evaluated for their ability to prevent cases of PID, using a decision model.[77] In a hypothetical cohort of 1000 male and 1000 female index patients, strategy 1 prevented 64 cases and strategy 2 prevented 20 cases of PID. Strategy 1 saved \$247 000 and strategy 2 saved \$33 000 over no partner notification.

The current guidelines for partner notification are that men who have had sexual contact with women later diagnosed with PID within 60 days of the onset of her symptoms should be evaluated for STIs. Alternatively, the CDC recommends that those partners may be treated empirically with regimens effective against *C. trachomatis* and *N. gonorrhoeae*.

COMPLEMENTARY AND ALTERNATIVE APPROACHES TO PELVIC INFLAMMATORY DISEASE

A variety of approaches other than anti-infectives have been proposed for the management of women with PID, and a few of those have been studied and published in the English-language literature.

Given that this infection has a significant inflammatory component, and that, particularly in those cases in which *C. trachomatis* is involved, pro-inflammatory cytokines may be the mechanism of tubal damage, many have advocated the use of anti-inflammatory therapy in the management of PID. Early investigators added steroids to antimicrobial therapy and noted excellent tubal patency rates on follow-up HSG.[41] In 1993, Landers and colleagues[75] reported that the use of ibuprofen, prostaglandin E_1 (PGE_1), or hydrocortisone, beginning 2 days after inoculation of the ovarian bursae of mice with the pneumonitis strain of *C. trachomatis*, did not change the degree of inflammation or subsequent fertility, although mean antichlamydial immunoglobulin G (IgG) titers were significantly lower compared with infected untreated mice.[78] More recently, Patton and colleagues conducted a triple-arm randomized controlled trial using the macaque model for chlamydial PID; they found that adding anti-inflammatory agents to doxycycline had a deleterious effect, rendering doxycycline no more efficacious than placebo.[79] This group has also shown that azithromycin appears to outperform doxycycline in the same animal model,[80] probably as a result of the drug's immunomodulatory effect in reducing the typical damage of chlamydial infection in the fallopian tube.

Balneotherapy, a range of interventions including mud baths, mud packs, mineral baths, electrotherapies, and gynecologic exercises provided under German sanatorium conditions, has been shown to reduce the occurrence of post-infection low abdominal pain.[81] In a more recent uncontrolled study in 39 Polish women with chronic PID who had failed prior treatment, acupuncture performed three times weekly for 4 weeks resulted in significant reductions in erythrocyte sedimentation rates, IgM levels, and pain scores, and a rise in IgG levels.[82] Finally, in an uncontrolled study of manual soft-tissue physical therapy among women with infertility due to pelvic adhesive disease, some of whom had had PID, there was a trend suggesting that this therapy facilitates fertility.[83]

UNUSUAL FORMS OF PELVIC INFLAMMATORY DISEASE

Actinomyces israelii is a Gram-positive anaerobe that has been identified as an etiologic agent in some women with PID. Women with PID caused by actinomycetes appear to have a higher clinical acuity when compared with women with other etiologic agents. In one study, 87.5% of women with actinomycetes PID had a TOA, compared with 28.9% of women without actinomycetes.[84] It is not known whether this microbe is associated with a typical polymicrobial milieu in those who have PID or its precise mechanism of action. TOAs with this microbe most often require surgical excision. Actinomycetes are difficult to isolate, hearty, and require prolonged antimicrobial therapy for eradication. Six to twelve weeks of penicillin, cephalosporins, cefoxitin, and clindamycin is considered appropriate therapy.

In areas of the world in which tuberculosis is endemic, genital tuberculosis is a common manifestation in women. Its primary presentation is salpingitis, and it is implicated in up to 10% of cases of infertility in those regions. Tuberculous salpingitis is treated with the same long-term, combined drug therapy that is used in pulmonary and extrapulmonary tuberculosis. Surgery with preservation of one ovary in women of reproductive age should be undertaken only after continuous drug treatment of 12–18 months' duration. Successful pregnancy is unlikely, however, even after appropriate anti-infective or surgical intervention.[85]

TUBO-OVARIAN ABSCESSES

See Chapter 7 for a detailed description of the management of TOAs.

THE ROLE OF SURGERY IN TREATING PELVIC INFLAMMATORY DISEASE

Surgery can be contemplated at several points during the care of a woman with PID. Many have advocated peritoneal lavage to reduce the potential for pelvic scar formation in women with PID. A recent study of laparoscopic lavage in a rabbit PID model compared two different solutions of povidone–iodine, chlorhexidine gluconate, saline, and no lavage. Subsequent histology revealed significantly more peritoneal inflammation with the active solutions than with saline or no lavage.[86]

Most surgical intervention is reserved for women with complicated presentations, including TOAs. In the study of 232 women with TOAs published by Lander and Sweet in 1983, only 59 (25%) underwent surgery.[87] Of those women who underwent surgery, 5 were drained, 19 had a unilateral adnexectomy, and 33 had a bilateral adnexectomy. These low rates for surgical intervention after antimicrobial treatment failure have been replicated in subsequent studies.[88,89] Laparoscopy was not a common gynecologic procedure at that time. Now, it has replaced laparotomy in many settings, and it is being used more and more among women with PID and TOAs.

Percutaneous or laparoscopic drainage of TOAs has been recommended by some as first-line therapy to improve response to anti-infective therapy. A prospective study of 40 women with TOAs measuring less than 10 cm randomized subjects to clindamycin and gentamicin alone or in association with early ultrasound-guided vaginal drainage.[90] The short-term (48–72 hours) response was 90% in women treated with antibiotics plus drainage vs 65% in the control group. In the medium-term (4 weeks) follow-up, 1 patient in the study group and 3 in the control group had a persistent adnexal mass.

More common is percutaneous drainage of a TOA, usually under computed tomography (CT) or ultrasound guidance, as an adjunt to antimicrobial treatment, particularly when therapy appears to be failing. The approach may be transabdominal, transvaginal, or transgluteal.[91,92]

Whereas laparoscopy is still considered the gold standard for diagnosing PID, its role in the treatment of PID remains uncertain. Technical developments and improvements in endoscopic provider skills have increased the use of laparoscopy in women with TOAs. Surgical approaches may include incision and drainage, unilateral or bilateral adnexectomy, or subtotal or total vaginal hysterectomy. In experienced hands, open laparoscopy appears to be as safe as exploratory laparotomy, and may have advantages. One non-comparative study reported that when compared with 37 women who underwent laparotomy for management for TOAs, 19 women who underwent open laparoscopy had shorter hospital stays (5.37 ± 1.38 days vs 8.92 ± 2.59 days, $p = 0.0001$), had a lower percentage of wound infections, and had a shorter time for fever to subside (25.79 ± 11.45 vs 39.46 ± 17.47 hours, $p = 0.003$).[93]

In a recent non-randomized study of 60 women with TOAs who underwent surgery, the authors reported significantly more complications in those women who underwent gynecologic organ removal.[94] They found open laparoscopy to be safe as laparotomy, and recommended that when laparoscopic treatment of TOA is performed, organ-preserving treatment should be chosen irrespective of the patient's age or desire to have children, because of the risk of complications.

Laparotomy is typically reserved for persistent or ruptured TOAs and treatment failures following a reasonable course of appropriate anti-infective therapy. As in laparoscopy, surgical approaches may include incision and drainage, unilateral or bilateral adnexectomy, or subtotal or total vaginal hysterectomy.[87] In addition, given the high frequency of genital tract malignancy in postmenopausal women with TOAs, conservative management is not appropriate.[68] Surgical exploration is recommended in these women.

REFERENCES

1. Curtis AH. Bacteriology and pathology of fallopian tubes removed at operation. Surg Gynecol Obstet 1921;33:621.
2. Kahn JG, Walker CK, Washington AE, et al. Diagnosing pelvic inflammatory disease. A comprehensive analysis and considerations for developing a new model. JAMA 1991;266:2594–604.
3. Centers for Disease Control and Prevention. Sexually transmitted diseases treatment guidelines 2002. MMWR Recomm Report 2002;51(RR–6):1–78.
4. Wolner-Hanssen P. Silent pelvic inflammatory disease: is it overstated? Obstet Gynecol 1995;86:321–5.
5. Eschenbach DA, Wolner-Hanssen P, Hawes SE, et al. Acute pelvic inflammatory disease: associations of clinical and laboratory findings with laparoscopic findings. Obstet Gynecol 997;89:184–92.
6. Peipert JF, Boardman L, Hogan JW, et al. Laboratory evaluation of acute upper genital tract infection. Obstet Gynecol 1996;87:730–6.
7. Patton DL, Moore DE, Spadoni LR, et al. A comparison of the fallopian tube's response to overt and silent salpingitis. Obstet Gynecol 1989;73:622–30.
8. Sweet RL. Pelvic inflammatory disease and infertility in women. Infect Dis Clin North Am 1987;1:199–215.
9. Wasserheit JN, Bell TA, Kiviat NB, et al. Microbiological causes of proven pelvic inflammatory disease and efficacy of clindamycin and tobramycin. Am Intern Med 1986;104:187–93.
10. Heinonen PK, Teisala K, Punnonen R, et al. Anatomic sites of upper genital tract infection. Obstet Gynecol 1985;66:384–90.
11. Paavonen J, Teisala K, Heinonen PK, et al. Microbiological and histopathological findings in acute pelvic inflammatory disease. Br J Obstet Gynaecol 1987;94:454–60.
12. Brunham RC, Binns B, Guijon F, et al. Etiology and outcome of acute pelvic inflammatory disease. J Infect Dis 1988;158:510–17.
13. Soper DE, Brockwell NJ, Dalton HP, et al. Observations concerning the microbial etiology of acute salpingitis. Am J Obstet Gynecol 1994;170:1008–17.
14. Hillier SL, Kiviat NB, Hawes SE, et al. Role of bacterial vaginosis-associated microorganisms in endometritis. Am J Obstet Gynecol 1996;175:435–41.
15. Carney FE Jr, Taylor-Robinson D. Growth and effect of *Neisseria gonorrhoeae* in organ cultures. Br J Vener Dis 1973;49:435–40.
16. McGee ZA, Johnson AP, Taylor-Robinson D. Pathogenic mechanisms of *Neisseria gonorrhoeae*: observations on damage to human fallopian tubes in organ culture by gonococci of colony type 1 or type 4. J Infect Dis 1981;143:413–22.
17. McGee ZA, Jensen RL, Clemens CM, et al. Gonococcal infection of human fallopian tube mucosa in organ culture: relationship of mucosal tissue TNF-alpha concentration to sloughing of ciliated cells. Sex Transm Dis 1999;26:160–5.
18. Melly MA, Gregg CR, McGee ZA. Studies of toxicity of *Neisseria gonorrhoeae* for human fallopian tube mucosa. J Infect Dis 1981;143:413–22.
19. Patton DL, Sweeney YT, Kuo CC. Demonstration of delayed hypersensitivity in *Chlamydia trachomatis* salpingitis in monkeys: a pathogenic mechanism of tubal damage. J Infect Dis 1994;169:680–3.
20. Morrison RP, Belland RJ, Lyng K, et al. Chlamydial disease pathogenesis. The 57-kD chlamydial hypersensitivity antigen is a stress response protein. J Exp Med 1989;170:1271–83.
21. Brunham RC, Peeling RW. *Chlamydia trachomatis* antigens: role in immunity and pathogenesis. Infect Agents Dis 1994;3:218–33.
22. Eckert LO, Hawes SE, Wolner-Hanssen P, et al. Prevalence and correlates of antibody to chlamydial heat shock protein in women attending sexually transmitted disease clinics and women with confirmed pelvic inflammatory disease. J Infect Dis 1997;175:1453–8.
23. Patton DL, Landers DV, Schachter J. Experimental *Chlamydia trachomatis* salpingitis in mice: initial studies on the characterization of the leukocyte response to chlamydial infection. J Infect Dis 1989;159:1105–10.
24. Kiviat NB, Wolner-Hanssen P, Peterson M, et al. Localization of *Chlamydia trachomatis* infection by direct immunofluorescence and culture in pelvic inflammatory disease. Am J Obstet Gynecol 1986;154:865–73.
25. Sweet RL, Mills J, Hadley KW, et al. Use of laparoscopy to determine the microbiologic etiology of acute salpingitis. Am J Obstet Gynecol 1979;134:68–74.
26. Lip J, Burgoyne X. Cervical and peritoneal bacterial flora associated with salpingitis. Obstet Gynecol 1966;28:561–3.
27. Chow AW, Malkasian KL, Marshall JR, et al. The bacteriology of acute pelvic inflammatory disease. Am J Obstet Gynecol 1975;122:876–9.
28. Eschenbach DA, Buchanan TM, Pollock HM, et al. Polymicrobial etiology of acute pelvic inflammatory disease. N Engl J Med 1975;293:166–71.
29. Monif GR, Welkos SL, Baer H, et al. Cul-de-sac isolates from patients with endometritis–salpingitis–peritonitis and gonococcal endocervicitis. Am J Obstet Gynecol 1976;126:158–61.
30. Cunningham FG, Hauth JC, Gilstrap LC, et al. The bacterial pathogenesis of acute pelvic inflammatory disease. Obstet Gynecol 1978;52:161–4.
31. Eschenbach DA. Epidemiology and diagnosis of acute pelvic inflammatory disease. Obstet Gynecol 1980;55(5 Suppl):142–53S.
32. Sweet RL, Draper DL, Schachter J, et al. Microbiology and pathogenesis of acute salpingitis as determined by laparoscopy: what is the appropriate site to sample? Am J Obstet Gynecol 1980;138:985–9.

33. Thompson SE 3rd, Hager WD, Wong KH, et al. The microbiology and therapy of acute pelvic inflammatory disease in hospitalized patients. Am J Obstet Gynecol 1980;136:179–86.
34. Haggerty CL, Hillier SL, Bass DC, et al. Bacterial vaginosis and anaerobic bacteria are associated with endometritis. Clin Infect Dis 2004;39:990–5.
35. Walker CK, Workowski KA, Washington AE, et al. Anaerobes in pelvic inflammatory disease: implications for the Centers for Disease Control and Prevention's guidelines for treatment of sexually transmitted diseases. Clin Infect Dis 1999; 28(Suppl 1):S29–36.
36. Sweet RL, Schachter J, Robbie MO. Failure of beta-lactam antibiotics to eradicate *Chlamydia trachomatis* in the endometrium despite apparent clinical cure of acute salpingitis. JAMA. 1983;250:2641–5.
37. Crombleholme WR, Schachter J, Ohm-Smith M, et al. Efficacy of single-agent therapy for the treatment of acute pelvic inflammatory disease with ciprofloxacin. Am J Med 1989;87:142–7S.
38. Eckert LO, Thwin SS, Hillier SL, et al. The antimicrobial treatment of subacute endometritis: a proof of concept study. Am J Obstet Gynecol 2004;190:305–13.
39. Ness RB, Soper DE, Holley RL, et al. Effectiveness of inpatient and outpatient treatment strategies for women with pelvic inflammatory disease: results from the Pelvic Inflammatory Disease Evaluation and Clinical Health (PEACH) Randomized Trial. Am J Obstet Gynecol 2002;186:929–37.
40. Holtz F. Klinische studien uber die nicht tuberkulose salpingoophoritis. Acta Obstet Gynecol 1930;10(Suppl):5.
41. Falk V. Treatment of acute non-tuberculous salpingitis with antibiotics alone and in combination with glucocorticoids. A prospective double blind controlled study of the clinical course and prognosis. Acta Obstet Gynecol Scand 1965;44(Suppl 6):3–118.
42. Hedberg E, Anberg A. Gonorrheal salpingitis: views on treatment and prognosis. Fertil Steril 1965;16:125–9.
43. Falk V, Krook G. Do results of culture for gonococci vary with sampling phase of menstrual cycle? Acta Derm Venereol 1967;47:190–3.
44. Westrom L, Joesoef R, Reynolds G, et al. Pelvic inflammatory disease and fertility. A cohort study of 1,844 women with laparoscopically verified disease and 657 control women with normal laparoscopic results. Sex Transm Dis 1992;19:185–92.
45. Walker CK, Kahn JG, Washington AE, et al. Pelvic inflammatory disease: metaanalysis of antimicrobial regimen efficacy. J Infect Dis 1993;168:969–78.
46. Peipert JF, Sweet RL, Walker CK, et al. Evaluation of ofloxacin in the treatment of laparoscopically documented acute pelvic inflammatory disease (salpingitis). Infect Dis Obstet Gynecol 1999;7:138–44.
47. Amsden GW. Anti-inflammatory effects of macrolides – an underappreciated benefit in the treatment of community-acquired respiratory tract infections and chronic inflammatory pulmonary conditions? J Antimicrob Chemother 2005;55:10–21.
48. Bevan C, Ridgway G, Rothermel C. Efficacy and safety of azithromycin as monotherapy or combined with metronidazole compared with two standard multidrug regimens for the treatment of acute pelvic inflammatory disease. J Int Med Res 2003;31:45–54.
49. Aldridge KE, Ashcraft D, Cambre K, et al. Multicenter survey of the changing in vitro antimicrobial susceptibilities of clinical isolates of *Bacteroides fragilis* group, *Prevotella*, *Fusobacterium*, *Porphyromonas*, and *Peptostreptococcus* species. Antimicrob Agents Chemother 2001;45:1238–43.
50. Matsuda S, et al. Clinical study of levofloxacin (LVFX) on the infectious diseases in the field of obstetrics and gynecology. Chemotherapy 1992;40:311–23.
51. Arredondo JL, Diaz V, Gaitan H, et al. Oral clindamycin and ciprofloxacin versus intramuscular ceftriaxone and oral doxycycline in the treatment of mild-to-moderate pelvic inflammatory disease in outpatients. Clin Infect Dis 1997;24:170–8.
52. Dunbar-Jacob J, Sereika SM, Foley SM, et al. Adherence to oral therapies in pelvic inflammatory disease. J Womens Health 2004;13:285–91.
53. Kane BG, Degutis LC, Sayward HK, D'Onofrio G. Compliance with the Centers for Disease Control and Prevention recommendations for the diagnosis and treatment of sexually transmitted diseases. Acad Emerg Med 2004;11:371–7.
54. Ratelle S, Yokoe D, Blejan C, et al. Predictive value of clinical diagnostic codes for the CDC case definition of pelvic inflammatory disease (PID): implications for surveillance. Sex Transm Dis 2003;30:866–70.
55. Velebil P, Wingo PA, Xia Z, et al. Rate of hospitalization for gynecologic disorders among reproductive-age women in the United States. Obstet Gynecol 1995;86:764–9.
56. Nathwani D, Zambrowski JJ; AdHOC Workshop. Advisory group on Home-based and Outpatient Care (AdHOC): an international consensus statement on non-inpatient parenteral therapy. Clin Microbiol Infect 2000;6:464–76.
57. Leggett JE. Ambulatory use of parenteral antibacterials: contemporary perspectives. Drugs 2000;59 (Suppl 3):1–8.
58. Yip L, Sweeny PJ, Bock BF. Acute suppurative salpingitis with concomitant intrauterine pregnancy. Am J Emerg Med 1993;11:476–9.
59. Blanchard AC, Pastorek JG 2nd, Weeks T. Pelvic inflammatory disease during pregnancy. South Med J 1987;80:1363–5.
60. Lardaro HH. Spontaneous rupture of tubo-ovarial abscess into the free peritoneal cavity. JAMA 1954;156:699–701.
61. Franklin EW 3rd, Hevron JE Jr, Thompson JD. Management of the pelvic abscess. Clin Obstet Gynecol 1973;16:66–79.
62. Cerha HT, Collins CG, Nix FJ. Ruptured tuboovarian abscess. Am J Obstet Gynecol 1956;72:820–9.
63. Centers for Disease Control and Prevention. 1998 guidelines for treatment of sexually transmitted diseases. MMWR Recommend Rep 1998;47(RR–1):1–11.
64. Hemsel DL, Ledger WJ, Martens MG, et al. Concerns regarding the Centers for Disease Control's published guidelines for pelvic inflammatory disease. Clin Infect Dis 2001;32:103–7.
65. Gonik B, Pokorny S, Garcia S, et al. Pelvic inflammatory disease in the adolescent. Tex Med 1987;83:25–6.
66. Jamieson DJ, Duerr A, Macasaet MA, et al. Risk factors for a complicated clinical course among women hospitalized with pelvic inflammatory disease. Infect Dis Obstet Gynecol 2000;8:88–93.
67. Halperin R, Levinson O, Yaron M, et al. Tubo-ovarian abscess in older women: is the woman's age a risk factor for failed response to conservative treatment? Gynecol Obstet Invest 2003;55:211–15.
68. Protopapas AG, Diakomanolis ES, Milingos SD, et al. Tubo-ovarian abscesses in postmenopausal women: gynecological malignancy until proven otherwise? Eur J Obstet Gynecol Reprod Biol 2004;114:203–9.
69. Korn AP. Pelvic inflammatory disease in women infected with HIV. AIDS Patient Care STDS 1998;12:431–4.
70. Cohen CR, Sinei S, Reilly M, et al. Effect of human immunodeficiency virus type 1 infection upon acute salpingitis: a laparoscopic study. J Infect Dis 1998;178:1352–8.
71. Bukusi EA, Cohen CR, Stevens CE, et al. Effects of human immunodeficiency virus 1 infection on microbial origins of pelvic inflammatory disease and on efficacy of ambulatory oral therapy. Am J Obstet Gynecol 1999;18:1374–81.
72. Irwin KL, Moorman AC, O'Sullivan MJ, et al. Influence of human immunodeficiency virus infection on pelvic inflammatory disease. Obstet Gynecol 2000;95:525–34.
73. Swenson CE, Schachter J. Infertility as a consequence of chlamydial infection of the upper genital tract in female mice. Sex Transm Dis 1984;11:64–7.

74. Hillis SD, Joesoef R, Marchbanks PA, et al. Delayed care of pelvic inflammatory disease as a risk factor for impaired fertility. Am J Obstet Gynecol 1993;168:1503–9.
75. Viberg L. Acute inflammatory conditions of the uterine adnexa. Clinical, radiological and isotopic investigations of non-gonococcal adnexitis. Acta Obstet Gynecol Scand 1964;43:(Suppl 4):1–86.
76. Eschenbach DA, Holmes KK. Acute pelvic inflammatory disease: current concepts of pathogenesis, etiology, and management. Clin Obstet Gynecol 1975;18:35.
77. Howell MR, Kassler WJ, Haddix A. Partner notification to prevent pelvic inflammatory disease in women. Cost-effectiveness of two strategies. Sex Transm Dis 1997;24:287–92.
78. Landers DV, Sung ML, Bottles K, et al. Does addition of anti-inflammatory agents to antimicrobial therapy reduce infertility after murine chlamydial salpingitis? Sex Transm Dis 1993:20;121–5.
79. Patton DL, Sweeney YC, Bohannon NJ, et al. Effects of doxycycline and antiinflammatory agents on experimentally induced chlamydial upper genital tract infection in female macaques. J Infect Dis 1997;175:648–54.
80. Patton DL, Cosgrove-Sweeney YT, Stamm WE. Azithromycin vs doxycycline vs placebo for resolution of chlamydial infection and associated inflammation in the pig-tailed macaque model. In: Schachter J, Christianson G, Clarke IN, et al, eds. Chlamydial Infections – Proceedings of the Tenth International Symposium on Human Chlamydial Infections. San Francisco: International Chlamydia Symposium; 2002, 365–8.
81. Gerber B, Wilken H, Barten G, et al. Positive effect of balneotherapy on post-PID symptoms. Int J Fertil Menopausal Stud 1993;38:296–300.
82. Wozniak PR, Stachowiak GP, Pieta-Dolinska AK, et al. Anti-phlogistic and immunocompetent effects of acupuncture treatment in women suffering from chronic pelvic inflammatory diseases. Am J Chin Med 2003;31:315–20.
83. Wurn BF, Wurn LJ, King CR, et al. Treating female infertility and improving IVF pregnancy rates with a manual physical therapy technique. Med Gen Med 2004;6:51.
84. Burkman R, Schlesselman S, McCaffrey L, et al. The relationship of genital tract actinomycetes and the development of pelvic inflammatory disease. Am J Obstet Gynecol 1982;143:585–9.
85. Chowdhury NN. Overview of tuberculosis of the female genital tract. J Indian Med Assoc 1996;94:345–6, 361.
86. Roberts LM, Sanfilippo JS, Raab S. Effects of laparoscopic lavage on adhesion formation and peritoneum in an animal model of pelvic inflammatory disease. J Am Assoc Gynecol Laparosc 202;9:503–7.
87. Landers DV, Sweet RL. Tubo-ovarian abscess: contemporary approach to management. Rev Infect Dis 1983;5:876–84.
88. Reed SD, Landers DV, Sweet RL. Antibiotic treatment of tuboovarian abscess: comparison of broad-spectrum beta-lactam agents versus clindamycin-containing regimens. Am J Obstet Gynecol 1991;164:1556–61.
89. McNeeley SG, Hendrix SL, Mazzoni MM, et al. Medically sound, cost-effective treatment for pelvic inflammatory disease and tuboovarian abscess. Am J Obstet Gynecol 1998;178(6):1272-8.
90. Perez-Medina T, Huertas MA, Bajo JM. Early ultrasound-guided transvaginal drainage of tubo-ovarian abscesses: a randomized study. Ultrasound Obstet Gynecol 1996;7:435–8.
91. Caspi B, Zalel Y, Or Y, et al. Sonographically guided aspiration: an alternative therapy for tubo-ovarian abscess. Ultrasound Obstet Gynecol 1996;7:439–42.
92. Harisinghani MG, Gervais DA, Maher MM, et al. Transgluteal approach for percutaneous drainage of deep pelvic abscesses: 154 cases. Radiology 2003;228:701–5.
93. Yang CC, Chen P, Tseng JY, et al. Advantages of open laparoscopic surgery over exploratory laparotomy in patients with tubo-ovarian abscess. J Am Assoc Gynecol Laparosc 2002;9:327–32.
94. Buchweitz O, Malik E, Kressin P, et al. Laparoscopic management of tubo-ovarian abscesses: retrospective analysis of 60 cases. Surg Endosc 2000;14:948–50.

10. Prevention

Richard L. Sweet

INTRODUCTION

As reviewed in previous chapters, acute pelvic inflammatory disease (PID), one of the most common and important complications of sexually transmitted diseases (STDs), is a substantial public health problem adversely affecting the health of women. Worldwide, acute PID affects millions of women, and in the United States over 1 million women develop acute PID annually. Of major concern are the significant short-term and long-term complications and/or sequelae associated with PID. It is well recognized that women who develop acute PID are at substantial risk for tubal factor infertility (TFI), ectopic pregnancy, recurrent PID, and chronic pelvic pain. The Centers for Disease Control and Prevention (CDC) estimates that, on an annual basis, over 100 000 women become infertile and 150 women die as the result of acute PID.[1]

In addition, the economic impact of acute PID is staggering, with an estimated cost in the United States of $5.5 billion during the 1990s.[2] A more recent estimate placed the direct medical cost of PID and its sequelae within 1 year of diagnosis at $2 billion.[3] Projection of economic cost to 5 years after diagnosis of PID resulted in estimated average per-person lifetime cost of PID ranging from $1060 to $3180.[4] However, those cost estimates were based on clinically apparent PID and do not take into account the impact of subclinical PID, which is at least as common as clinically recognized PID.[5]

Several studies have demonstrated an association between lower genital tract infection with gonorrhea and chlamydia and histologic endometritis (subclinical PID). Paavonen et al reported that histologic endometritis was correlated with chlamydial and/or gonococcal cervicitis.[6] Korn et al demonstrated that over 50% of women with gonococcal or chlamydial infection of the cervix had plasma cell endometritis.[7] Wiesenfeld and coworkers demonstrated that subclinical PID was detected in 27% of women with chlamydial infection, 26% of those with gonococcal infection.[8] Similarly, investigations have demonstrated an association between bacterial vaginosis (BV) and subclinical PID. Korn et al reported that nearly one-half of women with BV in the absence of *Neisseria gonorrhoeae* or *Chlamydia trachomatis* had plasma cell endometritis.[9] Wiesenfeld et al detected histologic endometritis in 16% of asymptomatic women with BV.[8] Thus, the economic cost of PID is substantially greater than previous estimates. These economic costs make screening and presentation strategies cost-effective.

One in four women develop major sequelae, including TFI, ectopic pregnancy, and chronic pelvic pain, following a single episode of PID, and with recurrent episodes nearly 50% of women suffer major sequelae.[10] Several areas of investigation support the concept that the development of strategies for the prevention of PID is critically important to improving the health of women worldwide. First, the most important factor in the development of TFI is the number of PID episodes.[11] Thus, preventing recurrent episodes of PID is a high priority. Secondly, treatment of PID, in hopes of preventing the associated long-term sequelae, has resulted in unacceptable rates of fertility preservation.[12–16] Thirdly, delay in diagnosing and initiating treatment for PID beyond 72 hours from onset of symptoms is associated with poor prognosis for future fertility.[17,18] Lastly, and maybe most important, the elucidation of subclinical PID as a definite entity associated with adverse effects on future fertility similar to that of clinically recognized PID speaks loudly to the importance of prevention. In response to concerns over the short-term and long-term medical and economic consequences of PID, reducing the incidence of

PID is a goal of the Public Health Service Healthy People Program.[19] However, as summarized by Scholes et al, these efforts have been thwarted by:

- the variety of microorganisms (including normal vaginal flora) recognized as pathogens in PID
- uncertainties in the diagnosis of PID
- frequency of subclinical PID
- lack of adequate surveillance systems for PID.[20]

PREVENTION STRATEGIES

Prevention of PID incorporates two major goals:

- a short-term goal to prevent the morbidity, lost work time, pain, suffering, medical costs, and uncommon mortality associated with acute PID
- prevention of the long-term sequelae of PID, which include infertility, ectopic pregnancy, chronic pelvic pain, and recurrent infection.[21]

Knowledge of the risk factors and risk markers for PID is key to developing successful prevention strategies for PID and its sequelae.[22] The determinants of risk for PID include:

- inoculum size of putative pathogen(s)
- number of infecting pathogens
- virulence of infecting organism(s)
- host susceptibility
- environmental factors.[22]

Prevention and intervention strategies (except vaccine development) are generally based on the last two factors. These risk factors are discussed in detail in Chapter 1 and will be briefly summarized here. As noted by Washington et al,[22] these factors may be assessed relative to increased risk of exposure to an infectious pathogen, risk of acquiring infection when exposed, risk of developing disease when infected, and risk of progression to adverse sequelae (Table 10.1). These authors further identi-

Table 10.1 Health outcome affected by demographic variables and individual behaviours and practices

Risk variable	Acquisition of STD	Development of PID	Development of PID sequelae
Demographic and social indicators			
Age	↑	↑	↓
Socioeconomic status	↑	↑	–
Marital status	↑	↑	–
Residence (urban, rural)	↑	–	–
Individual behavior and practices			
Sexual behavior:			
No. of partners	↑	–	–
Age at first sexual intercourse	↑	–	–
Frequency of sexual intercourse	↑	–	–
Rate of acquiring new partners	↑	–	–
Contraceptive practice:			
Barrier	↓	↓	↓
Oral contraceptives	↑	↓	–
Intrauterine device	–	↑	↑
Healthcare behavior:			
Evaluation of symptoms	↑	↑	↑
Compliance with treatment	↑	↑	↑
Sex partner referral	↑	↑	↑
Others:			
Douching	–	↑	–
Substance abuse	↑	↑	–
Smoking	↑	–	–
Menstrual cycle	↑	↑	–

STD = sexually transmitted disease; PID = pelvic inflammatory disease; ↑ = increased risk; ↓ = decreased risk; – = no association.
Reprinted with permission from Washington AE, Aral SO, Wolner Hamsen P, et al. Assessing risk for pelvic inflammatory disease and its sequelae. JAMA 1991;266:2581–6.

Table 10.2 Probable risk category and summary of quality of evidence supporting association between risk factor and pelvic inflammatory disease

Health outcome	Risk marker	Risk factor	Quality of evidence[a]
Acquisition of STD	Age[b]	Age[b]	II
	Socioeconomic status	Sexual behavior	II
	Residence	Contraceptive practice (barrier and OC)	II
	Substance abuse	Healthcare behavior	III
		Smoking	III
Development of PID	Age[b]	Age[b]	II
	Socioeconomic status	Contraceptive practice (OC and IUD)	II
	Contraceptive practice (barrier)	Healthcare behavior	III
	Smoking	Douching[c]	II
Development of PID sequelae	Age[b]	Age[b]	II
	Contraceptive practice (barrier and IUD)	Healthcare behavior	III

STD = sexually transmitted disease; PID = pelvic inflammatory disease; OC = oral contraceptive; IUD = intrauterine device.
[a]Grading scheme refers to risk factors only and is based on US Preventive Services Task Force: I, evidence from at least one randomized controlled trial; II, evidence from well-designed cohorts or case–control studies; and III, opinions of respective authorities.
[b]Age may be a risk factor, risk marker, or both.
[c]Data suggestive but not conclusive.
Reprinted with permission from Washington AE, Aral SO, Wolner Hamsen P, et al. Assessing risk for pelvic inflammatory disease and its sequelae. JAMA 1991;266:2581–6.

fied risk markers that are surrogates for risk factors (Table 10.2). Whereas both risk factors and risk markers are useful in determining clinical risk for disease, only risk factors identify where to focus prevention/intervention strategies. Risk markers, on the other hand, are important for identifying target populations in which to implement prevention strategies. A major focus of prevention strategies related to PID involves prevention of sexually transmitted diseases.[21,22] This is not surprising

Table 10.3 Recommendations for individuals to prevent sexually transmitted disease and pelvic inflammatory disease

General preventive measures	Specific recommendations	Quality of evidence supporting effectiveness of intervention
Maintain healthy sexual behavior	1. Postpone initiation of sexual intercourse until 2–3 years post menarche	III
	2. Limit number of sexual partners	II
	3. Avoid casual sex and sex with high-risk partners	III
	4. Question potential sex partners about STD and inspect genitals for lesions or discharge	III
Use barrier methods	Use condoms (diaphragms and/or vaginal spermicides) consistently and correctly throughout all sex for protection against STD, even if contraception not needed	II
Adopt healthy medical care-seeking behavior	1. Seek medical treatment promptly after having unprotected sex with someone suspected of having an STD	
	2. Seek medical care immediately when genital lesions or discharge appear	III
	3. Seek routine checkups for STD if in nonmutually monogamous relationship(s)	III
Comply with management instructions	1. Take all medication as directed, regardless of symptoms	I
	2. Return for follow-up evaluation as directed	III
	3. Abstain from sex until symptoms disappear and treatment completed	III
Ensure examination of sex partners	1. When diagnosed as having an STD, notify all sex partners in need of medical assessment	III
	2. If preferred, assist health providers in identifying and notifying sex partners	III

STD = sexually transmitted disease.
Reprinted with permission from Washington AE, Cates W Jr, Wasserheit JN. Preventing pelvic inflammatory disease. JAMA 1991;266:2574–80.

Table 10.4 Recommendations for health providers to prevent sexually transmitted disease and pelvic inflammatory disease

General preventive measures	Specific recommendations
Maintain up-to-date knowledge on prevention and treatment of STD/PID	1. Develop an accurate base of information or diagnosis, treatment, and prevention of STD/PID 2. Complete continuing education courses to update knowledge on STD/PID prevention and treatment
Provide effective patient education and counseling	1. Educate patients about STD/PID and their potential complications 2. Encourage individuals to maintain healthy sexual behavior, use condoms, and adopt healthy medical care-seeking behavior
Promote appropriate preventive medicine services	1. Screen patients for chlamydial and gonococcal infections per published guidelines. 2. Consider screening for BV in select patient groups 3. Provide epidemiologic treatment for STD/PID per recommended guidelines
Provide appropriate medical management for illness	1. Diagnose STD/PID promptly 2. Treat STD/PID promptly with effective antibiotics 3. Encourage patients to comply with treatment instructions
Ensure examination of sex partners	1. Encourage infected patients to refer all sex partners in need of medical assessment 2. Examine and treat sex partners appropriately

STD = sexually transmitted disease; PID = pelvic inflammatory disease, BV = bacterial vaginosis.
Reprinted with permission from Washington AE, Cates W Jr, Wasserheit JN. Preventing pelvic inflammatory disease. JAMA 1991;266:2574–80.

because, as discussed in Chapter 2, the sexually transmitted pathogens *N. gonorrhoeae* and *C. trachomatis* have been implicated in up to 65–75% of acute PID episodes.

Prevention of PID and its associated sequelae involves three levels: primary, secondary, and tertiary prevention.[23] In turn, these are further divided into prevention strategies for individuals (Table 10.3), healthcare providers (Table 10.4), and communities.

PRIMARY PREVENTION

Primary prevention addresses interventions for avoiding exposure to STDs or acquisition of infection after exposure has occurred.[23] For PID, this involves *C. trachomatis* and *N. gonorrhoeae*, the primary STD pathogens associated with development of acute PID.[24] BV, a disequilibrium of the vaginal flora in which the hydrogen peroxide-producing lactobacillus-dominated flora is replaced with substantial increases of anaerobic (especially Gram-negative) bacteria, *Gardnerella vaginalis*, *Mobiluncus* species, and genital mycoplasmas, has also been implicated in the development of PID.[25] More recently, a role has also been demonstrated for BV in the development of subclinical PID.[8,9,26] Examples of primary prevention of STDs and/or PID include:

- delayed onset of sexual activity
- monogamous sexual relationships
- use of barrier methods of contraception, especially condoms (Table 10.3).

In addition to behavioral changes, which form the cornerstone of current primary prevention, two possible medical interventions hold great potential as future primary prevention approaches. When effective vaccines are developed and available against *N. gonorrhoeae* and *C. trachomatis*, immunization against infection caused by these STD pathogens will be possible and could play an important role in prevention of these pathogens and, as a result, prevent up to 65–75% of cases of PID. Unfortunately, it does not seem likely that effective vaccines for gonococcal or chlamydial infections will become available soon.[21] A second biologic preventive measure, which has received a great deal of recent attention, is the use of microbicides placed intravaginally. Although microbicides are very attractive, especially because they empower women to protect themselves from STDs, development and clinical testing are still in their infancy.

SECONDARY PREVENTION

Secondary prevention is directed at precluding lower genital tract infection with STDs such as *N.*

gonorrhoeae and *C. trachomatis* or BV from ascending to the upper genital tract to produce PID, clinically apparent and subclinical. Similar to primary prevention efforts, strategies for secondary prevention of PID involve many of the concepts utilized for STD prevention, including disease detection, appropriate treatment, and partner notification and treatment.[21–23] Cates and Meheus pointed out that efforts at early disease detection are critical to PID (and STD) prevention and/or intervention programs.[27] These strategies include:

- targeted and general screening programs for gonorrhea and chlamydia
- presumptive diagnosis of lower genital tract infection(s) based on symptoms and signs (i.e. a syndromic approach)
- assessment and/or treatment of sex partners of persons diagnosed with gonococcal and/or chlamydial infection.

Screening programs for chlamydia were endorsed by Hillis and Wasserheit as a pivotal step in attempts to prevent PID.[28] With the recent recognition of the key role played by chlamydia in subclinical (and thus inapparent) PID, this approach takes on even greater importance. The first suggestion that detection and treatment of lower genital tract chlamydial infection results in decreased risk for development of PID was provided by Stamm et al.[29] These authors noted that in a group of women treated for gonorrhea with penicillin and co-infected with cervical chlamydial infection (culture-proven), nearly 40% of the women developed PID during the ensuing 7 days. In contrast, among women treated with tetracycline for gonorrhea, no cases of PID were detected. Subsequent reports have provided convincing evidence that screening programs for detection and treatment of chlamydial infection are effective in preventing PID.[20,28,30] Implementation of regional, state, and local programs of chlamydial prevention have led to dramatic decreases in the prevalence of chlamydial infection.[28] In a bell weather study, Scholes et al undertook a prospective, randomized, controlled clinical trial in which selective screening of women at high risk for chlamydial infection was compared with the usual approach of only testing symptomatic women for chlamydia.[20] Among the women in the screening group, there was a nearly 60% reduction in PID relative risk = 0.44; 95% confidence interval (CI) 0.20–0.90). Similarly, Kamwendo et al, in a study from Sweden, demonstrated that concerted efforts to screen for chlamydia and gonorrhea – and a reduction in IUD (intrauterine device) use in sexually active, nulliparous women – resulted in a substantial decrease in PID.[30]

Two technological advances have augmented prevention efforts for chlamydial infection. First, the availability of DNA-amplification tests has enhanced our diagnostic abilities. These tests are more sensitive than culture or antigen-detection tests and thus detect a greater number of chlamydial-infected persons. Perhaps more importantly, DNA-amplification tests can be used on urine specimens and vaginal swabs, thus expanding screening programs into hard-to-reach populations.[28] For women, the availability of vaginal swab diagnostics, including self-collected specimens, has the potential to revolutionize our efforts at secondary prevention of PID due to chlamydial and gonorrheal infection.[31,32]

Controversy has surrounded the role of BV in the development of acute PID. Retrospective and cross-sectional studies have demonstrated an association between BV and PID.[8,9,25,26,33] In contradistinction, Ness et al, in a multicenter study in which predominantly young, African-American women at risk of acquiring sexually transmitted infections (STIs) were followed longitudinally for a median of 3 years, did not demonstrate an association between BV, characterized by findings on microscopy, and development of PID.[34] However, in a more recent analysis of this large longitudinal study (n = 1140) utilizing bacteriologic cultures, Ness et al noted that women with heavy growth (highest textile) of BV-associated microorganisms (e.g. anaerobic Gram-negative rods, *Mycoplasma hominis*, and *Gardnerella vaginalis* plus absence of hydrogen peroxide-producing lactobacilli) were at increased risk for PID (adjusted rate ratio = 2.03; 95% CI 1.16–3.53).[35] Moreover, women with heavy growth of BV-associated microorganisms and a new sexual partner were at substantial high risk to develop PID (adjusted rate ratio = 8.77; 95% CI 1.11–69.2).[35] This latter finding raises the question of whether a subset of BV-associated microorganisms, especially the anaerobic Gram-negative rods, may be sexually transmitted. Whether sexually transmitted or (as previously believed) sexually associated, no data have yet been presented that assess the efficacy of screening and treatment of BV in an attempt to prevent development of PID. Such studies should be undertaken.

Other examples of potential secondary prevention approaches include:

- limiting IUD use in young, nulliparous women, especially those at risk for STIs
- screening of *C. trachomatis* and BV (and possibly *N. gonorrhoeae*) prior to elective abortion
- decreased use of vaginal douching
- cessation of smoking.

TERTIARY PREVENTION

Tertiary prevention is directed at strategies that prevent upper genital tract infection from resulting in chronic sequelae such as infertility, ectopic pregnancy, and chronic pelvic pain. As noted by Washington et al, tertiary prevention has produced disappointing and unacceptable results.[23] Whereas antibiotic therapy has improved the prognosis and alleviates the symptoms of acute PID compared with the pre-antibiotic era, currently recommended treatment regimens have had little impact on the long-term sequelae of PID.[14,36] This is particularly true if treatment is commenced prior to 72 hours after onset of symptoms.[17,18] Viberg reported that no cases of involuntary infertility occurred among patients treated within 2 days of the onset of symptoms, and all had patent fallopian tubes on follow-up hysterosalpingogram.[17] In those women where treatment was not instituted until $\geq$7 days after onset of symptoms, 30% of the women had blocked fallopian tubes. In an analysis of the large Lund cohort of laparoscopically confirmed cases of acute PID, Hillis et al demonstrated that women treated $\geq$3 days after onset of symptoms were at significantly increased risk for infertility compared with those treated within 3 days of symptom onset (19.7% vs 8.3%).[18] Thus, it seems clear that early diagnosis and treatment within the initial 48–72 hours of symptomatic acute PID is a crucial component of tertiary prevention strategies and emphasizes the importance for healthcare providers of maintaining a high index of suspicion for the diagnosis of PID.

Concerns have been voiced over the ability of outpatient (oral) treatment of PID to optimally prevent chronic sequelae, especially among adolescents and nulliparous patients.[37] The Pelvic Inflammatory Disease Evaluation And Clinical Health (PEACH) study, a randomized clinical trial comparing the CDC-recommended inpatient and outpatient antibiotic regimens for women with mild and moderate PID, demonstrated no differences between treatment groups in the rates of pregnancy, time to pregnancy, recurrence of PID, chronic pelvic pain, or ectopic pregnancy.[15] More recently, an updated analysis, with a longer follow-up period, of the PEACH study revealed that outpatient treatment did not adversely impact the occurrence of a follow-up pregnancy, live birth, or ectopic pregnancy; time to pregnancy; infertility; recurrent PID; or chronic pelvic pain.[35] These findings held true for women of various ages and races; with and without a prior birth; with or without previous PID; with or without baseline *N. gonorrhoeae* and/or *C. trachomatis*; and with or without high-temperature/white blood cell count/pelvic tenderness score.[35]

On the other hand, no tertiary prevention strategies have been either proposed for or demonstrated to be effective in the case of subclinical PID, an area that research needs to urgently address. Weisenfeld et al reported that subclinical PID (histologic endometritis) was present in one-fourth and 16% of women with lower genital tract infection with chlamydia and gonorrhea or BV, respectively.[8] Perhaps longer courses of treatment (i.e. 14 days), with regimens appropriate for PID, for these lower genital tract infections would have a positive effect on prevention of the long-term sequelae associated with PID. Another area that requires research is development of diagnostic tests for detection of subclinical PID that do not require invasive procedures such as endometrial biopsy. This is a key step if we are to institute treatment before subclinical PID has initiated the process of tubal scarring and obstruction.

Whether the use of immune and/or inflammatory response modulators would enhance the efficacy of antibiotic therapy in preventing the long-term sequelae of acute PID is an interesting but unanswered question. In an early prospective study assessing the efficacy of adjunctive steroid administration, Falk noted that the use of steroids in the treatment of acute salpingitis failed to improve the outcome as determined by hysterosalpingogram, findings at follow-up laparoscopy, or fertility rates.[38] Whether the use of higher, pharmacologic doses of steroids would demonstrate a more beneficial effect is unknown. It is an attractive hypothesis that concomitant use of anti-inflammatory agents such as nonsteroidal anti-inflammatory drugs (NSAIDs) or immune modulators, including macrolide antibiotics, would lead to improved outcomes, especially in the case of chlamydial PID, where the cell-mediated immune response plays a pivotal role in the tubal scarring and obstruction.[39–41] Recently, Patton et al, utilizing the macaque model of chlamydial PID, demonstrated that treatment with the macrolide antibiotic azithromycin dramatically reduced the inflammatory response, as well as more effectively eradicating *C. trachomatis* from the lower and upper genital tract, compared with doxycycline or placebo.[42] Moreover, azithromycin more effectively prevented progression of inflammation and fibrosis in the upper genital tract after repeated chlamydial infection. Azithromycin significantly reduced evidence of transforming growth factor-beta (TGF-β), a cytokine indicative of fibrosis, in the tissues of the genital tract. Other studies have demonstrated that azithromycin inhibits the production of the proinflammatory cytokines interleukin (IL)-1β, IL-6, and IL-8 and tumor necrosis factor-alpha (TNFα).[43–46] Thus, azithromycin may provide anti-inflammatory effects that would enhance the treatment efficacy for PID and reduce adverse long-term sequelae. Addressing this issue is a fruitful area for future research.

COMMUNITY-BASED PREVENTION

Rolfs suggested that PID prevention strategies require an increased emphasis on community-based, public health approaches.[46] Health education is an important component of a community-based approach to STD and PID intervention and includes the use of mass media and culturally appropriate messages that target high-risk populations such as adolescents and minorities.[46] In addition, communities must be assured access to adequate medical care.[23] Prevention of lower genital tract infection and PID requires effective clinical STD services and laboratory support.[23] Unfortunately, as noted by Washington et al, development and maintenance of high-quality, widely available, and easily accessible care for STDs and STIs has been difficult in the United States.[23]

CONCLUSION

In summary, prevention of PID must remain a high priority because of its adverse effect on the reproductive health of women and its associated substantial medical and economic costs. Our prevention efforts require involvement of individuals, healthcare providers, and communities.[23] In addition, new prevention strategies, such as vaccine development and microbicides, and innovative health promotion and education programs need to be developed and assessed. Hopefully, in the near future, strategies for PID prevention will be forthcoming that will alleviate the public health burden of PID and ameliorate the adverse reproductive health impact of this disease that afflicts millions of women worldwide.

REFERENCES

1. Centers for Disease Control and Prevention. Sexually Transmitted Disease Surveillance 2003: Last update September 2004. Accessed August 30, 2005. http:www.cdc.gov/std/stats
2. Washington AE, Katz P. Cost of and payment source for pelvic inflammatory: trends and projections, 1983 through 2000. JAMA 1991;266:2565–9.
3. Rein DB, Kassler WJ, Irwin KL, et al. Direct medical cost of pelvic inflammatory disease: decreasing but still substantial. Obstet Gynecol 2000;95:397–402.
4. Yeh JS, Hook EW, Goldie SJ. A refined estimate of the average lifetime cost of pelvic inflammatory disease. Sex Transm Dis 2003;30:369–78.
5. Westrom L, Eschenbach DA. Pelvic inflammatory disease. In: Holmes KK, Sparling PF, Mardh P-A, et al (eds). Sexually transmitted diseases. New York: McGraw-Hill, 1999:783–809.

6. Paavonen J, Kiviat N, Brunham RC, et al. Prevalence and manifestations of endometritis among women with cervicitis. Am J Obstet Gynecol 1985;152:280–6.
7. Korn AP, Hessol NA, Padian N, et al. Risk factors for plasma cell endometritis among women with cervical *Neisseria gonorrhoeae*, cervical *Chlamydia trachomatis*, or bacterial vaginosis. Am J Obstet Gynecol 1998;178:987–90.
8. Wiesenfeld HC, Hillier SL, Krohn M, et al. Lower genital tract infection and endometritis: insight into subclinical pelvic inflammatory disease. Obstet Gynecol 2002;100:456–63.
9. Korn AP, Bolan G, Padian N, et al. Plasma cell endometritis in women with symptomatic bacterial vaginosis. Obstet Gynecol 1995;85:387–90.
10. Westrom L. Incidence, prevalence, and trends of acute pelvic inflammatory disease and its consequences in industrialized countries. Am J Obstet Gynecol 1980;138:880–92.
11. Westrom L, Joesoef R, Reynolds G, et al. Pelvic inflammatory disease and fertility: a cohort study of 1844 women with laparoscopically verified disease and 657 control women with normal laparoscopic results. Sex Transm Dis 1992;19:185–92.
12. Westrom L. Influence of sexually transmitted diseases on sterility and ectopic pregnancy. Acta Eur Fertil 1985;16:21–4.
13. Svensson L. Mardh P-A, Westrom L. Infertility of the acute salpingitis with special reference to *Chlamydia trachomatis*. Fertil Steril 1983;40:322–9.
14. Westrom L, Iosif S, Svensson L, et al. Infertility after acute salpingitis: Results of treatment with different antibiotics. Curr Ther Res 1979;26:752–9.
15. Ness RB, Soper DE, Holley RL, et al. Effectiveness of inpatient and outpatient treatment strategies for women with pelvic inflammatory disease: Results from the pelvic inflammatory disease evaluation and clinical health (PEACH) randomized trial. Am J Obstet Gynecol 2002;186:929–37.
16. Safrin S, Schachter J, Dahrouge D, Sweet RL. Long-term sequelae of acute pelvic inflammatory disease: a retrospective cohort study. Am J Obstet Gynecol 1992;166:1300–5.
17. Viberg I. Acute inflammatory conditions of the uterine adnexa. Acta Obstet Gynecol Scand 1964;43(Suppl 4):5.
18. Hillis SD, Joesoef R, Marchbanks PA, et al. Delayed care of pelvic inflammatory disease as a risk factor for impaired fertility. Am J Obstet Gynecol 1993;168:1503–9.
19. Department of Health and Human Services. Healthy People 2000: National Health Promotion and Disease Prevention Objectives 1990. Washington: US Government Printing Office, 1991. DHHS Publication No. 91–50212.
20. Scholes D, Stergachis A, Heidrich FE, et al. Prevention of pelvic inflammatory disease by screening for cervical chlamydial infection. N Engl J Med 1996;334:1362–6.
21. Schachter J. Prevention of pelvic inflammatory disease. In: Landers DV, Sweet RL (eds). Pelvic inflammatory disease. New York: Springer-Verlag, 1997:146–51.
22. Washington AE, Aral SO, Wolner-Hanssen P, et al. Assessing risk for pelvic inflammatory disease and its sequelae. JAMA 1991;266:2581–6.
23. Washington AE, Cates W Jr, Wasserheit JN. Preventing pelvic inflammatory disease. JAMA 1991;266:2574–80.
24. Sweet RL, Gibbs RS. Pelvic inflammatory disease. In: Sweet RL, Gibbs RS, (eds). Infectious diseases of the female genital tract. Philadelphia: Lippincott, Williams & Wilkins, 2002:368–412.
25. Sweet RL. Role of bacterial vaginosis in pelvic inflammatory disease. Clin Infect Dis 1995;20:S271–5.
26. Hillier SL, Kiviat NB, Howes SE, et al. Role of bacterial vaginosis-associated microorganisms in endometritis. Am J Obstet Gynecol 1996;175:435–41.
27. Cates W Jr, Meheus A. Strategies for development of sexually transmitted diseases control programs. In: Holmes KK, Sparling PF, Wiesner PJ (eds). Sexually Transmitted Diseases. New York: McGraw-Hill, 1990:1023–30.
28. Hillis SD, Wasserheit JN. Screening for chlamydia – a key to the prevention of PID. N Engl J Med 1996;334:1399–401.
29. Stamm WE, Guinan ME, Johnson C, et al. Effect of treatment regimens for *Neisseria gonorrhoeae* on simultaneous infection with *Chlamydia trachomatis*. N Engl J Med 1984;310:545–51.
30. Kamwendo F, Forslin L, Bodin I, et al. Programs to reduce pelvic inflammatory disease – the Swedish experience. Lancet 1998;351(Suppl III):25–8.
31. Wiesenfeld HC, Heine RP, Rideout A, et al. The vaginal introitus: a novel site for *Chlamydia trachomatis* testing in women. Am J Obstet Gynecol 1996;174:1542–6.
32. Wiesenfeld HC, Lowry DL, Heine RP, et al. Self-collection of vaginal swabs for the detection of chlamydia, gonorrhea and trichomonas: opportunity to encourage sexually transmitted disease testing among adolescents. Sex Transm Dis 2001;28:321–5.
33. Peipert JR, Montagno AB, Cooper AS, et al. Bacterial vaginosis as a risk factor for upper genital tract infection. Am J Obstet Gynecol 1997;177:1184–7.
34. Ness RB, Hillier SL, Kip KE, et al. Bacterial vaginosis and risk of pelvic inflammatory disease. Obstet Gynecol 2004;104:1–9.
35. Ness RB, Kip KE, Hillier SL, et al. A cluster analysis of bacterial vaginosis-associated microflora and pelvic inflammatory disease. Am J Epidem 2005;162:585–90.
36. Teisala K, Heinonen PK, Aine R, et al. Second laparoscopy after treatment of acute pelvic inflammatory disease. Obstet Gynecol 1987;69:343–46.
37. Hemsell DL, Ledger WJ, Martens M, et al. Concerns regarding the Centers of Disease Control's published guidelines for pelvic inflammatory disease. Clin Infect Dis 2001;32:103–7.
38. Falk V. Treatment of acute nontuberulous salpingitis with antibiotics alone and in combination with glucocorticoids. Acta Obstet Gynecol Scand 1965;44 (Suppl 16):65.
39. Morrison RP, Manning DS, Caldwell HD. Immunology of Chlamydia trachomatis infections: immunoprotective and immunopathogenic responses. In: Gallin JI, Fauci AS, Quinn TC, eds. Advances in Host Defense Mechanisms: Sexually Transmitted Diseases, Vol 8. New York: Raven Press, 1992:57–84.
40. Patton DL, Cosgrove-Sweeney YT, Kuoa CC. Demonstration of delayed hypersensitivity in *Chlamydia trachomatis* salpingitis in monkeys: a pathologic mechanism of tubal damage. J Infect Dis 1994;169:680–3.
41. Brunham RC, Peeling RW. *Chlamydia trachomatis* antigens: role in immunity and pathogenesis. Infect Agents Dis 1994;3:218–23.
42. Patton DL, Cosgrove Sweeney YT, Stamm WE. Significant reduction in inflammatory response in the macaque model of chlamydial pelvic inflammatory disease with azithromycin treatment. J Infect Dis 2005;192:129–35.
43. Culie O, Erakovic V, Cepelak I, et al. Azithromycin modulates neutrophil function and circulating inflammatory mediators in healthy human subjects. Eur J Pharmacol 2002;450:277–89.
44. Ohara T, Kojio S, Taneike I, et al. Effects of azithromycin on shiga toxin production by *Escherichia coli* and subsequent host inflammatory response. Antimicrob Agents Chemother 2002;46:3478–83.
45. Anderson JL, Muhlestein JB, Carlquist J, et al. Randomized secondary prevention trial of azithromycin in patients with coronary artery disease and serological evidence for *Chlamydia pneumoniae* infection. Circulation 1999;99:1540–7.
46. Rolfs RT. "Think PID". New directions in prevention and management of pelvic inflammatory disease. Sex Transm Dis 1991;18:131–32.

Index

Note: Page numbers in **bold** text refer to figures in the text; those in *italic* to tables and boxed material